Aesthetic Facial Reconstruction

Guest Editor

STEFAN O.P. HOFER, MD, PhD, FRCS(C)

CLINICS IN PLASTIC SURGERY

www.plasticsurgery.theclinics.com

July 2009 • Volume 36 • Number 3

SAUNDERS an imprint of ELSEVIER, Inc.

W.B. SAUNDERS COMPANY
A Division of Elsevier Inc.

1600 John F. Kennedy Boulevard • Suite 1800 • Philadelphia, Pennsylvania 19103-2899

http://www.theclinics.com

CLINICS IN PLASTIC SURGERY Volume 36, Number 3
July 2009 ISSN 0094-1298, ISBN-13: 978-1-4377-1264-3, ISBN-10: 1-4377-1264-9

Editor: Barbara Cohen-Kligerman

Clinics in Plastic Surgery (ISSN 0094-1298) is published quarterly by Elsevier Inc., 360 Park Avenue South, New York, NY 10010-1710. Months of issue are January, April, July, and October. Business and Editorial Offices: 1600 John F. Kennedy Blvd., Suite 1800, Philadelphia, PA 19103-2899. Periodicals postage paid at New York, NY and additional mailing offices. Subscription prices are $352.00 per year for US individuals, $510.00 per year for US institutions, $177.00 per year for US students and residents, $400.00 per year for Canadian individuals, $596.00 per year for Canadian institutions, $454.00 per year for international individuals, $596.00 per year for international institutions, and $224.00 per year for Canadian and foreign students/residents. To receive student/resident rate, orders must be accompanied by name of affiliated institution, date of term, and the *signature* of program/residency coordinator on institution letterhead. Orders will be billed at individual rate until proof of status is received. Foreign air speed delivery is included in all *Clinics* subscription prices. All prices are subject to change without notice. **POSTMASTER:** Send address changes to *Clinics in Plastic Surgery*, Elsevier Periodicals Customer Service, 11830 Westline Industrial Drive, St. Louis, MO 63146. **Customer Service: 1-800-654-2452 (US). From outside of the United States, call 314-453-7041. Fax: 314-453-5170. E-mail: JournalsCustomerService-usa@elsevier.com (for print support); JournalsOnlineSupport-usa@elsevier.com (for online support).**

Reprints. For copies of 100 or more of articles in this publication, please contact the Commercial Reprints Department, Elsevier Inc., 360 Park Avenue South, New York, New York 10010-1710. Tel.: (+1) 212-633-3812; Fax: (+1) 212-462-1935; E-mail: reprints@elsevier.com.

Clinics in Plastic Surgery is covered in *Current Contents, EMBASE/Excerpta Medica, Science Citation Index, MEDLINE/ PubMed (Index Medicus), ASCA,* and *ISI/BIOMED.*

Contributors

GUEST EDITOR

STEFAN O.P. HOFER, MD, PhD, FRCS(C)
Wharton Chair in Reconstructive Plastic
Surgery; Associate Professor, University
of Toronto; and Chief, Division of Plastic
Surgery, Department of Surgery and
Department of Surgical Oncology, University
Health Network, Toronto, Ontario, Canada

AUTHORS

OLEH M. ANTONYSHYN, MD, FRCSC
Head, Adult Craniofacial Program and
Associate Professor, University of Toronto,
Sunnybrook Health Sciences Centre, Toronto,
Ontario, Canada

JUAN P. BARRET, MD, PhD
Professor and Head, Department of Plastic
Surgery and Burns, University Hospital Vall
d'Hebron, Universidad Autonoma de
Barcelona; and Centro Medico Teknon,
Barcelona, Spain

LAWRENCE J. GOTTLIEB, MD
Professor of Surgery; Director, Burn and
Complex Wound Center; and Director,
Reconstructive Microsurgery Fellowship,
Section of Plastic and Reconstructive
Surgery, The University of Chicago, Chicago,
Illinois

NELIDA GRANDE, MD
Plastic Surgery Associates, Centro Medico
Teknon, Barcelona, Spain

E. HAJDARBEGOVIC, MD
Resident, Department of Dermatology,
Erasmus Medical Center, Rotterdam,
The Netherlands

K. DE ROON HERTOGE, MD
Resident, Department of Ophthalmology,
Erasmus Medical Center, Erasmus University
Rotterdam, Rotterdam, The Netherlands

STEFAN O.P. HOFER, MD, PhD, FRCS(C)
Wharton Chair in Reconstructive Plastic
Surgery; Associate Professor, University
of Toronto; and Chief, Division of Plastic
Surgery, Department of Surgery and
Department of Surgical Oncology, University
Health Network, Toronto, Ontario, Canada

BENOÎT G. LENGELÉ, MD, PhD
Professor of Anatomy and Surgery; Head,
Department of Experimental Morphology,
Université catholique de Louvain; and Clinical
Chief, Reconstructive Surgery, Faculty
of Medicine, Cliniques Universitaires
Saint-Luc, Brussels, Belgium

JON A. MATHY, MD
Chief Resident, Harvard Combined Plastic
Surgery Training Program, Division of Plastic
Surgery, Department of Surgery, Harvard
Medical School, Brigham and Women's
Hospital, Boston, Massachusetts

FREDERICK J. MENICK, MD
Chief, Division of Plastic Surgery, St. Joseph's
Hospital; Clinical Associate Professor,
University of Arizona College of Medicine;
and Private Practice, Tucson, Arizona

K. MUNTE, MD
Dermatologist, Department of Dermatology,
Erasmus Medical Center, Rotterdam,
The Netherlands

MARC A.M. MUREAU, MD, PhD
Assistant Professor and Head, Oncological
Reconstructive Surgery, Department of Plastic
and Reconstructive Surgery, Erasmus
University Medical Center, Rotterdam,
The Netherlands

**PETER C. NELIGAN, MB, FRCS(I), FRCSC,
FACS**
Professor of Surgery and Director, Center
for Reconstructive Surgery, Division of Plastic
Surgery, University of Washington Medical
Center, Seattle, Washington

H.A.M. NEUMANN, MD, PhD
Professor of Dermatology, Department
of Dermatology, Erasmus Medical Center,
Rotterdam, The Netherlands

JOSE M. PALACIN, MD
Plastic Surgery Associates, Program Director,
Aesthetic Plastic Surgery, Centro Medico
Teknon, Barcelona, Spain

BRIAN M. PARRETT, MD
Clinical Fellow in Surgery, Division of Plastic
Surgery, Harvard Medical School, Brigham
& Women's Hospital, Boston, Massachusetts

RENÉ M.L. POUBLON, MD, PhD
Associate Professor of Medicine, Department
of Otorhinolaryngology and Head and Neck
Surgery, Erasmus Medical Center, Erasmus
University Rotterdam, Rotterdam, The
Netherlands

JULIAN J. PRIBAZ, MD
Professor, Division of Plastic Surgery,
Department of Surgery, Harvard Medical
School, Brigham and Women's Hospital,
Boston, Massachusetts

NEUS SAROBE, MD
Plastic Surgery Associates, Centro Medico
Teknon, Barcelona, Spain

IRIS A. SEITZ, MD, PhD
Resident, Section of Plastic and
Reconstructive Surgery, The University
of Chicago, Chicago, Illinois

JOHN D. STEIN, MD, FRCSC
Clinical Fellow, Craniofacial Surgery, University
of Toronto, Sunnybrook Health Sciences
Centre, Toronto, Ontario, Canada

H.B. THIO, MD, PhD
Dermatologist, Department of Dermatology,
Erasmus Medical Center, Rotterdam,
The Netherlands

R.J.T. VAN DER LEEST, MD
Intern, Department of Dermatology, Erasmus
Medical Center, Rotterdam, The Netherlands

DELIA VILA, MD
Plastic Surgery Associates, Centro Medico
Teknon, Barcelona, Spain

JOHN WALDRON, MD
Staff Radiation Oncologist and Assistant
Professor, University of Toronto, Radiation
Medicine Program, Princess Margaret
Hospital, Toronto, Ontario, Canada

YONGJIN WANG, MD
Clinical Fellow, University of Toronto, Radiation
Medicine Program, Princess Margaret
Hospital, Toronto, Ontario, Canada

WOODROW WELLS, MD
Staff Radiation Oncologist and Assistant
Professor, University of Toronto, Radiation
Medicine Program, Princess Margaret
Hospital, Toronto, Ontario, Canada

Contents

Neoplasms of the skin are found most often on the face. Malignant tumors of the facial skin pose a challenge in treatment, prohibiting compromises between oncologically responsible surgery and functional plus cosmetic outcome. The incidence of melanoma and nonmelanoma skin cancers is rising. Not all malignancies of the skin need to be treated by surgery. For in situ variants there are other options, such as photodynamic therapy and medical treatment. Knowledge of the clinical manifestation, behavior, and prognosis and histopathologic analysis lead to correct diagnosis and choice of suitable treatment. This article presents a synopsis of nonmelanoma, melanoma, and other cancers of the skin.

Radiation therapy is an important option for the treatment of skin cancer. Its advantages are preserving normal tissues, noninvasive outpatient treatment, and no need for anesthesia. Radiation therapy is used for deeper and extensive tumor and anatomic sites where it is difficult to obtain clear surgical margins. Radiation therapy is used as adjuvant treatment of patients who have positive surgical margins, perineural invasion, or regional node metastasis. It is useful for elderly patients who are unwilling or unable to undergo surgery. Radiation therapy is an effective treatment in eradicating gross and microscopic skin cancer, with a 5-year cure rate of 90% to 95%.

Aesthetic facial reconstruction is a challenging art. Improving outcomes in aesthetic facial reconstruction requires a thorough understanding of the basic principles of the functional and aesthetic requirements for facial reconstruction. From there, further refinement and attention to detail can be provided. This paper discusses basic principles of aesthetic facial reconstruction.

Reconstruction of scalp and forehead defects is a complex field with a broad variety of reconstructive options. The thought process and techniques used for reconstruction of scalp and forehead defects are the subject of this article.

John D. Stein and Oleh M. Antonyshyn

The eyelids are critical in the protection of the conjunctiva and sclera of the globe and, in turn, the preservation of vision. Aesthetically, the position and shape of the eyelids define a distinctive frame for the eyes, and disproportions in any given individual are immediately obvious. Reconstruction of the eyelids must address both functional and aesthetic requirements. This article emphasizes eyelid morphology and discusses the principles and key reconstructive methods used to achieve optimal results for upper and lower eyelid defects, defects of the medial and lateral canthi, and complex combined defects.

René M.L. Poublon and K. de Roon Hertoge

Reconstructive surgery of the nasolacrimal duct, or dacryocystorhinostomy, can be performed via an external or endonasal approach. For almost a century external dacryocystorhinostomy was the gold standard for correction of lacrimal duct obstruction. The endonasal approach became a safe surgical procedure using endoscopes and has the same anatomic and functional success rate as the external approach. It can be performed in adults and in children with close collaboration between a rhinologist and an ophthalmologist. An overview is given of the literature and of the authors' experience in this field.

Brian M. Parrett and Julian J. Pribaz

Nasal defects are common after cancer resection, and the goal of treatment is to appropriately define the defect and then to select the best reconstructive options. The plastic surgeon must reestablish all deficient layers of the nose (support, lining, and external cover). The authors' algorithm is based on defect location and orientation, with the nose divided transversely into three zones, and then into subunits. In this article, using the aforementioned algorithm, the authors simplify the complex topic of nasal reconstruction, concentrating on local and regional flap reconstruction. The appropriate treatment for full-thickness defects, including options for reconstruction of lining and support, is also discussed.

Frederick J. Menick

Historically, external skin is the most obvious tissue deficiency after nasal trauma or skin cancer excision. The loss of underlying support and lining is less apparent and practically speaking has been considered an afterthought in the repair of nasal defects. The importance of lining was initially recognized by Keegan and Gillies. Modern surgeons can effectively employ both traditional techniques and more modern methods to successfully combine thin, supple covering skin; a shaped, supportive mid layer; and thin, conforming lining to re-create the form and function of a nose.

Frederick J. Menick

The tint of forehead skin so exactly matches that of the face and nose that a forehead flap must be the first choice for reconstruction of a nasal defect. The forehead flap makes by far the best nose. With some plastic surgery juggling, the forehead defect can be camouflaged effectively. This article describes the author's technique in two-stage and three-stage forehead flap procedures.

Maximizing Results in Reconstruction of Cheek Defects

461

Marc A.M. Mureau and Stefan O.P. Hofer

The face is exceedingly important, as it is the medium through which individuals interact with the rest of society. Reconstruction of cheek defects after trauma or surgery is a continuing challenge for surgeons who wish to reliably restore facial function and appearance. Important in aesthetic facial reconstruction are the aesthetic unit principles, by which the face can be divided in central facial units (nose, lips, eyelids) and peripheral facial units (cheeks, forehead, chin). This article summarizes established options for reconstruction of cheek defects and provides an overview of several modifications as well as tips and tricks to avoid complications and maximize aesthetic results.

Strategies in Lip Reconstruction

477

Peter C. Neligan

Injury or surgical trauma can result in significant alterations of normal lip appearance and function that can profoundly impact the patient's self-image and quality of life. Neuromuscular injury can lead to asymmetry at rest and during facial animation, and distressing functional disabilities are common. Loss of labial competence may interfere with the ability to articulate, whistle, suck, kiss, and contain salivary secretions. For smaller defects, reconstruction can be very effective. Reconstructing an aesthetically pleasing and functional lip is more difficult with larger defects.

Maximizing Results for Lipofilling in Facial Reconstruction

487

Juan P. Barret, Neus Sarobe, Nelida Grande, Delia Vila, and Jose M. Palacin

Lipostructure (also known as structural fat grafts, lipofilling, or fat grafting) has become a technique with a good reputation and reproducible results. The application of this technology in patients undergoing reconstruction is a novel surgical alternative. Obtaining good results in this patient population is very difficult, but the application of small fat grafts with a strict Coleman technique produces long-term cosmetic effects. Adult-derived stem cells have been pointed out as important effectors of this regenerative technology, and future research should focus in this direction.

Prefabrication and Prelamination Applications in Current Aesthetic Facial Reconstruction

493

Jon A. Mathy and Julian J. Pribaz

Prefabrication and prelamination techniques can offer significant advantage in aesthetic facial reconstruction. Specifically, they can be applied to expand the recruitment and assembly of optimal tissues for better approximation of aesthetic ideals. Some of their unique abilities are presented, and their advantages, limitations, and technical pointers are provided. The place for prelamination and prefabrication in the burgeoning era of composite tissue transplantation is addressed. Some of the relevant features and interdependencies among these procedures as they relate to aesthetic facial reconstruction are discussed.

Facial allotransplantation has become a surgical reality. The first successful segmental human face transplants have demonstrated that facial allografts are reliable,
their rejection can be prevented by low-dose immunosuppression, and their neurologic recovery enables oral and expressive functions of the face to be restored. Clinical facts have shown that the risk-benefit balance is acceptable in the medium term,
that at the neurocognitive level the allograft is reintegrated in the body scheme of the
recipient, and that it does not engender a donor identity transfer. This article presents a classification of facial allografts and discusses the technical, immunologic,
and ethical challenges that lie ahead.

Clinics in Plastic Surgery

THE CLINICS ARE NOW AVAILABLE ONLINE!

Access your subscription at:
www.theclinics.com

Clinics in Plastic Surgery

Preface

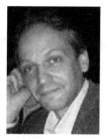

Stefan O.P. Hofer, MD, PhD, FRCS(C)
Guest Editor

Aesthetic facial reconstruction is an exciting area that speaks to everyone's imagination. The combination of increased anatomic knowledge and the concept of aesthetic facial units and subunits has made it possible over time to enhance reconstructive outcomes. We can continue improvement of our outcomes, building on the knowledge and solutions from creative surgeons who faced similar reconstructive challenges before us.

This issue of *Clinics in Plastic Surgery* tries to give a comprehensive overview of aesthetic facial reconstruction. I am grateful and honored to be given the opportunity to host this issue. Experts in aesthetic facial reconstruction from around the globe have put in their time to share with us their wealth of knowledge. The result of all their efforts is worthwhile. A comprehensive update on the current practice of surgical and nonsurgical treatments for skin cancer gives a perspective on possible causes of facial defects. The different aesthetic units and subunits that are involved in facial reconstruction are reviewed in separate articles. The basic principles are systematically presented, interwoven with many pearls to improve one's aesthetic reconstructive outcomes. Proven and state-of-the-art principles and techniques are intermixed with cutting edge practices and new frontiers that are currently being challenged.

I am confident that this issue of *Clinics in Plastic Surgery* will be not only interesting to read but also a valuable resource for the surgeon faced with difficult facial reconstructions in the clinic and operating theater.

Stefan O.P. Hofer, MD, PhD, FRCS(C)
Department of Surgery and Department
of Surgical Oncology
University Health Network
200 Elizabeth Street, 8N-865
Toronto, Ontario, Canada M5G 2C4

E-mail address:
stefan.hofer@uhn.on.ca (S.O.P. Hofer)

Clin Plastic Surg 36 (2009) xi
doi:10.1016/j.cps.2009.02.012
0094-1298/09/$ – see front matter

Neoplasms of the Facial Skin

E. Hajdarbegovic, MD*, R.J.T. van der Leest, MD, K. Munte, MD,
H.B. Thio, MD, PhD, H.A.M. Neumann, MD, PhD

KEYWORDS

- Skin tumors • Face • Melanoma
- Non-melanoma • Synopsis

Neoplasms of the skin are found most often on the face. Cosmetically, the face is the most important anatomic area for most patients. Because of this, malignant tumors of the facial skin pose a great challenge in treatment, prohibiting compromises between oncologically responsible surgery and functional plus cosmetic outcome. The incidence of melanoma and nonmelanoma skin cancers is still rising, which commonly is attributed to increased exposure to UV light in white populations. An increased elderly population also contributes to this increase in incidence of nonmelanoma skin cancer. In addition, many patients develop more than one nonmelanoma skin cancer after the first one.

Basal cell carcinoma (BCC) is by far the most prevalent skin cancer. Eighty percent of BCCs affect the facial skin. The greatest challenge is removing all tumor cells to prevent a recurrence in complicated cases, as recurrent tumors are more difficult to cure. Slightly less prevalent is squamous cell carcinoma (SCC), also seen most frequently on the face. This type of skin cancer is known to metastasize if left untreated. The most feared neoplasm is the malignant melanoma because of its aggressiveness and its occurrence at a younger age. Adherence to the treatment guidelines is of paramount importance in these cases.

Whenever a skin cancer is suspected on the basis of history and clinical findings, a biopsy should be performed. This helps make the correct diagnosis and determine the subtype of the tumor so that correct treatment can be initiated.

Similar to most other cancers, the most suitable treatment for neoplasms of the skin is surgery. The goal of treatment is curing the disease with the lowest percentage of recurrence and with the best functional and cosmetic result possible. Mohs' micrographic surgery (MMS) is proved to aid in achieving this twofold goal with best results in cases of difficult BCCs.

Not all malignancies of the skin need to be treated by surgery. For in situ variants of nonmelanoma skin cancers there are other options, such as photodynamic therapy (PDT) and medical treatment. Good knowledge of the clinical manifestation, behavior, and prognosis of a tumor together with histopathologic analysis lead to correct diagnosis and choice of the most suitable treatment modality. This article presents a short synopsis for nonmelanoma, melanoma, and other cancers of the skin.

BASAL CELL CARCINOMA
Background

Nonmelanoma skin cancer is the most common cancer in white populations worldwide and its incidence continues to rise. BCC is the most common type of nonmelanoma skin cancer, with SCC being the second most common.[1–3] BCC is the easiest cancer to diagnose and treat. Although a BCC rarely metastasizes, some BCCs (especially large and neglected or incompletely treated primary and recurrent tumors) may cause substantial morbidity and even mortality, posing a therapeutic challenge.[3,4] BCCs occur in 1 of 5 to 6 persons in a lifetime and the incidence is rising every year.[1,5,6] Every year 500,000 BCCs are diagnosed in the United States. Incidence rate of BCC in Rochester,

Department of Dermatology, Erasmus Medical Center, Burg. 's Jacobplein 51, 3015 NL, Rotterdam, The Netherlands
* Corresponding author.
E-mail address: e.hajdarbegovic@erasmusmc.nl (E. Hajdarbegovic).

Clin Plastic Surg 36 (2009) 319–334
doi:10.1016/j.cps.2009.02.007
0094-1298/09/$ – see front matter © 2009 Elsevier Inc. All rights reserved.

Minnesota, is 146 per 100,000 person-years; Tucson, Arizona, has an incidence of 317 per 100,000.[7] In some areas of Australia, incidence rate is rising to 1 per 100 persons.[8] These geographic differences in incidence reflect the role of exposure to UV radiation, the causative agent implied in all skin cancers. Because approximately 80% of all BCCs are located in the face and neck (sun-exposed areas), preservation of healthy skin and an excellent functional and cosmetic outcome are important in treatment of BCC.[1,9–11]

BCCs are slowly growing, malignant (usually nonmetastazing) follicular tumors that develop in the epithelium of the skin appendages. Several factors (tumor size, invasion depth, and intrinsic factors) are associated with metastasis and aggressive growth of BCC. Poor accuracy of data results in incidence of metastatic BCC varying from 0.003% to 0.55%. BCCs are reported with metastases to lymph nodes, bone, bone marrow, and lungs.[4] Known risk factors for development of BCCs are white race, sun exposure, age, male gender, radiation therapy, immunosuppressive medication, albinism, xeroderma pigmentosum, DNA polymorphisms and mutations, and familiar syndromes (Bazex, Rombo, and Gorlin syndromes). Because there are several criteria, BCC can be classified as a genuine type, as premalignant, as hamartoma, and as part of certain syndromes (**Table 1**). Some genetic syndromes, of which the basal cell nevus syndrome (Gorlin syndrome) is best known, are associated with higher risk for developing skin malignancies. BCC often plays a part in these syndromes.

Clinical Presentation

Early tumors can be recognized as small, translucent, light-colored eminences of the skin, completely covered by a thin epidermis through which telangiectases are noticeable (**Fig. 1**). On dermatoscopy, subtle pigment granules often are observed. Sporadically BCCs are pedunculated and when they present with telangiectases they can be confused with telangiectatic granuloma. As a result of continuous growth the tumor slowly becomes a nodus with a typical pearly aspect and telangiectasis (nodular type). Subsequently ulceration appears (nodo-ulcerative type). Sometimes the lesion can be saturated with pigment (pigmented type) so that confusion with a melanoma is possible. The classical ulcus rodens is an extensive nodo-ulcerative BCC. The designation, ulcus terebrans, is reserved for extraordinarily large and ulcerating BCCs. Furthermore, there is a superficial type (BCC of the trunk or pagetoid type), often confused with eczema (**Fig. 2**). At the border of this tumor, translucent papules with a pearly aspect and telangiectases, a characteristic morphologic aspect of BCC, can be localized.

Table 1
Classification of basal cell carcinoma

Type	Description
Premalignant	Fibroepithelioma (Pinkus tumor)
Primary	Genuine or primary BCC
Genetic	Basal cell nevus syndrome (OMIM 109,400) Xeroderma pigmentosum (XP), complementation groups: XPA (OMIM 278,700) XPB (OMIM 610,651) XPC (OMIM 278,720) XPD (OMIM 278,730) XPE (OMIM 278,740) XPF (OMIM 278,760) XPG (OMIM 278,780) XP dominant (OMIM 194,400) XP variant (OMIM 278,750) XP IX (OMIM 278,810) Oley-Sharpe-Chenevix-Trench syndrome (OMIM 109,390)[12] Twin pairs[13] Bazex syndrome (OMIM 301,845) Rombo syndrome (OMIM 180,730)
Hamartoma	Primary: hamartomatous form of BCC Secondary: BCC developed from sebaceous nevus[14]

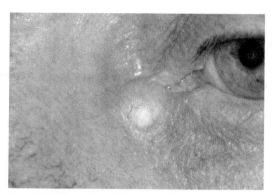

Fig. 1. Nodular BCC in the medial canthus of the left eye. Note the pearly aspect and telangiectasia.

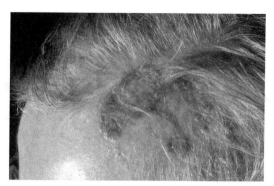

Fig. 3. Morpheaform BCC on the forehead. It emulates cutaneous sclerosis and atrophy.

The morphea or sclerodermiform type has a low prevalence but its course is highly aggressive (**Fig. 3**). The average age of patients developing a primary BCC is 63 years. The age of patients who have metastases of a primary BCC is relatively young, with an average of 45 years.[15] The younger age of patients who have a metastatic BCC can be explained by death of patients who have BCC before metastasis of the tumor or by a different oncologic behavior of BCCs originating at younger age.[16] The biologic behavior of BCCs in younger patients presents with an aggressive character.[16,17] Differential diagnosis of BCC is listed in **Box 1**.

Histologically, BCC can be divided into six subtypes (**Table 2**). Superficial BCCs show irregular proliferation of tumor cells attached to the undersurface of the epidermis. The peripheral cells show palisading and there is little penetration into the dermis. Nodo-ulcerative BCCs appear solid, keratotic, or adenoid. Micronodular BCC is symmetric and circumscribed with an infiltrative element; nodular BCCs show peripheral palisading in the islands of tumor cells. Infiltrative BCCs show more atypia and tumor cells infiltrating the dermis. Basosquamous carcinomas have a prominent element of squamous differentiation, but the architecture is that of a BCC.

Histology

Histopathologic examination shows epithelial islands, characterized by dark cells with a small volume of cytoplasm. Nuclear palisades surround these cells, the same way as in the stratum basale and around the hair papilla. The tumor cells, included in the palisade layer, appear disorganized. The cells resemble cells of the basal lamina in the epidermis and matrix cells of the adnexa.[18] The cells in the palisade arrangement present minimal signs of organization and differentiation and, likewise, mitoses occasionally are observed. The nuclei have a regular, large, oval, or elongated and uniform aspect with relatively little cytoplasm. The clumping of nuclei is variable. Incidentally compact cell masses occur without recognizable structure and look like hair roots. Sometimes they appear like adenoid structures (eccrine,

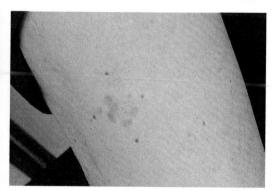

Fig. 2. Superficial BCC. The lesion resembles inflammatory skin diseases, such as psoriasis or eczema. On the basis of history, its isolated occurrence, or failure of medical therapy, suspicion of malignancy is raised.

Box 1
Differential diagnosis of basal cell carcinoma
SCC
Adnexal tumor, especially trichoepithelioma, nonpigmented nevus cell nevus, and sebaceous gland hypertrophy
Melanoma
Bowen's disease
Actinic keratosis (AK)

Table 2
Histologic subtypes of basal cell carcinoma

Histology	Clinical Presentation	Risk of Recurrence
Superficial	BCC of the trunk	High
Solid	Nodo-ulcerative	Low
Micronodular	Flat, papulous	High
Adenoid	Nodular	High
Spiky	Morphea, poorly circumscribed	Severe
Squamous differentiation	Keratosis	Low

apocrine, or sebaceous gland-like). The connective tissue seems to grow together with the tumor cells. In transplant experiments, BCCs hardly survived without connective tissue.[19] At first, little overgrowth arises from the epidermis/adnexa,[20] which soon changes. A 3-D reconstruction model demonstrated the existence of a contiguous tumor with a reticular pattern.[20,21]

Treatment

There are many treatment options for BCC, including surgical excision (SE), cryosurgery, radiotherapy, imiquimod, 5-fluorouracil (5-FU), PDT, curettage and electrocoagulation, and MMS. SE and MMS have the advantage of histopathologic margin control and, therefore, are gold standards. Other modalities should be reserved for patients who cannot undergo surgery. Superficial BCC can be treated medically or with PDT. Although most BCCs are well treated by traditional methods, such as standard excision and cryosurgery, some BCCs require a more specialized technique, such as MMS. MMS aims to achieve almost a 100% margin control and has been shown to have a high cure rate.[22–24]

Because a BCC rarely metastasizes, the main goal for treatment is radical tumor removal, with preservation of uninvolved skin. Indication for MMS is a nonmelanoma skin cancer, which has a high risk for local recurrence or is located in cosmetically and functionally important areas. The indications for BCCs are listed in **Box 2**.

BCCs with clinically undefined borders are more difficult to treat with conventional methods. BCCs with aggressive histopathologic subtypes are known for their extensive subclinical spread.[25,26] Examples are morphea, sclerosing, micronodular, and trabecular BCCs and BCCs with a squamous differentiation. Spiky tumor extension can easily be missed using standard histopathology. Large BCCs (>2 cm) cause problems, such as incomplete excision and subsequent recurrences, when managed with other treatments. Prediction

of tumor-free margins in large tumors is difficult. Unsuspected deep and lateral extensions are common in the H zone of the face (**Fig. 4**). Especially in the nasolabial fold and in the medial canthal area, tumor tends to invade deep before it spreads laterally.[27] An explanation for higher recurrence rates in the H zone is that it is a cosmetically and functionally important area. Therefore, surgeons may be more conservative in trying to preserve these sensitive structures at the expense of adequate tumor resection. Recurrence rates are high after incompletely excised BCCs. Incompletely excised BCCs require a re-excision, because a recurrence generally is more difficult to treat than the primary tumor and often results in mutilating surgery. Clinical margins of tumors with perineural growth extend further. When a BCC reaches a nerve sheath it can easily spread along the nerve trunk with an axial extension rate exceeding that of concentric growth. Patient age also is an important factor. In younger patients, prevention of a recurrence is even more important than in the elderly. Moreover younger patients tend to have BCCs with more aggressive histopathologic subtypes. Besides prevention of recurrence, these patients also are more concerned about cosmetics and consequently more

Box 2
Indications for treatment with Mohs' micrographic surgery for basal cell carcinoma

Undefined borders

Aggressive histopathologic subtype

Larger than 2 cm

Localized to the H zone

Incompletely excised

Perineural invasion

Recurrent BCC

Younger patients

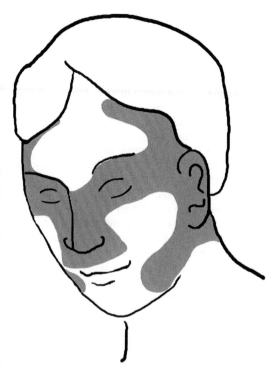

Fig. 4. H zone of the face.

demanding. Older age, however, should not be an excuse for suboptimal treatment.

Primary BCCs (<2 cm and solid histology) should be excised with 3-mm margins.[28,29] Primary BCCs larger than 2 cm with a solid growth,

infiltrative BCCs, and recurrent BCCs should be excised with 0.5-cm margins (**Fig. 5**).

Mohs' Micrographic Surgery

The first step in MMS is debulking of the tumor. After debulking, the first Mohs' stage is performed. A Mohs' stage is a circumferential incision on a 45° angle, the so-called round saucer-shaped incision. After the incision is made, the excision continues perpendicularly to the surface. In this way a somewhat bowl-shaped tissue specimen is obtained. The tissue specimen is divided into smaller pieces, with color staining of the edges of each piece. For precise orientation of the tumor, the Mohs' map is accordingly color-coded. All pieces are taken to the cryostat where they are put upside-down on a cryostat chuck with a few drops of tissue-tech. The tissue pieces then are crushed and, because of the bowl shape of the tissue pieces, the lateral tissue edges are brought into the same plane as the base of the specimen. After freezing of the tissue pieces, horizontal sections of 5 or 10 μm are made and stained with toludine blue or hematoxylin-eosin. By constructing orientation points in vivo (dye or a suture) and on digital images, a full digital model of the excised tissue is constructed (**Fig. 6**). When the procedure is performed properly, almost all of the surgical margins are visible under the microscope. The procedure for color-coding and horizontal sectioning is repeated until tumor-free margins are obtained. After complete

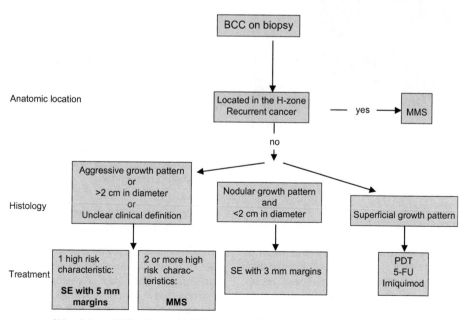

Abbreviations: MMS, micrographic Mohs' surgery, SE, standard excision, PDT, photodynamic light therapy, 5-FU, 5-flururacil cream

Fig. 5. Therapeutic algorithm for facial basal cell carcinoma (BCC).

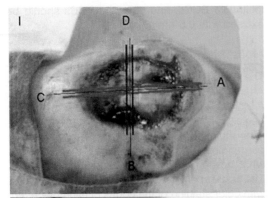

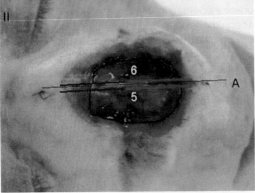

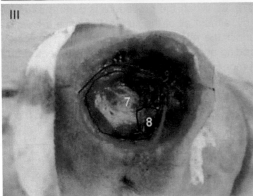

Fig. 6. Sequential digital mapping images made in real time during Mohs' surgery for a recurrent BCC on the nose. To aid in the orientation an axis system is set up. Different colors and numbers enable more detailed mapping of the borders so that remaining tumor tissue can be removed.

tumor removal, surgeons have to decide how best to reconstruct the defect.

MMS is preferred over SE for the treatment of facial recurrent BCCs because of significantly fewer recurrences after MMS. The lower recurrence rate is largely attributable to more extensive oncologic control of the excision margins as all of them are visualized in Mohs' sections. On normal histopathologic examination, less than 1% of the excision area is examined.

In primary cases of BCC, however, treatment with SE probably is sufficient in most cases.[24] Almost one fourth of all aggressive carcinomas of 1-cm or more diameter and approximately one third of all recurrent carcinomas were excised incompletely with a 3-mm margin. MMS is preferable to use for these tumors to avoid larger defects, a poor aesthetic outcome, and functional problems (see **Box 2**).[3]

Recurrent BCCs are larger at presentation than primary BCCs;[30] 64% of recurrences after incomplete excision of the primary tumor consisted of multiple tumor nests.[31] This may be because of scar tissue, which can act as a barrier, preventing upward migration of malignant cells and encouraging tumor cells to spread in a horizontal and deep direction. This emphasizes the importance of excising the whole scar in recurrent BCCs because residual tumor can be buried underneath or within it. Recurrent BCC after radiotherapy results in many incurable tumors, some of which metastasize.

Cosmetic results after treatment with MMS and SE are similar. For those facial BCCs that run an increased risk for being excised incompletely, however, MMS results in a significantly smaller defect and, therefore, provides a better cosmetic outcome. Performing MMS requires trained doctors and laboratory technicians. Creating horizontal frozen sections is more time consuming than a traditional pathologic examination after SE. Cook and Zitelli performed a cost analysis and concluded, however, that MMS is a method that still is cost-effective compared with traditional SE.[32] This is because recurrence rates after MMS are lower and defects often are closed in a simpler fashion, because more uninvolved skin is preserved. A 5-year follow-up of patients in a prospective trial comparing MMS to SE showed that MMS was equally cost-effective for at least recurrent BCCs.[24] MMS should be performed in well-equipped centers with surgeons trained and experienced with MMS. In this fashion, several patients can be treated at the same time, maintaining cost-efficiency. Strict indications are important in keeping costs limited.

SKIN SQUAMOUS CELL CARCINOMA AND ITS PRECURSORS
Background

Like BCC, SCC of the skin typically is found in older, fair-skinned individuals. As with BCC, cases are not recorded in cancer registries, but the American Cancer Society estimated that 200,000 new cases were diagnosed in 2001. In the Netherlands, the incidence for men was 25.4 and for women 11.7 per 100,000 in 2000.[33] SCC is more prevalent in southern states of the United States reflecting its etiologic relationship with exposure to sunlight. An incidence of 118 per 100,000 has been reported in Hawaii.[34] Other risk factors are suppression of the immune system, chronic ulcerating disease, scars from burns, albinism, xeroderma pigmentosum, previous skin cancer, and AK. Recently, human papilloma virus has been found to play a role especially in non–sun-exposed body parts, such as the genitals and perianal area.[35]

SCCs of skin and adjacent mucosal surfaces are true carcinomas in origin and behavior. They arise from keratinocytes and show features of keratinization. SCCs are more likely to metastasize than BCCs but less likely compared with melanoma. Approximately 5% of SSCs metastasize.[36] Unlike BCC, SCC usually arises from precursors, such as AK and other in situ variants.

Precursors

Actinic keratosis

SCC has a highly prevalent progenitor in AK. It is widespread in white individuals who have a history of sunlight exposure. These neoplasms are found mostly on the face, ears, and dorsum of the hands. They represent solar damage to the keratinocytes, which clinically manifests itself as a small (usually <6 mm) erythematous patch covered with rigid, adherent scales (**Fig. 7**). The lesions are more easily palpated than seen. They can be solitary but also occur in groups. Patients usually complain when they induce a traumatic ulcer or erosion through scratching of the AKs. Younger patients usually present earlier with cosmetic complaints. The risk for progression of AK to SCC is estimated to be 8%, with mean time until conversion of approximately 2 years.[37,38]

A special type of AK occurs on the lower lip, called actinic cheilitis (**Fig. 8**). When it transforms

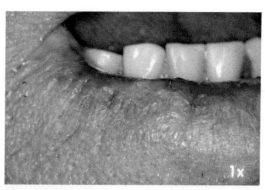

Fig. 8. Actinic cheilitis is an AK of the lower lip. The normal texture of the lip is lost; there is hyperkeratosis and the lesion feels indurated.

into SCC it is more likely to metastasize than SCC arising from AK anywhere else on the body.[39]

Other clinical variants are spreading pigmented AK (SPAK) and hypertrophic AK or cutaneous horn (**Figs. 9** and **10**). SPAK consists of a light brown to black, variegated plaque, which easily can be mistaken for lentigo maligna. Different from lentigo maligna, it has a more verrucous surface, which gives the same "AK feel" as common AKs. The cutaneous horn is exactly what the name insinuates, a horn made of keratin. This bizarrely shaped outgrowth hides a plain AK or even a SCC underneath.

When biopsied, AKs show overlying hyper- and parakeratosis and dysplasia at the level of germinative layer and stratum corneum, which sometimes extends into the papillary dermis as smalls nests of keratinocytes. Solar damage always is found in reticular dermis. The moment of transition from AK to SCC is a subject of debate among pathologists. To some the difference lies in the degree of dysplasia whereas others state that invasion of the reticular dermis should be regarded as a cutoff point. It is argued that groups of

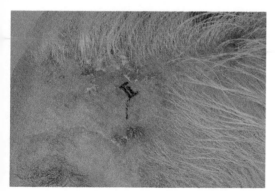

Fig. 7. AK in the temporal area. There is erythema and adherent yellowish scaling.

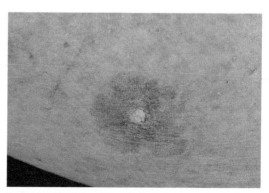

Fig. 9. SPAK with a hyperkeratotic center. It is distinguished from lentigo maligna by the absence of a pigment network on dermatoscopy.

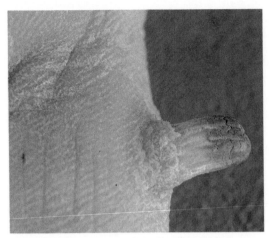

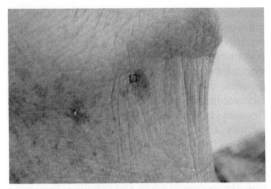

Fig. 11. Bowen's disease under the chin. This intraepi-thelial carcinoma presents as an erythematous macula with scaling.

Fig. 10. Cutaneous horn of the hand. A bizarre kera-totic outgrowth on the palm of the hand.

atypical keratinocytes, which are found in papillary dermis not in continuity with the overlying epidermis, should be classified as SCC. Nevertheless, there is consensus of regarding the advanced AKs as SCC in situ.

Treatment

There are many therapeutic options for AK. All clinical variants can be treated essentially in same fashion. The most common modality is cryosurgery. Medical treatment consisting of 5-FU or imiquimod cream also is widely used. PDT is an option especially if multiple grouped lesions can be treated simultaneously. In transplant patients in whom multiple and recurrent AKs often are found, preventive systemic treatment with retinoids yields good results.

Patients should be followed up regularly, at least twice every year, unless no new lesions develop. This allows for a safety margin if a SCC is missed.

Bowen's disease (intraepithelial carcinoma)

Bowen's disease is another clinical variant of SCC in situ. Clinically it manifests as a sharply defined erythematous plaque sometimes covered with scales. As such it resembles eczema and psoriasis (**Fig. 11**). It is rarely found on the face and occurs more frequently on the trunk and the extremities. When found in anogenital region it is called erythroplasia of Queyrat.

The aberration usually involves full thickness of the epidermis where different degrees of dysplasia can be seen. The cells show atypical mitoses but as a rule no invasion of the dermis is found. Full involvement of adnexal epithelium differentiates it from AK.

Treatment

Although SE does cure this in situ carcinoma, nonsurgical treatments might be more elegant. Treatment with imiquimod and 5-FU gives good success rates without cosmetic problems. PDT also is one of the nonsurgical methods regularly used by dermatologists. As with AKs, cryotherapy also gives good results.

Invasive Squamous Cell Carcinoma

SCCs usually present with hyperkeratosis, which makes it easy to tell them apart from BCCs. Like BCCs, they have a polymorph-presenting pattern, which varies from ulceration to tumors (**Fig. 12**). The distribution is similar to that of AK. Approximately two thirds of SCCs are found on the head.

Five percent of all SCCs metastasize even after treatment.[36] In 95% of cases, they take fewer than 5 years to become apparent. SCCs arising de novo or from radiation injury, chronic ulcers, or burn scars have the most potential to metastasize

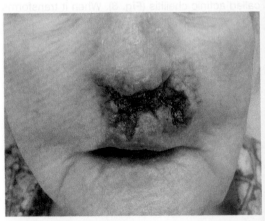

Fig. 12. A relatively large ulcer representing a SCC between nose and the lips.

compared with SCCs developing from AKs.[36,39] The likelihood of metastasis seems to depend on a few factors. A tumor size greater than 2 cm doubles the recurrence rate and triples the prevalence of metastases.[40] Tumor thickness, degree of histologic differentiation, tumor variants, perineural invasion, recurrence, and patient immunosuppression all also seem to play a role.

SCCs on non–sun-exposed sites have a greater potential to metastasize than SCC found on the face or extremities.[36] Considering the head, SCC on ears, nose, and lips are more likely to produce metastases than tumors occurring elsewhere on the face or scalp. The first route for dissemination is via lymphatic vessels into regional lymph nodes. These usually are the submandibular and parotid glands. Hematogenous spread does not seem to play a role. Probably more important means of advancement are the in-transit metastases. These are clusters of tumor cells found in the close vicinity of the primary tumor without direct contact. It is possible that this phenomenon accounts for recurrence after micrographic surgery.

Treatment

Conventional SE or excision by MMS always should be the first choice in treatment of primary cutaneous SCC. Other modalities, such as cryosurgery, excochleation, or radiotherapy, offer no histopathologic control (**Table 3**).

The British multidisciplinary guidelines (2003) advise a minimum of 4 mm of surgical margin in tumors less than 2 cm in diameter. For tumors larger than 2 cm or with a Broders' grade higher than 2 and those at high-risk locations (ear, lip, scalp, eyelids, and nose), a margin of 6 mm or more seems more appropriate.[39,41]

These rules are only applicable, however, when a tumor can be clinically defined. This is why the guidelines recommend MMS in these cases and at difficult sites where wider margins could result in functional impairment.

MMS results in highest cure rates and as such deserves an important place in treatment of high risk SCCs.[42] Indications for MMS in SCC are the same as for BCC (**Box 3**). There is no evidence of benefit of prophylactic lymph node dissection. Advanced stages with involvement of other tissues should be discussed within multidisciplinary teams before treatment.

MELANOMA AND BENIGN MELANOCYTIC LEASIONS
Background

Embryonically, melanocytes are derived from the neural crest; unlike BCCs and SCCs, which are pure epithelial tumors, melanomas are not carcinomas. Another, clinically more important difference is the potential to metastasize. Melanoma is one of the most aggressive tumors and virtually incurable after metastasis. It is known for its rapid growth and ability to rapidly metastasize hematogenously or through lymphatics.

The incidence of melanoma in the United States is 3 in 100,000 and it has been rising during the past 30 years.[43] Fortunately, the rise in incidence has been accompanied by a 39% decrease in overall mortality rates.[44] This is due to early detection, which is probably attributable to increased awareness among patients and physicians.

Risk factors for development of melanoma are fair skin, history of melanoma in index patients or family members, having atypical moles, sunburns, and exposure to UV radiation not only during childhood but also in adult life.[45,46] Genetics also play a role and, more specifically, individuals who have mutation of the CDKN2A gene are susceptible to development of melanoma. Patients who have xeroderma pigmentosum also are at high

Table 3 Treatment of squamous cell carcinoma and its precursors	
Neoplasm with Squamous Differentiation	**Treatment Options**
AK/in situ SCC	Cryotherapy 5-FU topical therapy Imiquimod Photodynamic therapy Laser resurfacing Systemic retinoids
Bowen's disease/erythroplasia of Queyrat	Cryotherapy 5-FU topical therapy Imiquimod Photodynamic therapy
SCC	MMS Conventional surgery

Box 3
Indications for Mohs' micrographic surgery for squamous cell carcinoma

SCC in the H zone of the face and the lip

Perineural growth

Tumor size >2 cm

Clinically hard to define tumor

Recurrent cancer

risk. Recently a role for vitamin D receptor polymorphism has been implied.[47]

Benign and Borderline Melanocytic Lesions

The vast majority of patients do not present with full-blown melanomas but with precursor forms or with concerns about pigmented lesions. Therefore, it is important to be able to recognize various forms of melanocytic lesions to prevent unnecessary excisions or treatment delay.

Melanocytes are found throughout the skin as single, dendritic cells surrounded by keratinocytes in the basal layer. In cases of hyperplasia, such as lentigo simplex and lentigo solaris, the relative number of normal melanocytes is increased. In neoplasms they are found as a group of cells or a nest and then are called nevus cells. Neoplasms of melanocytic origin can be classified approximately as benign, borderline, or malignant, with the borderline group represented by atypical moles.

Congenital Melanocytic Nevus

Congenital melanocytic nevi, or brown birthmarks, are present from birth. They represent local overgrowth of melanocytes (**Fig. 13**). They are classified arbitrarily according to size as small (<1.5 cm in diameter), medium (up to 10 cm), large (between 10 and 20 cm), and giant (>20 cm) melanocytic nevi. These lesions sometimes become darker with age or start exophytic growth. It is not unusual to observe hypertrichosis within these nevi. A 2.8% to 8.5% rate of malignant transformation is reported in giant nevi.[48,49] The nevus cells are not necessarily limited to the skin and sometimes are observed in subcutaneous tissues. The lesions can be treated for cosmetic reasons. Excision of these moles is not always an option because of their size. Early curettage (second or sixth week after birth) is the first choice of treatment but these nevi also can be treated with erbium lasers.

Blue Nevus

Blue nevus is a solitary bluish or black subepidermal dome-shaped node, which usually appears after the second decade but then never grows (**Fig. 14**). It is a variant of the common mole but appears blue because of its deeper location and subsequent Tyndall effect.

Clinical differential diagnosis of these moles includes nodular melanoma, Kaposi's sarcoma, and fibroangioma. Dendritic and spindle form melanocytes can be found at any level of the skin but usually reside deep in the dermis around skin adnexes.

Spindle Cell Melanocytic Nevus

The obsolete name for this neoplasia is juvenile melanoma. Patients are young children who have a firm, smooth surfaced papule with a color that can vary from pink to black (**Fig. 15**). It usually occurs on the face and patients present with parents concerned with the rapid growth.

Also known as Spitz tumor, this neoplasm can pose a great diagnostic challenge to pathologists as differentiation from frank melanoma can be difficult because almost all features of a melanoma sometimes are found. The cells usually show no atypical mitoses, and architectural arrangement is in neat, uniform, ovoid nests. Pagetoid spread of cells found in melanoma always is absent. Necrosis and a lymphocytic infiltrate further differentiate a melanoma form spindle cell melanocytic nevus.

Nevus Spilus

Nevus spilus consists of a light brown macula of several centimeters in diameter, which is filled

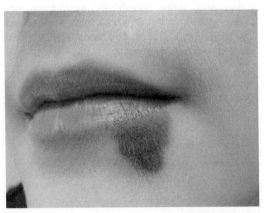

Fig. 13. Congenital nevus. A pigmented macula with hypertrichosis is seen under the lower lip.

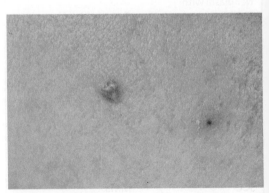

Fig. 14. A blue nevus. A gray bluish papule on the cheek.

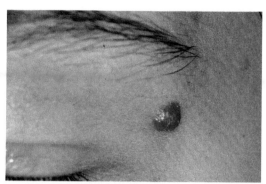

Fig. 15. Spindle cell melanocytic nevus. This boy presented with a growing red papule under the left eyebrow.

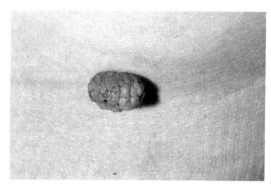

Fig. 16. Moles sometimes can grow into polypoid tumors. This one has become pedunculated. Its appearance has similarities to a berry.

with darker smaller maculas. The big macula often exists from birth whereas the smaller spots may emerge later in life. In these two areas, nevus spilus shows resemblance to lentigo solaris and junctional nevi.

Nevomelanocytic Nevus

Nevomelanocytic nevus (NMN) is the technical term for moles. They are acquired after birth and usually before the second decade. Nevus cells are melanocytes with a less dendritic morphology and arranged in small nests. There are three types of NMNs: dermal nevus, junction nevus, and compound nevus. This is a histopathologic classification: in dermal nevus, the nevus cells reside deep in the dermis; in junction nevus, cells are found in dermoepidermal junction; and compound nevus represents a hybrid form of the other two types. The dermal form is found almost exclusively on the face, where a firm flesh-colored papule can be seen. Sometimes telangiectases can be found over these moles, which add BCC to the differential diagnosis. In women, they may give rise to cosmetic concerns, and in men, frequent cutting during shaving may be a problem.

The other two forms can be a colored macula or a colored papule or sometimes appear papilomatous and pedunculated. The latter two types can pose mechanical and cosmetic problems (**Fig. 16**).

NMNs sometimes are surrounded by a halo of hypopigmentation. Although this phenomenon sometimes is seen in melanoma it has no diagnostic value.

Atypical Nevomelanocytic Nevus

Atypical melanocytic nevi (AMN) are the most important differential diagnosis of NMN. Approximately 5% of the white population has them. Their presence significantly raises the lifetime risk for

melanoma and they are regarded as potentially malignant. Patients who have familial multiple mole/melanoma syndrome (ie, individuals who have two first- or second-degree family members who have a history of melanoma) and who have atypical moles are especially at risk.

AMNs are an intermediate entity between NMN and superficial spreading melanoma (SSM). It can be difficult to distinguish between these types of melanocytic outgrowths but a few characteristics can be helpful. AMNs usually are acquired after puberty and measure more than 5 mm in diameter. When examined visually, asymmetry found in any of the aspects of the mole should alert clinicians. The aspects that can be appreciated by the naked eye are asymmetry in level or color distribution and circumscription of the mole (**Fig. 17**).

In dermatology it is a good practice to examine all pigmented lesions using a dermatoscope. This tool aids in diagnostic accuracy and in trained hands sensitivities and specificities of up to 90% are

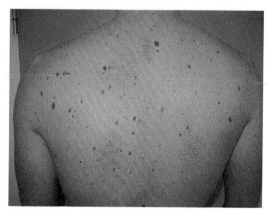

Fig. 17. Multiple AMN on the back of a young man. Note the size, variegation, and asymmetry.

reported.[50,51] On dermatoscopy the mole is examined systematically using the ABCD rule (**Fig. 18**).

ABCD Rule

The letters, ABCD, represent different aspects of a pigmented lesion that can be visualized with a dermatoscope (**Box 4**). The anomalies found in these aspects can be quantified further by scoring them linearly to the total area of the mole that is involved in it.

AMN resemble normal compound nevi histologically, except that they show cellular atypia (large nuclei and substantial quantities of cytoplasm) and abnormal nevus nests. The atypia varies in individual cells much more than what is seen in melanoma. Because of a high degree of proliferation, the rete ridges can be "bridged" by melanocytes. There is no pagetoid spread of melanocytes as in melanoma. A lymphocytic infiltrate sometimes is visualized.

Whenever there is suspicion of malignancy as a result of a high ABCD score, an atypical mole should be excised with 2-mm margins and sent for histopathologic examination.

Malignant Melanocytic Lesions

History and clinical manifestations

Suspicion of melanoma is raised not only by the clinical appearance but also by information from a patient's history. Growing, color changing, or itching moles are highly suspect. Also, bleeding or ulceration in an existing mole is suspicious. Family history of melanoma should be assessed in every patient as should risk factors, such as previous exposure to sun, sunburns, or other UV sources.

The archetypical bleeding mole with a history of rapid growth is not always found. Moreover, approximately 1.8% to 8.1% of melanomas are hypopigmented or fully amelanotic.[52]

Whenever pigment is seen, use of a dermatoscope should not be omitted. It also is important to palpate all probable draining lymph nodes, as this is an easy way of discovering advanced disease. Clinically, melanoma can be classified into four different variants: lentigo maligna, SSM, nodular melanoma, and acral lentiginous melanoma. Pathologists also use other divisions on the basis of tissue architecture, appearance of individual cells, and production of melanin.

Lentigo maligna and lentigo maligna melanoma

Lentigo maligna is the most relevant form of melanocytic neoplasm in facial surgery as it arises most frequently on sun-exposed areas, such as the hands and face. Clinically lentigo maligna melanoma is an irregularly pigmented brownish macula, usually in older patients, that keeps growing radially. Flat seborrheic keratosis and SPAK are main clinical differentials. Histologically, it is regarded as a melanoma in situ as it is characterized by proliferation of atypical melanocytes into the basal layers of the epidermis and hair follicles. It could be regarded as a lentigo senilis that has become malignant because they share many features.

The melanocytes usually form no nests and epidermis is unaffected. After some time the

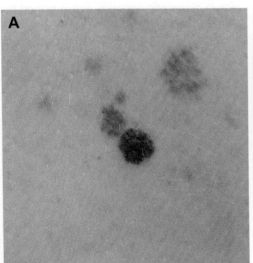
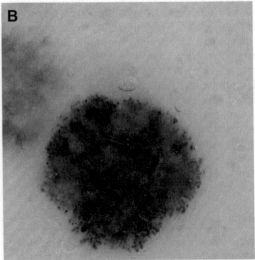

Fig. 18. (*A*) High-risk mole. (*B*) Same mole viewed through a dermatoscope. Dermatoscopy reveals more details; here variegation, globules, a gray veil, and streaks can easily be seen.

> **Box 4**
> **The ABCD rule**
>
> *Asymmetry:* asymmetry of the shape, texture, and color distribution
>
> *Border:* sharpness of demarcation, radial streaming
>
> *Color:* variegation, blue-white veil
>
> *Differential structures:* pigment network, globules, dots, and vascularization

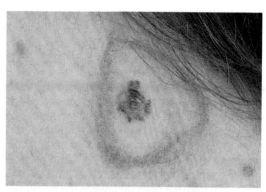

Fig. 20. SSM on the neck. This usually is a macular lesion although a papulous component can be observed in this example. This lesion also exhibits regression seen at the 9-o'clock position.

macula can thicken and become an invasive melanoma. Then it is called lentigo maligna melanoma (**Fig. 19**).

Superficial spreading melanoma

SSM usually originates from AMN. It is the most diagnosed melanocytic neoplasm. Up to 70% of all melanomas are SSMs. In men it frequently is found on the back and in women the legs usually are affected. Its growth is divided in two phases, radial and vertical. The radial phase is the first to start. After months or years, thickening of the lesion or vertical growth ensues. Even in the early phase it does not leave the epidermis unaffected so it easily can be distinguished from lentigo maligna (**Fig. 20**). Alternatively it shows many features exhibited by AMN. The melanocytes are arranged near the tips of rete ridges and show atypia, atypical mitoses, and pagetoid growth pattern. Individual cells or nests of cells invade the epidermis. A lymphocytic infiltrate is seen in the upper dermis.

Nodular melanoma

Nodular melanoma presents without a radial growth phase. This rapid growing tumor materializes de novo or originates from AMN and represents the most aggressive form (**Fig. 21**). Approximately 15% to 30% of melanomas are nodular. Because of its sometimes papulous and amelanotic appearance, it easily can be mistaken for a pyogenic granuloma or a hemangioma. Highly atypical cells infiltrate the epidermis and deep dermis. The tumor usually is encircled by lymphocytes. Perivascular extension often is seen.

Acral lentiginous melanoma

This type of melanoma is seen on the palms and soles and under the nails. It does not occur on the face. It is the most prevalent form in Asian and black populations. Subungual melanomas easily can be missed as they can manifest with subtle signs as brown streaks on the nails.

New hyperpigmentation in these areas, especially in Asian and black people, that are not present bilaterally or on two or more nails, should be perceived as a red flag. Its histology is similar

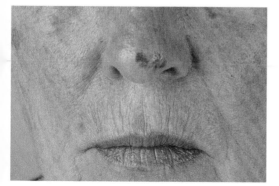

Fig. 19. Lentigo maligna of the nose. It presents as a sharply demarcated pigmented macula with variegation.

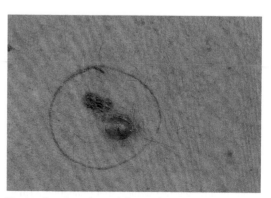

Fig. 21. Amelanotic nodular melanoma arising at the periphery of AMN.

to SSM as dendritic melanocytes predominate over spindle form ones.

Assessment of the melanoma

The first step in assessing a melanoma is measuring its thickness. This can be done using the method according to Breslow or Clark. Currently, the American Joint Committee on Cancer incorporates the Breslow method in T staging of the TNM system because of its higher accuracy and reproducibility. The Breslow thickness is the depth that the melanoma reaches measured from the granular layer in the epidermis. In conjunction with the consideration of ulceration it is the most prognostic factor for survival (**Table 4**). Excision margins also are determined using Breslow thickness.

Treatment

After a pathologist has found a malignancy, a re-excision has to be performed. Although currently trials with imiquimod for in situ variants are being conducted, the standard of care for all melanocytic malignancies is SE.

With histopathologic information obtained, minimal surgical margins can be used. For in situ melanomas this should be 5 mm. For tumors up to 2 mm in Breslow thickness, a margin of 1 cm should be applied and, in cases of thicker tumors, a re-excision of 2 cm is advisable (**Table 5**).[53–56]

Approximately 5% of patients who have melanoma with a diameter of 10 mm or less have positive sentinel nodes on biopsy.[57] Having a positive sentinel node influences the survival rate greatly and sentinel node procedure, therefore, has been a point of great interest. Its value has been subject of many debates but it seems that it has only prognostic value and does not contribute to disease-free survival.[58] Imaging diagnostics are only of prognostic value and in cases of clinically local disease the yield is too low to justify their deployment.[59]

Table 5
Surgical margins for excision of melanoma

Breslow Thickness	Surgical Margin (Cm)
In situ melanoma or excisional biopsy	0.5
≤2 mm	1.0
>2 mm	2.0

OTHER SKIN NEOPLASMS

Besides BCCs, SCCs, and melanomas, there are a variety of other cancers arising in the skin. The spectrum of the tumors of skin appendages is too vast to be discussed in detail in this article.

Skin appendages are eccrine and apocrine sweat glands and hair follicles. Tumors originating in them are classified considering the appendage, type of cell they resemble, degree of differentiation, and malignancy.

One of the cancers worth mention is the Merkel cell tumor. It accounts for less than 1% of all skin cancers and usually is found in older white patients. The survival rates are low, even compared with melanoma. Merkel's cells are believed to have a neuroendocrine function in the skin. They are normal residents found in skin of lips and hands. Merkel cell carcinomas usually are found in the head and neck region. They present as firm livid papules (**Fig. 22**). Microscopically the cells and their arrangement resemble those found in small cell lung carcinoma and sometimes they are confused with lymphomas. Special immunohistochemical stains are necessary to make the correct diagnosis. Treatment should be discussed in a multidisciplinary setting.

Cancers from subcutaneous and noncutaneous tissues can present in the skin, including Kaposi's

Table 4
Five-year survival rates for patients who have ulcerating and nonulcerating melanoma in relation to Breslow thickness

	Breslow Thickness in Millimeters			
	<1	1.01–2.0	2.01–4.0	>4
Nonulcerated	95%	89%	79%	67%
Ulcerated	91%	77%	63%	45%

Data from Balch CM, Soong SJ, Smith T, et al. Long-term results of a prospective surgical trial comparing 2 cm vs. 4 cm excision margins for 740 patients with 1–4 mm melanomas. Ann Surg Oncol 2001;8:101.

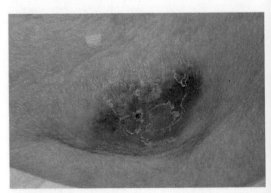

Fig. 22. Merkel cell carcinoma measuring 5 cm on the left hip.

sarcoma, lymphanigitis carcinomatosa, angiosarcoma, leimyoma, and myosarcoma. Also metastases from distant sites sometimes are found in the skin. Furthermore hematologic tumors, such as B- and T-cell lymphomas, are known to sometimes reside in the skin.

REFERENCES

1. Holme SA, Malinovszky K, Roberts DL. Changing trends in non-melanoma skin cancer in South Wales, 1988–98. Br J Dermatol 2000;143:1224–9.

2. Ko CB, Walton S, Keczkes K, et al. The emerging epidemic of skin cancer. Br J Dermatol 1994;130:269–72.

3. Smeets NW, Krekels GA, Ostertag JU, et al. Surgical excision vs Mohs' micrographic surgery for basal-cell carcinoma of the face: randomised controlled trial. Lancet 2004;364:1766–72.

4. Robinson JK, Dahiya M. Basal cell carcinoma with pulmonary and lymph node metastasis causing death. Arch Dermatol 2003;139:643–8.

5. Rigel DS, Friedman RJ, Kopf AW. Lifetime risk for development of skin cancer in the U.S. population: current estimate is now 1 in 5. J Am Acad Dermatol 1996;35:1012–3.

6. Smeets NW, Kuijpers DI, Nelemans P, et al. Mohs' micrographic surgery for treatment of basal cell carcinoma of the face—results of a retrospective study and review of the literature. Br J Dermatol 2004;151:141–7.

7. Chuang TY, Popescu A, Su WP, et al. Basal cell carcinoma. A population-based incidence study in Rochester, Minnesota. J Am Acad Dermatol 1990;22:413–7.

8. Giles GG, Marks R, Foley P. Incidence of non-melanocytic skin cancer treated in Australia. Br Med J (Clin Res Ed) 1988;296:13–7.

9. Coebergh JW, Neumann HA, Vrints LW, et al. Trends in the incidence of non-melanoma skin cancer in the SE Netherlands 1975–1988: a registry-based study. Br J Dermatol 1991;125:353–9.

10. Gallagher RP, Ma B, McLean DI, et al. Trends in basal cell carcinoma, squamous cell carcinoma, and melanoma of the skin from 1973 through 1987. J Am Acad Dermatol 1990;23:413–21.

11. Kumar P, Watson S, Brain AN, et al. Incomplete excision of basal cell carcinoma: a prospective multicentre audit. Br J Plast Surg 2002;55:616–22.

12. Oley CA, Sharpe H, Chenevix-Trench G. Basal cell carcinomas, coarse sparse hair, and milia. Am J Med Genet 1992;43:799–804.

13. Oettle AG. Rodent ulcers in identical twins. AMA Arch Derm 1956;74:167–72.

14. Schirren CG, Pfirstinger H [On the development of squamous cell carcinoma based Onjadassohn's nevus sebaceous.]. Hautarzt 1963;14:397–401 [in German].

15. von Domarus H, Stevens PJ. Metastatic basal cell carcinoma. Report of five cases and review of 170 cases in the literature. J Am Acad Dermatol 1984;10:1043–60.

16. Leffell DJ, Headington JT, Wong DS, et al. Aggressive-growth basal cell carcinoma in young adults. Arch Dermatol 1991;127:1663–7.

17. Cox NH. Basal cell carcinoma in young adults. Br J Dermatol 1992;127:26–9.

18. Kumakiri M, Hashimoto K. Ultrastructural resemblance of basal cell epithelioma to primary epithelial germ. J Cutan Pathol 1978;5:53–67.

19. Van Scott EJ, Reinertson RP. The modulating influence of stromal environment on epithelial cells studied in human autotransplants. J Invest Dermatol 1961;36:109–31.

20. Zackheim HS. Origin of the human basal cell epithelioma. J Invest Dermatol 1963;40:283–97.

21. Madsen A. Studies on basal-cell epithelioma of the skin.The architecture, manner of growth, and histogenesis of the tumours. Whole tumours examined in serial sections cut parallel to the skin surface. Acta Pathol Microbiol Scand Suppl 1965;177:163–73.

22. Rowe DE, Carroll RJ, Day CL Jr. Mohs surgery is the treatment of choice for recurrent (previously treated) basal cell carcinoma. J Dermatol Surg Oncol 1989;15:424–31.

23. Rowe DE, Carroll RJ, Day CL Jr. Long-term recurrence rates in previously untreated (primary) basal cell carcinoma: implications for patient follow-up. J Dermatol Surg Oncol 1989;15:315–28.

24. Mosterd K, Krekels GA, Nieman FH, et al. Surgical excision versus Mohs' micrographic surgery for primary and recurrent basal-cell carcinoma of the face: a prospective randomised controlled trial with 5-years' follow-up. Lancet Oncol 2008;9:1149–56.

25. Burg G, Hirsch RD, Konz B, et al. Histographic surgery: accuracy of visual assessment of the margins of basal-cell epithelioma. J Dermatol Surg 1975;1:21–4.

26. Breuninger H, Dietz K. Prediction of subclinical tumor infiltration in basal cell carcinoma. J Dermatol Surg Oncol 1991;17:574–8.

27. Panje WR, Ceilley RI. The influence of embryology of the mid-face on the spread of epithelial malignancies. Laryngoscope 1979;89:1914–20.

28. Smeets N. Workgroup basal cell carcinoma: Guideline Treatment of patients with basal cell carcinoma. In: Richtlijn Behandeling van patienten met basaalcelcarcinoom. Utrecht: Publication of the quality institute for healthcare CBO; 2003. p. 16–26. Available at: www.cbo.nl. Accessed February 2, 2009.

29. Verhaegh MEJM, Gruintjens FWG, Krekels GAM, et al. Surgical margins for excision of primary and recurrent basal cell carcinoma. [in. Maastricht] 1998;93–105.

30. Smith SP, Grande DJ. Basal cell carcinoma recurring after radiotherapy: a unique, difficult treatment subclass of recurrent basal cell carcinoma. J Dermatol Surg Oncol 1991;17:26–30.

31. Robinson JK, Fisher SG. Recurrent basal cell carcinoma after incomplete resection. Arch Dermatol 2000;136:1318–24.

32. Cook J, Zitelli JA. Mohs micrographic surgery: a cost analysis. J Am Acad Dermatol 1998;39:698–703.

33. de Vries E, van de Poll-Franse LV, Louwman WJ, et al. Predictions of skin cancer incidence in the Netherlands up to 2015. Br J Dermatol 2005;152:481–8.

34. Chuang TY, Reizner GT, Elpern DJ, et al. Squamous cell carcinoma in Kauai, Hawaii. Int J Dermatol 1995;34:393–7.

35. Hama N, Ohtsuka T, Yamazaki S. Detection of mucosal human papilloma virus DNA in bowenoid papulosis, Bowen's disease and squamous cell carcinoma of the skin. J Dermatol 2006;33:331–7.

36. Weinberg AS, Ogle CA, Shim EK. Metastatic cutaneous squamous cell carcinoma: an update. Dermatol Surg 2007;33:885–99.

37. Glogau RG. The risk of progression to invasive disease. J Am Acad Dermatol 2000;42:23–4.

38. Fuchs A, Marmur E. The kinetics of skin cancer: progression of actinic keratosis to squamous cell carcinoma. Dermatol Surg 2007;33:1099–101.

39. Motley R, Kersey P, Lawrence C. Multiprofessional guidelines for the management of the patient with primary cutaneous squamous cell carcinoma. Br J Plast Surg 2003;56:85–91.

40. Rowe DE, Carroll RJ, Day CL Jr. Prognostic factors for local recurrence, metastasis, and survival rates in squamous cell carcinoma of the skin, ear, and lip. Implications for treatment modality selection. J Am Acad Dermatol 1992;26:976–90.

41. Broders AC. Squamous-cell epithelioma of the skin: a study of 256 cases. Ann Surg 1921;73:141–60.

42. Neville JA, Welch E, Leffell DJ. Management of non-melanoma skin cancer in 2007. Nat Clin Pract Oncol 2007;4:462–9.

43. Ward EM, Thun MJ, Hannan LM, et al. Interpreting cancer trends. Ann N Y Acad Sci 2006;1076:29–53.

44. Geller AC, Miller DR, Annas GD, et al. Melanoma incidence and mortality among US whites, 1969–1999. JAMA 2002;288:1719–20.

45. Moan J, Porojnicu AC, Dahlback A. Ultraviolet radiation and malignant melanoma. Adv Exp Med Biol 2008;624:104–16.

46. Dennis LK, Vanbeek MJ, Beane Freeman LE, et al. Sunburns and risk of cutaneous melanoma: does age matter? A comprehensive meta-analysis. Ann Epidemiol 2008;18:614–27.

47. Mocellin S, Nitti D. Vitamin D receptor polymorphisms and the risk of cutaneous melanoma: a systematic review and meta-analysis. Cancer 2008;113:2398–407.

48. Watt AJ, Kotsis SV, Chung KC. Risk of melanoma arising in large congenital melanocytic nevi: a systematic review. Plast Reconstr Surg 2004;113:1968–74.

49. Quaba AA, Wallace AF. The incidence of malignant melanoma (0 to 15 years of age) arising in "large" congenital nevocellular nevi. Plast Reconstr Surg 1986;78:174–81.

50. Bafounta ML, Beauchet A, Aegerter P, et al. Is dermoscopy (epiluminescence microscopy) useful for the diagnosis of melanoma? Results of a meta-analysis using techniques adapted to the evaluation of diagnostic tests. Arch Dermatol 2001;137:1343–50.

51. Kittler H, Pehamberger H, Wolff K, et al. Diagnostic accuracy of dermoscopy. Lancet Oncol 2002;3:159–65.

52. Koch SE, Lange JR. Amelanotic melanoma: the great masquerader. J Am Acad Dermatol 2000;42:731–4.

53. Balch CM, Soong SJ, Smith T, et al. Long-term results of a prospective surgical trial comparing 2 cm vs. 4 cm excision margins for 740 patients with 1–4 mm melanomas. Ann Surg Oncol 2001;8:101–8.

54. Lens MB, Nathan P, Bataille V. Excision margins for primary cutaneous melanoma: updated pooled analysis of randomized controlled trials. Arch Surg 2007;142:885–91.

55. Haigh PI, DiFronzo LA, McCready DR. Optimal excision margins for primary cutaneous melanoma: a systematic review and meta-analysis. Can J Surg 2003;46:419–26.

56. Balch CM, Urist MM, Karakousis CP, et al. Efficacy of 2-cm surgical margins for intermediate-thickness melanomas (1 to 4 mm). Results of a multi-institutional randomized surgical trial. Ann Surg 1993;218:262–7.

57. Wright BE, Scheri RP, Ye X, et al. Importance of sentinel lymph node biopsy in patients with thin melanoma. Arch Surg 2008;143:892–9.

58. Koskivuo I, Talve L, Vihinen P, et al. Sentinel lymph node biopsy in cutaneous melanoma: a case-control study. Ann Surg Oncol 2007;14:3566–74.

59. Bergman W, Kruit WHJ, Nieweg OE, et al. Melanoma workgroup. Guideline Melanoma of the skin. In: Richtlijn Melanoom van de huid. Utrecht: Publication of the quality institute for healthcare CBO; 2004. p. 49–51. Available at: www.cbo.nl. Accessed February 2, 2009.

Indications and Outcomes of Radiation Therapy for Skin Cancer of the Head and Neck

Yongjin Wang, MD, Woodrow Wells, MD, John Waldron, MD*

KEYWORDS

- Skin cancer • Head and neck
- Radiation therapy • Indication • Outcome

Skin cancer is the most common malignancy. Basal cell carcinoma (BCC) and squamous cell carcinoma (SCC) account for approximately 95% of all primary malignant skin tumors and are the primary focus of this review. More than 1 million cases of BCC and SCC of the skin were expected to be newly diagnosed in United States in 2008.[1] Although BCC and SCC of the skin are common, they account for less than 0.1% of patient deaths caused by cancer.[2] Characteristically, skin cancer develops on sun-exposed areas of lighter-skinned individuals, with most lesions occurring on the head and neck.

For skin cancer of the head and neck the treatment options include surgery, radiation therapy, and in some instances a combination of both. Management decisions are guided by the extent of tumor, anatomic site, previous treatments, and the general medical condition of the patient. Cancer of the skin may be removed by conventional resection, Mohs' micrographic surgery, electrodesiccation, or curettage. Surgical resection of skin cancer is an expedient treatment that offers the advantage of pathologic assessment of the margins. Surgical resection usually achieves excellent local control rates of 90% to 95%. Higher risk for recurrence is correlated with larger tumor size, deep infiltration, poor histologic differentiation, location (ear, lip, and embryonic fusion zones), perineural invasion, recurrent cancer, and immunosuppression.[3–6] Radiation therapy represents an alternative to surgical resection for skin cancer of the head and neck. The advantages of radiation therapy include preservation of anatomy and avoidance of surgery, particularly in elderly patients who may not be suitable for general anesthesia. Irradiation can be administered with a variety of techniques, including orthovoltage x-ray, electrons, and megavoltage photons (x ray or γ ray). Orthovoltage x-rays are produced by x-ray tubes operating in the range of 150 to 500 kV. Orthovoltage x-rays have the advantages of full-radiation dose delivery at the skin surface with limited dose to deeper structures, sharply defined field edges because of sharp penumbra (a region at the edge of a radiation beam over which dose rate changes rapidly), and lower equipment costs. Electron and megavoltage photons are produced by linear accelerators and have the advantage of deeper penetration of dose for the treatment of tumors extending deeper than a few centimeters or involving regional nodes.

INDICATIONS FOR RADIATION THERAPY

Radiation therapy is an option in the primary treatment of skin cancer. It offers an advantage of tissue preservation in the treatment of large tumors where clear surgical margins may be difficult to obtain in the head and neck.[7,8] Tumors located along embryonic fusion planes of perinasal and periauricular regions have greater potential for deep invasion and may be managed better with primary irradiation.[9] Radiation therapy

Radiation Medicine Program, Princess Margaret Hospital, 610 University Avenue, 5th Floor, Toronto, Ontario M5G 2M9, Canada
* Corresponding author.
E-mail address: john.waldron@rmp.uhn.on.ca (J. Waldron).

Clin Plastic Surg 36 (2009) 335–344
doi:10.1016/j.cps.2009.02.008
0094-1298/09/$ – see front matter © 2009 Elsevier Inc. All rights reserved.

also may be used in a combined approach with surgery when it often is given postoperatively when there are concerns as to the potential for residual disease after resection.[10] Radiation therapy also may be considered when tumors are located at certain anatomic sites where surgery could cause cosmetic or functional impairment, such as the eyelid, nose, ear, or lip. Surgery for these sites can cause suboptimal cosmesis because of the need for excising some normal tissue around the tumor and surgical reconstruction. Radiation therapy treatment has the advantage of tissue preservation that may have better cosmesis, especially for medium- or large-sized tumors. When the normal tissue framework is not severely destroyed, reconstitution of these structures after tumor eradication usually is very good.

Primary radiation therapy offers an advantage for elderly, frail, or medically inoperable patients. Radiation therapy causes minimal discomfort for patients and avoids invasive procedures for patients who are unwilling to undergo or cannot tolerate surgery. It does not require anesthesia, and effective radiation dose fractionation can be designed to minimize the number of treatment fractions.[7]

In addition to primary radiation therapy, adjuvant postoperative radiation therapy may be indicated for patients who have close, indeterminate, or positive margins after surgical resection. The incidence of positive surgical margins varies from 5% to 31%.[11,12] Treatment decisions in the adjuvant setting need to be individualized and can be influenced by the histologic subtype of the primary tumor and margin status. Most patients who have positive surgical margins should be referred to a radiation oncologist for an opinion regarding the use of adjuvant radiation. Although selected patients who have small BCCs and positive margins may be observed, those who have more advanced disease or extensive margin involvement should be treated. For patients who have positive margins from SCC, adjuvant radiation therapy or re-excision usually is recommended because local control and survival can be improved with adjuvant irradiation compared with observation with salvage treatment at relapse.[13]

Radiation therapy often is used as adjuvant treatment of skin cancer with perineural invasion that has high risk for recurrence. Perineural invasion occurs in 2% to 6% of patients who have skin cancer.[14–16] It can be an incidental microscopic finding or clinical perineural invasion on imaging with or without cranial nerve deficits. The optimal treatment is surgical resection followed by postoperative radiation for patients who have resectable disease. Those who have unresectable tumors are treated with definitive radiation therapy. Patients who have gross perineural invasion have inferior outcome compared with patients who have microscopic perineural invasion. The local control rates in patients who have gross perineural invasion and microscopic perineural invasion were 50% to 55% and 78% to 87%, respectively.[17–19] MRI is the best imaging study for gross perineural invasion and can be used in radiation planning.[20] In cases of perineural invasion, radiation oncologists need to pay attention to the potential routes of perineural spread and include these in the irradiated volume. The radiation volumes usually encompass the primary site and the involved nerve up to the skull base. These patients may experience more treatment-related toxicity because of the larger volume of tissue irradiated.[19] The role of adjuvant radiation therapy for patients who have incidental microscopic perineural invasion found at biopsy is controversial. Adjuvant radiation may improve locoregional control in patients who have other additional risk features for recurrence. These high-risk features include anatomic location (midface), recurrent cancer, and extent of nerve involvement.[21]

Although lymph node metastases are rare for BCC, the risk of involvement is 5% 10% for SCC. Presentation with lymph node metastasis represents an aggressive disease presentation and is correlated with a less favorable prognosis. Patients presenting with nodal metastasis often have predisposing factors for aggressive disease, such as advanced age (ninth or tenth decade of life) or an immunosuppressed state (transplant patients). Such patients presenting with skin malignancies should have their neck examined carefully at the time of staging. Treatment options for positive lymph nodes include lymph node dissection, irradiation, or both. Patients who have multiple nodes involved or extracapsular extension of nodal metastasis should be considered for postoperative radiation to the neck. The 10-year survival rate is less than 20% for patients who have regional lymph node involvement.[22,23] The parotid area is the most commonly involved first echelon nodal site for skin cancer of the face and scalp. These nodes are particularly suited to treatment with combined surgical resection and adjuvant radiation therapy or radical radiation therapy alone. Combined treatment with surgery and irradiation has better nodal control compared with surgery alone or radiation therapy alone.[24] Patients who have high risk for microscopic metastasis to regional nodes but clinically negative nodes can be treated electively with surgery or radiation therapy.[19,25,26]

Prophylactic radiation therapy to a dose equivalent to 50 Gy in 25 fractions should be delivered to nodal regions considered at high risk.

In addition to curative intent, radiation therapy can be used in palliative treatment of patients who have metastatic skin cancer. Palliative irradiation is effective for stopping bleeding, improving pain control, or shrink tumoring for cosmetic and functional purposes. The indications of radiation therapy are summarized in **Box 1**.

The disadvantages of radiation therapy for the treatment of skin cancer include lack of full pathologic information, the inconvenience of attending daily radiation therapy for multiple fractions, potential worsening cosmesis over a long time, and risk for secondary malignancy. Radiation therapy usually is not recommended for treatment of skin cancer in young patients because of potential cosmetic deterioration over time and potential carcinogenic effect.[4,7] Patients younger than 50 years of age and who have small to medium-sized tumor amenable to resection without significant functional or cosmetic loss are treated better with surgery. The risk for secondary malignancy after radiation therapy for skin cancer is small. In a large retrospective study of 1188 patients, Caccialanza and colleagues[27] reported no radiation-induced malignancy; nevertheless, radiation-induced malignancies can occur. Skin cancer of the scalp usually is treated with surgery because

radiation causes permanent hair loss in the radiation field. Irradiation is contraindicated for xeroderma pigmentosum and basal cell nevus syndrome (Gorlin syndrome) because radiation may induce further malignancy.

RADIATION THERAPY TECHNIQUES

There are many specialized radiation therapy techniques for the treatment of skin cancer. The technique used is determined by tumor size, depth of invasion, and anatomic location of the tumor. By selecting the optimum radiation technique, adequate radiation dose is delivered to the target volume, but the surrounding normal tissues are spared. The dose fractionation regimen chosen depends on the total radiation dose required, desire for expedient treatment, expected toxicity, and cosmetic and functional considerations. Late effects on normal tissues are related to fraction size and can be minimized with a smaller dose per fraction. Small volume primary tumors requiring only a few square centimeters of skin irradiated can be treated with a shorter course of radiation with a larger dose per fraction, such as 35 Gy in 5 fractions, although for treatment of larger volumes, the dose often is delivered in smaller fractions to a higher total dose, such as 70 Gy in 35 fractions.

Patients usually are placed in a supine position on the bed of a treatment machine. The head and neck are immobilized with thermoplastic mask that is attached to the bed to achieve immobilization and good reproducibility of positioning day to day during the course of fractionated radiation therapy. Although a course of radiation therapy may be protracted over several weeks, daily treatment often requires only a few minutes. Treatment may be accelerated with excellent local control but with more side effects and poor cosmesis, including depigmentation, skin atrophy, fibrosis, and telangiectasia.

Most skin cancers are treated with orthovoltage x-rays or electron beams. Orthovoltage energies from 75 to 125 kV can treat targets up to 5-mm thick and higher energy of 200 to 250 kV beams used for thicker targets up to 1 cm. Orthovoltage x-rays deposit maximum dose at the skin surface, and the dose decreases exponentially at depth. Smaller radiation fields can be used because orthovoltage x-rays have the advantage of small penumbra of 1 to 2 mm. Because of these characteristics, orthovoltage x-rays often are used in the treatment of superficial small tumors, especially when the tumors are located on the eyelid, nose, or ear.

Box 1
Indications for radiation therapy

Primary radiation therapy

- Large tumors where clear surgical margins may be difficult to obtain
- Tumors located at certain anatomic sites where surgery could cause cosmetic or functional impairment (such as the eyelid, nose, ear, or lip)
- Tumors located along embryonic fusion planes
- Elderly, frail, or medically inoperable patients

Adjuvant postoperative radiation therapy

- Close, indeterminate, or positive margins after surgery
- Perineural invasion
- Multiple positive lymph nodes or nodal extracapsular extension

Palliative radiation therapy

- Symptomatic distant metastasis to soft tissue, bone, or lung
- Symptomatic (pain, bleeding, and/or mass effects) advanced incurable primary site disease

Electron beams are generated by a linear accelerator. Modern linear accelerators can produce a variety of electron beam energies, from 6 to 20 MeV. Electron beams offer the advantage of a relatively uniform dose superficially followed by a rapid dose fall-off at depth. The depth of tissue uniformly treated by an electron beam depends on beam energy, ranging from 1.5 cm for 6-MeV electron beam to 5 cm for 20-MeV electron beam. Beyond that depth, the rapid dose fall-off permits greater sparing of underlying normal structures. Electron beams can be modified with a bolus (tissue-equivalent material) on the skin surface to obtain full dose at skin in the treatment of skin cancer. Although there are a variety of reasons for choosing electron beam or orthovoltage x-ray for given patients, there is no difference in tumor control outcome between electron beam and orthovoltage x-ray therapy.[28,29]

Megavoltage photon beam irradiation is used for advanced tumors with deep penetration and large volumes, such as neck lymph node regions. Like electrons, megavoltage photons are generated by a linear accelerator. In modern radiation therapy of skin cancer of the head and neck, intensity-modulated radiation therapy (IMRT) with megavoltage photon is used to deliver highly conformal radiation dose to the target and spares surrounding critical normal structures. An example of conformal irradiation with IMRT technique is shown in **Fig. 1**.

For a typical course of radiation treatment, the volumes irradiated include gross tumor, a 0.5- to 1-cm normal tissue margin surrounding gross tumor volume to account for potential subclinical or microscopic extension of disease, and another 5-mm margin to account for variations in daily setup of the patient (defined as the planning target volume). For orthovoltage treatment, the radiation field edge usually is 1 to 1.5 cm from gross tumor. Radiation field is delineated carefully and lead cutouts are used to define the borders of the field. Protective shields may be used if necessary. For electron beams, the penumbra is wider (approximately 1 cm) and the field edge of electron beam usually is 2 to 2.5 cm from gross tumor.

Dose fractionation schemes depend on patient factors and tumor characteristics. The total radiation dose delivered varies with tumor size, depth of invasion, location, and dose fractionation. Higher dose per fraction (eg, 35 Gy in 5 fractions over 5 days) for shorter treatment times are used for small tumors, in frail elderly patients, and at locations where cosmesis is not a concern. For medium-sized tumors, 50 Gy in 20 fractions or 45 Gy in 10 to 15 fractions commonly is used. For large tumors, 60 to 70 Gy in 2 Gy per fraction is used. Similar dose and fractionation regimens are used for BCC and SCC.

TREATMENT OUTCOME WITH RADIATION THERAPY

Interpretation of the literature reporting the outcomes for skin cancer treatment with different modalities is challenging because of nonuniformity of endpoint reporting, treatment selection bias, varying length of follow-up in reported series,

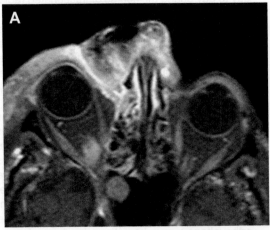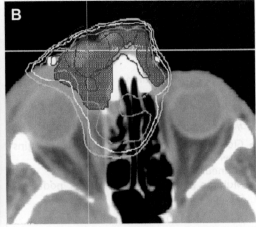

Fig. 1. (A) MRI of a patient who had SCC of bridge of the nose. The skin cancer was unresectable because of invasion of the orbit. (B) Radiation dose distribution in the same patient as in **Fig. 1**A. Conformal radiation therapy was administered with IMRT technique to deliver radiation to the gross tumor volume (*shaded red*) and surrounding tissues at risk for subclinical microscopic tumor extension with sparing of the surrounding critical structures (optic nerves, chiasm, brain, and eye globes). The yellow line and green lines were 95% and 90% isodose lines, respectively.

and the wide span of time periods over which case series were generated and reported.[5,30] Most patients have a favorable prognosis regardless of treatment selected. Care should be taken, however, to individualize treatment approach depending on tumor factors and patient characteristics. The treatment selected should offer high cure rate with acceptable cosmetic and functional results. Factors to be considered include tumor size, depth of invasion, anatomic location, involvement of adjacent cartilage or bone, previous treatment, and patient's general medical condition.

There has been only one randomized trial reported in the literature comparing the outcome of surgery versus radiation therapy. This randomized trial was designed to address the question whether or not conventional surgery or radiation therapy should be used in facial BCCs measuring less than 4 cm.[31] Radiation therapy was delivered using three techniques: "conventional" radiation therapy with 85 to 250 kV x-ray, superficial contact therapy with 50 kV x-ray, and brachytherapy with iridium-192 wire. The choice of the radiation technique was based on tumor size, location, and performance status, with small tumors receiving superficial contact therapy and the larger tumors receiving conventional radiation therapy. The 4-year actuarial local failure rate (persistence or recurrence) was lower in the surgery arm (0.7%) than the radiation therapy arm (8%). In this trial, surgery resulted in a dramatically low failure rate that was lower than published series, which ranged from 2% to 10%.[3] The tumor control with conventional surgery in this trial is similar to Mohs' micrographic surgery. Although radiation therapy had lower local control rate than surgery in the facial BCC in this trial, it can cure the majority of patients (92%).

There are many retrospective studies on treatment of skin cancer of the head and neck. Rowe and colleagues[3] conducted a comprehensive review of retrospective data in the literature. They examined all studies reporting local recurrence or metastasis data after surgical resection, radiation therapy, curettage and electrodesiccation, cryotherapy, or Mohs' micrographic surgery in SCC of the skin, lip, and ear. Eight clinical factors were found to correlate with increased risk for local recurrence or metastasis. These risk factors include tumor size greater than 2 cm, depth of 4 mm or greater, poor histologic differentiation, site (ear or lip), SCC within scar or on non–sun-exposed skin, recurrent tumor, perineural invasion, and immunosuppression. Long-term local recurrence rate was less for Mohs' micrographic surgery than any other treatment modalities. The non-Mohs' modalities (cryotherapy, curettage

and electrodesiccation, radiation therapy, and conventional surgery) had similar excellent cure rates (92%) in the absence of risk factors for local recurrence.[3] For BCC of the skin, the 5-year recurrence rates after conventional surgical excision (10%), radiation therapy (9%), curettage and electrodesiccation (8%), cryotherapy (8%), and Mohs' micrographic surgery (1%) were similar to the recurrence rates for SCC.[32]

Primary radiation therapy has been used to treat clinical T4 skin carcinoma of the head and neck. T4 skin cancer is defined as tumor that invades deep extradermal structures (eg, cartilage, skeletal muscle, or bone).[33] Radiation therapy alone results in 5-year local control rate of 47% to 53% and ultimate local control rate of 80% to 90% with salvage surgery.[8,34–36]

Patients who have positive lymph nodes generally are managed by nodal dissection and postoperative adjuvant radiation therapy. Veness and colleagues[37] reported on 167 patients who had nodal metastasis of skin cancer in the head and neck. Patients were treated with surgery alone or combined surgery and adjuvant radiation therapy. Adjuvant radiation therapy reduced locoregional recurrence from 43% to 20% and improved 5-year disease-free survival rates from 54% to 73%. Others have similarly reported that combined surgery and radiation therapy had more favorable results than either surgery alone or radiation therapy alone in patients who had positive nodes in parotid region.[38,39] The regional nodal control rates with surgery alone, irradiation alone, combined surgery and irradiation were 15% to 63%, 46% to 53%, and 80% to 90%, respectively.[24,38,39]

Eyelid

Medium to large-sized carcinomas of the eyelids most often are treated with irradiation because of difficulty in achieving adequate surgical margins. Attention to radiation technique is important to spare the anterior segment of the eye with appropriate shielding to minimize ocular complications. Surgery usually is the preferred treatment for eyelid tumors less than 0.5 cm.[40]

For radiation therapy for eyelid cancer, an eye shield is inserted over the conjunctiva daily using local anesthetic with eye drops. An eye shield can similarly protect the anterior segment when orthovoltage x-ray or electron beam irradiation is used. Orthovoltage x-rays are preferable to electron beam for skin cancer near the eye because of the ability to minimize radiation field size, sharper field edge, and ease of shielding.[41] When treating cancers located on the upper eyelid, if possible the lacrimal gland should be shielded to avoid late side effects of eye irritation and keratoconjunctivitis due to dry eye. Similarly, for lower eyelid cancers, protection of the lacrimal duct is desired to avoid stricture and overflow tearing. When tumor is located at medial canthus, ectropion and epiphora can occur because of inability to shield the lacrimal duct, but these complications are rare at 3% to 5%.[7,42] Epilation of eyelashes always occurs in the radiation field; hence, any uninvolved eyelid is shielded to prevent from epilation.

Fitzpatrick reviewed the Princess Margaret Hospital experience of treating BCC and SCC of the eyelid with orthovoltage x-rays. Of 1166 tumors, the 5-year tumor control rate was 95%. For most tumors with an average size of 1.2 cm in diameter, 35 Gy in 5 fractions over 5 days usually was used. Protracted fractionation schemes at small daily doses usually give better cosmetic and functional results, especially for large infiltrating tumors. The desire for good cosmesis should be weighed against the need for treatment expediency. When adequate shielding protected the eye, ocular complications did not occur. Epilation always occurred within the radiation field and most patients readily accepted this.[42] In another series of 128 patients who had periocular BCCs and who underwent radiation therapy, 100% local control at minimum 3 years' follow-up was achieved. There were no serious complications after radiation therapy.[43]

Nose

The nose is one of the most common sites for skin BCC and SCC. Nasal carcinoma can be treated effectively by radiation therapy with good local control and cosmesis even in the presence of cartilage invasion.[44] Careful attention to irradiation technique and dose fractionation is necessary. Contour variations of the nose could result in undesirable underdosing on the posterior area of the nose. This can be corrected by a compensating attenuator made of lucite or thin layers of aluminum. Electron or megavoltage photons also can be used to treat cancer of the nose. A wax bolus over the nose is used to ensure homogeneous radiation dose distribution over this otherwise uneven surface. Dose fractionation regimens depend on size and depth of the lesion, presence or absence of bone or cartilage involvement, radiation beam quality, and the general medical condition of patients. As with other sites, more fractionated treatment regimens are necessary for large tumors.[36] Cosmetic outcome depends on the amount of normal tissue

destroyed by tumor and treatment technique. When orthovoltage x-ray is used, lead cutouts are used to help define treatment field borders and spare surrounding normal tissues.

Caccialanza and colleagues[45] reported results in 405 skin cancers of the nose treated by radiation therapy. The total dose of radiation administered ranged from 40 to 85 Gy, with different dose fractionations according to the techniques used. The 5-year cure rate was 89%. Cosmetic results were evaluated as "good/acceptable" in 96% of the tumors that remained in complete remission. No severe radiation complications were observed. Radiation therapy was able to provide high rates of remission in the treatment of nose skin carcinoma without damaging the underlying cartilage. Although excellent local control and 5-year cancer-specific survival up to 96% can be achieved in patients who have skin cancers arising on the nose, overall survival of this patient cohort is poor because of advanced age and comorbidities.[46]

Ear

Skin cancers of the external ear can be treated successfully with radiation therapy. Smaller superficial lesions may be managed with orthovoltage x-ray or electron beam using more rapid dose fractionation. Extensive, deeply infiltrating tumors with bone or cartilage involvement require electron or megavoltage photon beam, with more protracted fractionation schemes. Irregular surface contour of the pinna can cause dose inhomogeneity, which can be eliminated with wax bolus to the ear.

Silva and colleagues[47] reported their experience of treating 334 cancers of the ear in 313 patients. Orthovoltage x-ray or electron beam was used. Dose fractionations were 35 Gy in 5 fractions, 42.5 to 45 Gy in 10 fractions, or 50 to 65 Gy in 20 to 30 fractions. Actuarial 5-year local control rate was 79%. Increased local failure rate was correlated to larger tumor size greater than 2 cm and lower biologic equivalent dose. For small tumors less than 2 cm in diameter, local control rates of 90% or more were achieved. Dose-fractionation schedules using fraction sizes less than 4 Gy can reduce the risk for cartilage necrosis and ulceration. Other investigators reported no cartilage necrosis of the ear when daily fraction size 3 Gy or less was used.[34]

Lip

Carcinoma of the lip can be treated with orthovoltage x-ray or electron beam. An intraoral lead shielding usually is used to protect the normal tissues of oral cavity. High local control rate in the range of 94% to 100% has been reported in SCC of the lip with tumor size of 4 cm or less. Patients usually tolerated radiation therapy well and the long-term cosmetic and functional results were good.[34,48] Petrovich and colleagues[34] reported 250 cases of cancer of the lip treated with radiation therapy. Some patients (2%) developed necrosis of mandible after radiation therapy, but all those patients had massive invasion of the mandible at diagnosis. Good cosmesis and function were observed in patients who had fractionation of 3 Gy or less per fraction.

ADJUVANT RADIATION THERAPY

Positive surgical margins are not uncommon in skin cancer of the head and neck. In a large retrospective review of 1833 patients, incidence of positive margins was 31% in the ear, 28% in the nose, 20% in the cheek, 18% in the lip, 17% in the periorbital area, and 12% in the neck.[12] Postoperative adjuvant radiation therapy is an effective treatment in the management of positive surgical margins in BCC and SCC.[49] For BCC of the skin, surveillance is an option for small BCCs in compliant patients willing to return for regular follow-up, for cancer not involving embryonic fusion planes, and for cancer not in the vicinity of sensitive areas for function and cosmesis. For patients who have positive margins in SCC of the skin, however, further immediate treatment with adjuvant radiation therapy or re-excision is recommended because recurrence could predispose patients to aggressive forms of tumor failure.

Salvage may be difficult if the recurrent tumor has extensive local failure, neurotropic invasion, or regional lymph node metastasis. Perez reported 87% local control and 10% to 15% nodal metastases in patients who had immediate radiation versus 65% local control and 39% nodal metastases in patients who had initial observation and salvage treatment at recurrence.[13]

PALLIATIVE RADIATION

Distant metastases in skin cancer are uncommon. The incidences of metastatic BCC and SCC are less than 0.1% and less than 5%, respectively.[3,50] Skin cancer can metastasize to the lung, bone, and liver. The diagnosis of distant metastasis represents an incurable state and the prognosis for such patients is poor, with median survival of 8 to 10 months.[51,52] Even though these metastases are incurable, radiation therapy can play a role in palliation for these patients to improve pain control, stop bleeding, or shrink tumor for cosmetic and functional purposes. Palliative radiation therapy with a short course of 20 Gy in 5 fractions or 30 Gy in 10 fractions can be used. For selected patients who have good performance status and minimal bulk of metastatic disease, higher doses (50–70 Gy) may be considered to prolong local control for palliative purposes.

COSMESIS AFTER RADIATION THERAPY

The early (acute) side effects of radiation therapy for skin cancer occur shortly after commencing a course of treatment, progress through treatment,

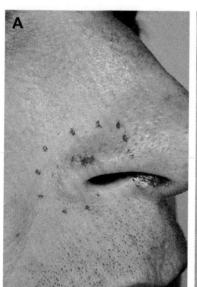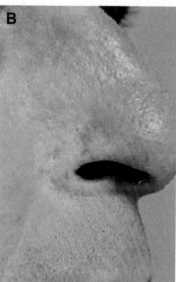

Fig. 2. (A) BCC of the nose (pretreatment). (B) Typical hypopigmentation and telangiectasia of the skin developed after radiation therapy. This photograph was taken 5 years after irradiation (same patient as in **Fig. 2A**).

and usually resolve within 90 days of completion of treatment. For areas of skin receiving full dose, these include skin erythema progressing to dry, then moist, desquamation and crusting. Areas of moist desquamation typically resolve within 6 weeks of completing treatment.

Late (chronic) side effects of radiation therapy include telangiectasia, depigmentation (hypopigmentation or hyperpigmentation), alopecia, skin atrophy, fibrosis, scar, ulcer, and necrosis. Late side effects may develop a few months to a few years after radiation therapy and may progress slowly over a few decades. Cosmetic results have been reported in retrospective studies. After radiation therapy, most patients have good to excellent cosmesis although mild hypopigmentation or telangiectasia develops in the radiation fields in the majority of patients (**Fig. 2**).[53] Cosmesis depends on tumor size, location, and radiation dose fractionation. Excellent or good cosmetic results were observed in 98% of patients who had tumor size 1 cm or less, 88% of patients who had tumor size 1 to 5 cm, and 82% of patients who had tumor size larger than 5 cm.[53] Radiation therapy schedules of lower dose per fraction can achieve equivalent tumor control and improved late cosmetic outcome compared with higher dose per fraction.[27,54]

For skin cancer of the eyelids, Fitzpatrick reported a special review of tumors less than 2 cm in diameter irradiated with 35 Gy in 5 daily fractions. A multidisciplinary audit was performed using the patients and members of an ocular oncology team that included an ophthalmologist, a radiation oncologist, and a nurse. There was remarkable agreement among the observers who scored independently using a scale from 1 to 10, with 1 indicating ugly/uncomfortable and 10 perfect. The average scores were 8 for cosmesis and for function at 5 years after radiation therapy.[42]

Small, uncomplicated skin cancers of the head and neck in young patients that can be excised easily are better treated with surgical excision because of possible higher local control rate and better long-term cosmetic results. In a randomized trial comparing outcome of surgery to radiation therapy in 347 patients who had facial BCC measuring less than 4 cm, cosmesis was assessed as a secondary endpoint. It was assessed by a level of patient satisfaction using a visual analog scale and questions to patients directed by a physician. A physician and three other individuals not involved in the trial, including a photographer, a data manager, and a medical secretary, also assessed cosmesis. Four years after treatment, the cosmetic results were good in 87% of patients after surgery and in 69% of patients after radiation therapy. The main chronic side effects of radiation therapy were depigmentation, telangiectasia, and skin atrophy.[31]

SUMMARY

Radiation therapy is an important option for the treatment of skin cancer. It has the advantages of preserving normal tissues, noninvasive outpatient treatment, and no need for anesthesia. Radiation therapy commonly is used for deeper and extensive tumor and anatomic sites where it is difficult to obtain clear surgical margins without functional or cosmetic loss (eg, eyelid, nose, ear, or lip). In addition, radiation therapy is used as adjuvant treatment for patients who have positive surgical margins, perineural invasion, or regional node metastasis. It is useful especially for elderly patients who are unwilling or unable to undergo surgery. Radiation therapy is an effective treatment in eradicating gross and microscopic skin cancer, with a 5-year cure rate of 90% to 95%.

REFERENCES

1. Jemal A, Siegel R, Ward E, et al. Cancer statistics, 2008. CA Cancer J Clin 2008;58(2):71–96.
2. Wagner RF, Casciato DA. Skin cancers. In: Casciato DA, Lowitz BB, editors. Manual of Clinical Oncology. Philadelphia: Lippincott, Williams, and Wilkins; 2000. p. 336–73.
3. Rowe DE, Carroll RJ, Day CL Jr. Prognostic factors for local recurrence, metastasis, and survival rates in squamous cell carcinoma of the skin, ear, and lip. Implications for treatment modality selection. J Am Acad Dermatol 1992;26(6):976–90.
4. Preston DS, Stern RS. Nonmelanoma cancers of the skin. N Engl J Med 1992;327(23):1649–62.
5. Thissen MR, Neumann MH, Schouten LJ. A systematic review of treatment modalities for primary basal cell carcinomas. Arch Dermatol 1999;135(10):1177–83.
6. Mikhail GR. Cancers, precancers, and pseudocancers on the male genitalia. A review of clinical appearances, histopathology, and management. J Dermatol Surg Oncol 1980;6(12):1027–35.
7. Morrison WH, Garden AS, Ang KK. Radiation therapy for nonmelanoma skin carcinomas. Clin Plast Surg 1997;24(4):719–29.
8. Al-Othman MO, Mendenhall WM, Amdur RJ. Radiotherapy alone for clinical T4 skin carcinoma of the head and neck with surgery reserved for salvage. Am J Otol 2001;22(6):387–90.
9. Panje WR, Ceilley RI. The influence of embryology of the mid-face on the spread of epithelial malignancies. Laryngoscope 1979;89(12):1914–20.

10. Fleming ID, Amonette R, Monaghan T, et al. Principles of management of basal and squamous cell carcinoma of the skin. Cancer 1995;75(Suppl 2): 699–704.

11. Miller SJ. Biology of basal cell carcinoma (part I). J Am Acad Dermatol 1991;24(1):1–13.

12. Talbot S, Hitchcock B. Incomplete primary excision of cutaneous basal and squamous cell carcinomas in the Bay of Plenty. N Z Med J 2004;117(1192): U848.

13. Perez CA. Management of incompletely excised carcinoma of the skin. Int J Radiat Oncol Biol Phys 1991;20(4):903–4.

14. Hassanein AM, Proper SA, Depcik-Smith ND, et al. Peritumoral fibrosis in basal cell and squamous cell carcinoma mimicking perineural invasion: potential pitfall in Mohs micrographic surgery. Dermatol Surg 2005;31(9 Pt 1):1101–6.

15. Leibovitch I, Huilgol SC, Selva D, et al. Cutaneous squamous cell carcinoma treated with Mohs micrographic surgery in Australia II. Perineural invasion. J Am Acad Dermatol 2005;53(2):261–6.

16. Leibovitch I, Huilgol SC, Selva D, et al. Basal cell carcinoma treated with Mohs surgery in Australia III. Perineural invasion. J Am Acad Dermatol 2005; 53(3):458–63.

17. McCord MW, Mendenhall WM, Parsons JT, et al. Skin cancer of the head and neck with incidental microscopic perineural invasion. Int J Radiat Oncol Biol Phys 1999;43(3):591–5.

18. McCord MW, Mendenhall WM, Parsons JT, et al. Skin cancer of the head and neck with clinical perineural invasion. Int J Radiat Oncol Biol Phys 2000; 47(1):89–93.

19. Garcia-Serra A, Hinerman RW, Mendenhall WM, et al. Carcinoma of the skin with perineural invasion. Head Neck 2003;25(12):1027–33.

20. Williams LS, Mancuso AA, Mendenhall WM. Perineural spread of cutaneous squamous and basal cell carcinoma: CT and MR detection and its impact on patient management and prognosis. Int J Radiat Oncol Biol Phys 2001;49(4):1061–9.

21. Han A, Ratner D. What is the role of adjuvant radiotherapy in the treatment of cutaneous squamous cell carcinoma with perineural invasion? Cancer 2007; 109(6):1053–9.

22. Cherpelis BS, Marcusen C, Lang PG. Prognostic factors for metastasis in squamous cell carcinoma of the skin. Dermatol Surg 2002;28(3):268–73.

23. Dinehart SM, Pollack SV. Metastases from squamous cell carcinoma of the skin and lip. An analysis of twenty-seven cases. J Am Acad Dermatol 1989; 21(2 Pt 1):241–8.

24. Mendenhall NP, Million RR, Cassisi NJ. Parotid area lymph node metastases from carcinoma of the skin. Int J Radiat Oncol Biol Phys 1985;11(4):707–14.

25. Mendenhall WM, Amdur RJ, Hinerman RW, et al. Skin cancer of the head and neck with perineural invasion. Am J Clin Oncol 2007;30(1):93–6.

26. Galloway TJ, Morris CG, Mancuso AA, et al. Impact of radiographic findings on prognosis for skin carcinoma with clinical perineural invasion. Cancer 2005; 103(6):1254–7.

27. Caccialanza M, Piccinno R, Beretta M, et al. Results and side effects of dermatologic radiotherapy: a retrospective study of irradiated cutaneous epithelial neoplasms. J Am Acad Dermatol 1999;41(4): 589–94.

28. Locke J, Karimpour S, Young G, et al. Radiotherapy for epithelial skin cancer. Int J Radiat Oncol Biol Phys 2001;51(3):748–55.

29. Griep C, Davelaar J, Scholten AN, et al. Electron beam therapy is not inferior to superficial x-ray therapy in the treatment of skin carcinoma. Int J Radiat Oncol Biol Phys 1995;32(5):1347–50.

30. Bath-Hextall F, Leonardi-Bee J, Somchand N, et al. Interventions for preventing non-melanoma skin cancers in high-risk groups. Cochrane Database Syst Rev 2007;(4): 005414.

31. Avril MF, Auperin A, Margulis A, et al. Basal cell carcinoma of the face: surgery or radiotherapy? Results of a randomized study. Br J Cancer 1997;76(1):100–6.

32. Rowe DE, Carroll RJ, Day CL Jr. Long-term recurrence rates in previously untreated (primary) basal cell carcinoma: implications for patient follow-up. J Dermatol Surg Oncol 1989;15(3):315–28.

33. Carcinoma of the skin (excluding eyelid, vulva, and penis). In: Green FL, Page DL, Flemming ID, et al, editors. American Joint Committee on Cancer. AJCC cancer staging manual. 6th edition. New York: Springer; 2002. p. 203–8.

34. Petrovich Z, Parker RG, Luxton G, et al. Carcinoma of the lip and selected sites of head and neck skin. A clinical study of 896 patients. Radiother Oncol 1987;8(1):11–7.

35. Mendenhall WM, Parsons JT, Mendenhall NP, et al. T2-T4 carcinoma of the skin of the head and neck treated with radical irradiation. Int J Radiat Oncol Biol Phys 1987;13(7):975–81.

36. Lee WR, Mendenhall WM, Parsons JT, et al. Radical radiotherapy for T4 carcinoma of the skin of the head and neck: a multivariate analysis. Head Neck 1993;15(4):320–4.

37. Veness MJ, Morgan GJ, Palme CE, et al. Surgery and adjuvant radiotherapy in patients with cutaneous head and neck squamous cell carcinoma metastatic to lymph nodes: combined treatment should be considered best practice. Laryngoscope 2005;115(5):870–5.

38. delCharco JO, Mendenhall WM, Parsons JT, et al. Carcinoma of the skin metastatic to the parotid area lymph nodes. Head Neck 1998;20(5):369–73.

39. Taylor BW Jr, Brant TA, Mendenhall NP, et al. Carcinoma of the skin metastatic to parotid area lymph nodes. Head Neck 1991;13(5):427–33.

40. Kaltreider SA, Callahan C. Oculoplastic surgery update: pathogenesis of malignant eyelid tumors. Ophthalmol Clin North Am 2000;13(4):557–69.

41. Amdur RJ, Kalbaugh KJ, Ewald LM, et al. Radiation therapy for skin cancer near the eye: kilovoltage x-rays versus electrons. Int J Radiat Oncol Biol Phys 1992;23(4):769–79.

42. Fitzpatrick PJ. Organ and functional preservation in the management of cancers of the eye and eyelid. Cancer Invest 1995;13(1):66–74.

43. Rodriguez JM, Deutsch GP. The treatment of periocular basal cell carcinomas by radiotherapy. Br J Ophthalmol 1992;76(4):195–7.

44. Mendenhall NP, Parsons JT, Cassisi NJ, et al. Carcinoma of the nasal vestibule treated with radiation therapy. Laryngoscope 1987;97(5):626–32.

45. Caccialanza M, Piccinno R, Moretti D, et al. Radiotherapy of carcinomas of the skin overlying the cartilage of the nose: results in 405 lesions. Eur J Dermatol 2003;13(5):462–5.

46. Tsao MN, Tsang RW, Liu FF, et al. Radiotherapy management for squamous cell carcinoma of the nasal skin: the Princess Margaret Hospital experience. Int J Radiat Oncol Biol Phys 2002;52(4):973–9.

47. Silva JJ, Tsang RW, Panzarella T, et al. Results of radiotherapy for epithelial skin cancer of the pinna: the Princess Margaret Hospital experience, 1982–1993. Int J Radiat Oncol Biol Phys 2000; 47(2):451–9.

48. Sykes AJ, Allan E, Irwin C. Squamous cell carcinoma of the lip: the role of electron treatment. Clin Oncol (R Coll Radiol) 1996;8(6):384–6.

49. Wilder RB, Kittelson JM, Shimm DS. Basal cell carcinoma treated with radiation therapy. Cancer 1991; 68(10):2134–7.

50. Robinson JK, Dahiya M. Basal cell carcinoma with pulmonary and lymph node metastasis causing death. Arch Dermatol 2003;139(5):643–8.

51. Raszewski RL, Guyuron B. Long-term survival following nodal metastases from basal cell carcinoma. Ann Plast Surg 1990;24(2):170–5.

52. Howle JR, Morgan GJ, Kalnins I, et al. Metastatic cutaneous squamous cell carcinoma of the scalp. ANZ J Surg 2008;78(6):449–53.

53. Lovett RD, Perez CA, Shapiro SJ, et al. External irradiation of epithelial skin cancer. Int J Radiat Oncol Biol Phys 1990;19(2):235–42.

54. Silverman MK, Kopf AW, Gladstein AH, et al. Recurrence rates of treated basal cell carcinomas. Part 4: X-ray therapy. J Dermatol Surg Oncol 1992;18(7): 549–54.

Improving Outcomes in Aesthetic Facial Reconstruction

Stefan O.P. Hofer, MD, PhD, FRCS(C)[a],*,
Marc A.M. Mureau, MD, PhD[b]

KEYWORDS

- Facial reconstruction • Aesthetic unit • Local flap
- Free flap • Skin cancer • Oncology

Facial reconstruction has mesmerized surgeons and the general public alike for many centuries. The earliest descriptions are of cheek flaps and later forehead flaps for nasal reconstruction done in ancient India.[1] The pioneering reconstructive work of Esser,[2] who at the beginning of the twentieth century was the first to have an understanding of vascularization in "arterial flaps," was fascinating. Current concepts of aesthetic facial reconstruction have again improved with the development of the aesthetic facial unit principle. The latest frontier in facial aesthetic reconstruction through facial transplantation is currently being challenged.

The focus of facial reconstruction has obviously always been restoration of function. With regard to aesthetics, however, facial reconstruction was considered successful when a hole was closed with a flap. Modern facial reconstruction has evolved with the help of detailed anatomic knowledge, which has made tissue transfer from local and distant sites very reliable. In recent decades, the concept of aesthetic facial reconstruction has been popularized. This concept honors the aesthetic facial units, the borders of which are made up of the transitional areas of light and shadow on the face as the facial surface changes from concave to convex (**Fig. 1**). These borders are the ideal locations to place scars. Central aesthetic facial units, such as nose or lips, can

be subdivided into subunits to further refine facial reconstruction.[3] The central facial subunits (ie. nose, eyes, and lips) are ideally replaced in their entirety, if feasible, when most of the unit is lost so as to have one inconspicuous reconstructed surface.

One of the cornerstones of aesthetic facial reconstruction is meticulous defect analysis. This holds true for all reconstructive surgery in which a restoration of function is sought. In aesthetic facial reconstruction, however, additional emphasis is placed on the different aesthetic units involved as well as the quality of the tissues and the possible structural support needed by those tissues. This analysis leads to the use of the reconstructive "elevator" rather than the reconstructive "ladder," in which the flap or combination of flaps are chosen that will give the most aesthetically pleasing as well as functional outcome.[4]

From an aesthetic viewpoint, one can consider donor-site morbidity to be a result of improper scar positioning. This is largely preventable by positioning scars in the borders of the aesthetic units. For instance, when looking at a person's face, the gaze is fixed on the eyes, cheekbones, nose, and mouth. Scars on the forehead or lateral to a vertical line through the lateral canthus are less conspicuous, and therefore also have less aesthetic donor-site morbidity, even if they run through an aesthetic unit. From the functional

[a] Division of Plastic Surgery, Department of Surgery and Department of Surgical Oncology, University Health Network, University of Toronto, 200 Elizabeth Street, 8N-865, Toronto, Ontario, Canada M5G 2C4
[b] Department of Plastic and Reconstructive Surgery, Erasmus University Medical Center Rotterdam, PO Box 2040, 3000 CA Rotterdam, The Netherlands
* Corresponding author. Division of Plastic Surgery, Department of Surgery, University Health Network, 200 Elizabeth Street, 8N-865, Toronto, Ontario, Canada M5G 2C4.
E-mail address: stefan.hofer@uhn.on.ca (S.O.P. Hofer).

Clin Plastic Surg 36 (2009) 345–354
doi:10.1016/j.cps.2009.02.009
0094-1298/09/$ – see front matter © 2009 Elsevier Inc. All rights reserved

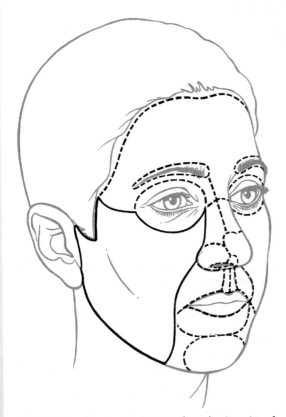

Fig. 1. Schematic representation of aesthetic units of the face.

perspective, the use of perforator flaps has greatly diminished donor-site morbidity because they save muscle function in those areas in which muscle was harvested previously to incorporate the blood supply that perfuses the overlying skin.

Aesthetic facial reconstruction is challenging and artistic. Reproducible and good outcomes can only be achieved by the use of detailed preoperative plans with possible back-up options. Proper planning is key to any good outcome. In many cases, consecutive stages need to be performed as part of the initial plan or as part of touch-ups. A perfect result will often need more than a single operation. This paper provides insight on how to prevent undesirable functional and aesthetic outcomes in facial reconstruction and gives solutions for the enhancement of functional and aesthetic outcomes using secondary procedures.

DEFECT ANALYSIS

Facial reconstruction is well beyond the period in which filling the hole or covering up the surface was a measure of success. Aesthetic facial reconstruction is only successful if normalcy and, if affected, symmetry are restored. Successful aesthetic facial reconstruction is largely dependent on the proper analysis of the defect. To properly analyze the defect, a list of the issues involved in functional impairment and the missing tissues from involved aesthetic units needs to be made. When all the requirements of the reconstruction have been identified, a plan can be made. Reconstruction of function should be the basis from which to start, after which the aesthetics of the reconstruction come in. As a general rule, aesthetic units should be reconstructed individually. For instance, a forehead flap used for nasal reconstruction should not be used to reconstruct part of a cheek because the cheek defect needs to be reconstructed separately from the nose.

FUNCTIONAL AND AESTHETIC OUTCOME ENHANCEMENT BY REGION
Forehead and Scalp

Forehead and scalp reconstruction first aims to cover exposed underlying skull bone or contents. Following successful defect coverage, the main focus of the reconstruction becomes one of a more an aesthetic nature. Successful coverage will not always result in good aesthetic outcome. Small- to medium-sized defects can be reconstructed satisfactorily using local scalp flaps (**Fig. 2**). In large defects, local tissue will not be of sufficient size to provide coverage, and free-tissue transfer will be required. The main concerns here generally are: (1) coverage that is too bulky or too thin, (2) incorrect skin color, (3) lack of hair, and (4) suboptimal scarring. In addition, sometimes a contour deficiency caused by missing bone may exist. There are a number of solutions to deal with these issues.

Suboptimal flap selection will usually result in excessive bulk after coverage of the forehead or scalp. Musculocutaneous flaps and thick fasciocutaneous flaps can result in bulky coverage. Skin on the forehead and scalp and related subcutaneous tissues are generally thinner than in most standard skin flap areas. Excising the skin paddle of a musculocutaneous flap and skin grafting the underlying muscle can thin excessive bulk of skin and subcutis. Alternatively, resection or liposuction of subcutaneous fat can further thin a flap.

When using a muscle flap with skin graft for coverage, the muscle will thin over time because it is no longer innervated. On the scalp, this will usually not be a major concern. These flaps, however, are less resilient to friction and can present with small areas of skin graft breakdown over time. On the forehead, thinning of a muscle flap can result in a skeletonized appearance, which accentuates the contour of the skull.

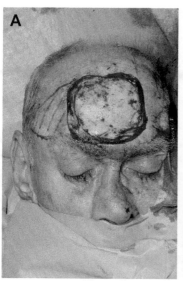 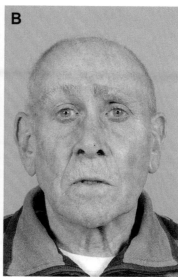

Fig. 2. Patient with defect on the forehead after radical full-thickness resection of squamous cell carcinoma. (*A*) Design of a scalp rotation flap, based on the superficial temporal and retroauricular vessels, with excision of a Burrow's triangle placing the final scar line at the superior brow line. (*B*) Final result after one operation. A large back cut and a split thickness skin graft were required on the posterior scalp to accommodate closure of the donor defect after scalp rotation.

Correction of this aesthetic problem can be solved by using reconstruction with a regional thin skin flap of appropriate skin color and texture, which, if unavailable, can be generated by flap prefabrication (**Fig. 3**).

The final skin paddle color of the flap used in a reconstruction is mostly hard to predict. Skin grafts will often change to a different color, which usually is not the color of the surrounding skin. Good results have been reported for skin grafting of the facial area using scalp skin grafts. This is a feasible option for forehead and facial skin reconstruction, but not for larger scalp reconstructions. Alternatively, skin grafting of a de-epithelialized, previously transferred, (distant) free flap using a scalp skin graft may improve skin color match.[5] An axiom states that skin flaps taken from sites closer to the face have better color match. This has not always been the authors' experience. Skin from areas that are primarily protected from the sun by clothes, like parascapular flap skin, is generally unpredictable in the way that it will color when transplanted to the facial area. For scalp reconstructions, it is less important to have an exact color match because many of these patients will wear hairpieces or wigs to cover the baldness.

Restoration of hair after scalp or forehead reconstruction can be addressed by using hair transplantation for smaller defects or eyebrows. Tissue expansion of remaining hair-bearing scalp to replace bald areas can be performed. When large hair-bearing scalp defects are present, men will have a bald head or a wig can be worn. The smaller the scalp defect, the more likely the area will be covered with a hairpiece or remaining hair as the easiest options. A simple alternative solution for eyebrow restoration can be tattooing.

Eyelids

The eyes are one of the areas of primary focus in social interaction. Eyelid defects, which cannot be closed primarily, should be reconstructed according to ocular plastic surgical principles. Eyelid reconstruction serves to prevent functional complications in this complex region and to preserve aesthetic harmony. Eyelid function, which is protection of the eye and maintaining hydration of the cornea, should be restored whenever feasible. The lateral and medial canthus and the tear duct system should be reconstructed, if affected. Without detailed knowledge of the anatomy of the periorbital region, it will not be possible to achieve a good functional and aesthetic result.

Incisions are preferably made parallel to the skin folds to minimize tension on the wound and vertical pull on the eyelid rim. Skin grafts should blend in with the recipient site. This can be achieved by using skin that has the same thickness, color, and texture. The opposite upper eyelid often makes for a good donor site. Disturbance of shape, contour, position, and symmetry of the

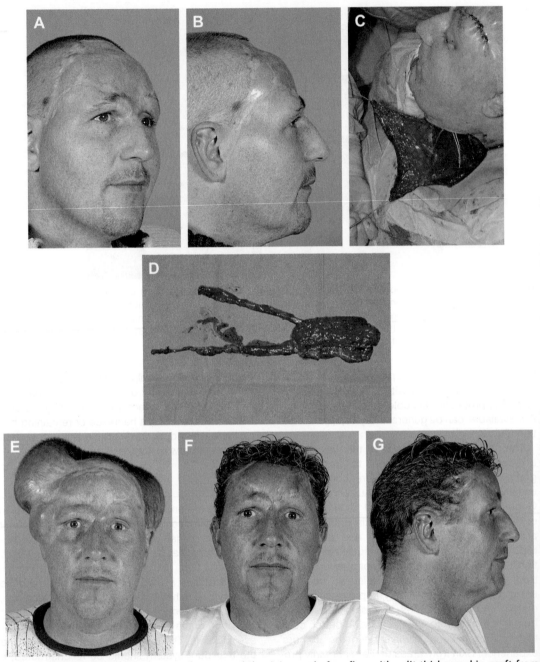

Fig. 3. Patient 9 months after the use of a rectus abdominis muscle free flap with split thickness skin graft from the thigh to reconstruct a defect after radical resection by an ENT surgeon of the outer table of the frontal bone in combination with all overlying soft tissues to treat severe sinusitis that had not resolved after more than 70 surgical attempts. (*A*) Three-quarter right view and (*B*) lateral view. Reconstruction of the forehead using an overlying skin graft was requested to improve the skeletonized appearance and the frequent breakdown of the atrophied muscle. The left-sided neck skin was prefabricated (*C*) by placing an adipofascial radial forearm free flap (*D*) under the neck skin. (*E*) At the same time, multiple tissue expanders were inserted under the scalp to restore the anterior hairline. End result after prefabricated neck skin free flap transfer and anterior hairline restoration in frontal (*F*) and lateral (*G*) view.

eyelid, eyebrow, and canthus should be avoided because this will effect social interaction.

Reconstruction of eyelid defects affecting up to 30% of the total length of the upper or lower lid can usually be performed by using primary closure in layers, with or without lateral cantholysis. Any defect that is reconstructed by means other than primary closure should therefore be one that affects 30% or more of the total length of the eyelid. A normal functioning eyelid is of paramount importance. Upper lid function requires adequate elevation to enable undisturbed vision. The upper lid needs to close sufficiently to prevent dehydration of the cornea. Dehydration of the cornea can lead to exposure keratitis, ulceration, and blindness.

A full-thickness skin graft (preferably from the upper eyelid) may be considered if only the skin is affected and primary closure is not possible. In complex defects with multiple tissue layers affected, use of a regional transposition flap with its own blood supply is indicated. Flaps from the periorbital region usually have excellent vascularization. They have the appropriate thickness,

texture, and color match. Conjunctival loss can be replaced with "like-for-like" tissue using mucosal grafts from the nasal septum or inner cheek. Eyelid support of the missing tarsal plate can be reconstructed using a nasal septum composite graft (**Fig. 4**), conchal cartilage with or without skin, or a tarsoconjunctival flap. If there is no severe lower-lid laxity or if most of the lower lid is not missing, reconstruction of the lower-lid tarsal plate is not always necessary, provided that a mucosal graft is sutured in tightly and covered with a local transposition flap from the upper lid. Reconstruction of full-thickness eyelid loss can be performed using a full-thickness flap of the upper or lower lid. In case of full-thickness upper-lid reconstructions, this is a good technique; however, it is generally not recommended to reconstruct full-thickness lower-eyelid defects because sacrificing part of the full-thickness upper eyelid may lead to serious functional problems.

Eyelid reconstruction has a very functional focus in which aesthetics are mostly governed by the goal of restoring symmetry.

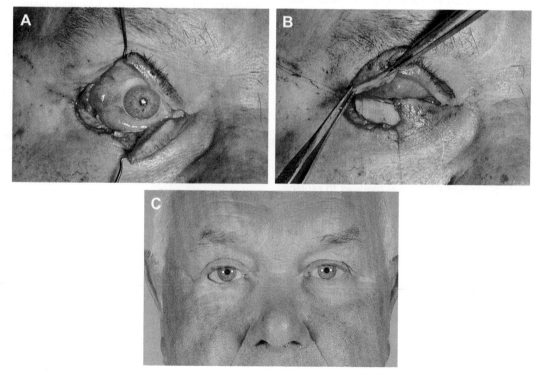

Fig. 4. Full-thickness re-resection for basal cell carcinoma of one third of the upper eyelid and one half of the lower eyelid on the right eye with destruction of the lateral canthus. (*A*) Reconstruction of the upper eyelid using a buccal mucosa graft for the inner lining and a musculocutaneous Tripier transposition flap for the external cover. (*B*) Reconstruction of the lower eyelid using a nasal composite septomucosal transposition for the inner lining and support with fixation to the lateral orbital wall and a cheek advancement flap for the external cover. (*C*) Result after 6 months with slightly detached lateral lower lid margin.

Nose

The nose naturally attracts the gaze of the onlooker because it is the center of the facial appearance. Nasal function has to act as a guide for the reconstruction. The reconstruction has to permit unobstructed airflow for normal breathing, speech, and smell.

Nasal reconstruction is based on the principle of restoration of anatomic structural layers. The nose is divided into three main layers: the mucosal lining (inner lining), the osteocartilaginous framework (structural support), and the external soft tissue and skin (outer lining).

Inner lining reconstruction is the first step in reconstructing the nose. Many options for inner lining reconstruction are available. It is important that the inner lining is thin to prevent obstruction of the nasal passage. In addition, nasal lining needs to be well vascularized to allow insertion of structural support in the process of nasal reconstruction. Inner lining materials include skin grafts, turnover flaps, mucosal flaps, folded parts of regional flaps, and free flaps. When secondary enhancement is needed, if initial inner lining reconstruction did not prove satisfactory, improvement of outcome mostly involves the use of local tissue rearrangement or the addition of skin grafts to add to the shortage of inner lining. Providing enough inner lining is of paramount importance during the first reconstructive procedure because correction of inner lining shortage during later stages is very hard to achieve.[6] In rare cases, the entire reconstruction has to be redone.

Structural support is vital in nasal reconstruction to maintain projection, restore the external and internal nasal valve, and allow for nasal air passage. Autologous materials such as auricular, septal, or costal cartilage are preferred materials. Structural support is not only required to replace the missing support but also to add support to previously unsupported areas such as the alar rim. This extra support is vital in most areas to withstand forces of wound contraction. In cases of secondary enhancement of structural support, the addition of extra cartilage to insufficiently supported areas (eg, columella) or unsatisfactorily projecting areas (eg, nasal tip) is generally undertaken. These cartilage grafts need to be thin to prevent too much bulk in the nose, yet strong to withstand all of the forces working on them.

The nose is given its external, three-dimensional appearance by its convex and concave surfaces. The surface contours are the basis of the nine-aesthetic subunit principle developed by Burget and Menick.[7] These contours have to be considered carefully when recreating or adapting the

defect. When providing the external skin cover, scars are placed in the boundaries of these units to make them less conspicuous. Generally, it is advisable to replace the entire subunit if 50% or more of that subunit is missing. Leaving smaller areas of a remaining subunit will result in an unsightly scar across a visual plane that should not have a scar and can easily result in distortion because of trapdooring and scar contraction.

The paramedian forehead flap is the workhorse flap for nasal reconstruction. Its use is best regarded as a three-stage operation, whether it is used to resurface a single-layer nasal defect or employed in a complex, three-layer nasal reconstruction. The first operation allows for laying the basis of the reconstruction by transferring the forehead flap, which has a very reliable blood supply without any thinning. The second stage allows for fine tuning of the flap and extensive thinning at week 3. At this time, the flap is fully detached from the nose and only left attached to its pedicle. Extensive thinning is tolerated at this time because the vascularity of this flap has improved during the first 3 weeks as the result of the delay phenomenon. The flap is still very pliable and moldable at this second stage because wound healing is still immature. In addition, there has also been no surgical trauma to the posterior surface of the dermis because the flap was initially raised in the plane underneath the frontalis muscle.

At this second stage, loosely placed quilting sutures in the thinned area will prevent seroma and hematoma formation. The third stage will take place 3 weeks after this second intermediate stage. This allows for vascularization of the flap from the surrounding tissue. The division of the pedicle is therefore performed 6 weeks after the original surgery (**Fig. 5**).

For secondary enhancement of outcomes, further touch-up operations will be postponed for at least 6 months to let wound healing occur, swelling disappear, and the nose soften. The procedures undertaken at that time are usually geared toward repositioning scars into the correct aesthetic units, thinning areas of excessive bulk, improving contour through shaping of subcutaneous tissue, or adding tissue to areas of tightness or contraction. When making these secondary enhancements, old scars can be disregarded, whereas new incisions should be placed exactly at the borders of aesthetic subunits.[8]

Cheeks

The cheek lies on the periphery of an onlooker's gaze in social interaction. As such, this area of the face falls to less critical appraisal when it

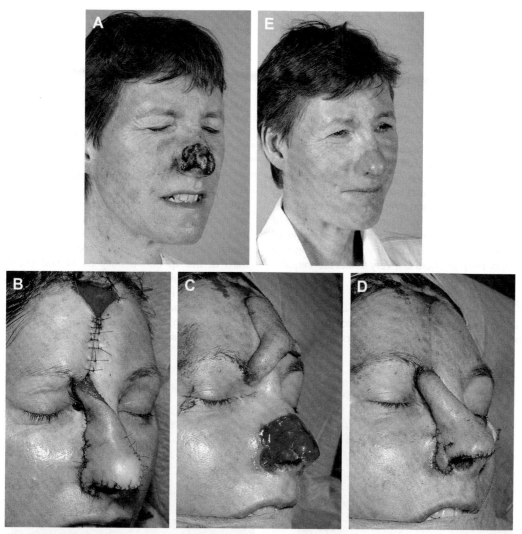

Fig. 5. (*A*) Skin defect of the nasal tip and ala, extending into the nasal dorsum and sidewall after Mohs' resection for basal cell cancer. (*B*) First stage paramedian forehead flap reconstruction. (*C*) Second stage thin lifting of paramedian forehead flap and sculpting of the nose with placement of delayed primary alar rim batten cartilage graft. (*D*) Repositioning of thin second stage paramedian forehead flap and placement of ala-defining quilting sutures. (*E*) Result one year after reconstruction.

comes to minor details, compared with appraisal of the nose, lips, and eyes. To achieve a good result in cheek reconstruction, it is important to restore normal facial surface appearance. This can be achieved by restoring a uniform skin color and texture, and is not so much dependent on contour and outline.

From a functional perspective, there are few requirements in cheek reconstruction unless there is a very extensive defect or a deeper lesion involving the facial nerve. In those cases, either distant or free flaps may be required to cover underlying structures or fill up cavities, or facial nerve repair or reconstruction is indicated.

In general, cheek defects that are not amenable to primary closure are preferably reconstructed using local tissues to prevent the color mismatch and inadequate bulk that distant tissues usually bring with them. In those cases in which only contour but no skin is lacking, the use of free-tissue transfer, local subcutaneous adipofascial flaps, or lipofilling for lesser bulk requirements can be very good options. Local flaps supplying "like-with-like" skin are either anterior-based, rotation-advancement flaps that are vascularized by the facial and submental vessels or posterior-based, rotation-advancement flaps supplied by the superficial temporal and preauricular vessels.

The use of free-tissue flaps, if required, will often lead to suboptimal aesthetic outcome.[9]

For obtaining an optimal aesthetic cheek reconstruction result, skin coverage of the defect should ideally be reconstructed using the aforementioned local or locoregional flaps, whenever possible. As mentioned before in this article, it is important to place scars in the aesthetic unit borders if possible. In addition, improved outcome is achieved if no scars run anterior to a vertical line drawn through the lateral canthus. The transposition of cheek skin often gives a downward pull on the lower eyelid. Attention should be directed at producing very strong support and overcorrection of the position of these flaps whenever there is a chance of downward pull to prevent ectropion. Fixation of the flap to the periorbital bony tissues using drill holes or bone anchors is a very useful technique.

Lips

The lips are important from a functional as well as from an aesthetic viewpoint. They play a vital role in facilitating speech and food intake and are a focal point of the central face during social contact. All the concepts of facial reconstruction play an equally important role in reconstructive surgery of the lips. Careful defect analysis is required to assess restorative options for function and loss of aesthetics. Any abnormality resulting from asymmetry in shape or movement will be picked up. This can be from such extreme cases as complete facial nerve palsy or total lip resection to as small as a step deformity in the white roll.

Lip defects are not different from other defects in that it is important to try to replace "like" tissue with "like" tissue. Lip tissue has such a specific anatomy and appearance that it is hard to replace it in a pleasing fashion using an alternate tissue source. Smaller lip defects of up to one third of the lip can usually be closed primarily without significant problems. Slightly larger defects may require the use of a lip shave or buccal mucosal advancement flaps for vermilion reconstruction, and lip switch flaps such as the Abbe and Estlander flaps for moderate-sized

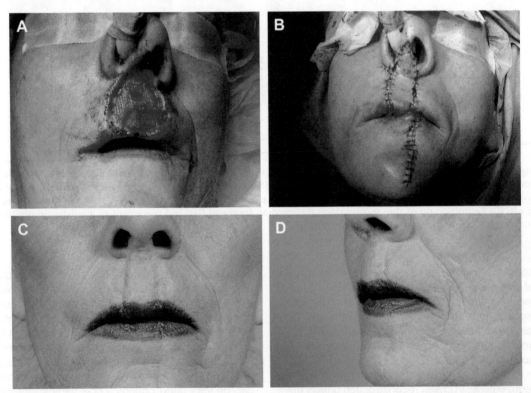

Fig. 6. Philtrum, medial borders of adjacent upper lip units, upper lip mid-vermilion, and partial columella defect after Mohs' resection for basal cell cancer. (*A*) Reconstruction of the defect after changing the defect into full-thickness defect. Bilateral medial advancement of the lateral upper lip units was performed to bring back the defect to a philtrum and columella defect. (*B*) Reconstruction of the philtrum and partial columella defect using an Abbe flap from the lower lip. (*C*) Anterior and (*D*) three-quarter view of the end result after 2 years, with an intermediate operation to separate the columella and philtrum units using thinning and quilting.

(less than one half of the lip length), full-thickness lip reconstruction (**Fig. 6**). If the defect lies centrally or more laterally with involvement of the commissure and no new lip tissue is required, the Karapandzic flap provides the ideal reconstruction because it preserves the neurovascular supply and the integrity of the oral sphincter. The need for new lip tissue and the necessity to avoid microstomia are the best indications for the use of the modified Bernard-Burrow's procedures. For large lower-lip defects measuring more than two thirds of the lip without sufficient cheek tissue available to execute these perioral flaps, distant or free flaps such as a free radial forearm flap with palmaris longus sling[10] or an innervated gracilis free flap are required.[11] These flaps will give less satisfactory outcomes from a functional and aesthetic view. Patients should be educated that postoperative oral function can be compromised because of tightness or impaired lip sensation.

Specific considerations to improve outcomes in lip reconstruction need to be considered. The aesthetic unit lines should be marked and incorporated in the plan of reconstruction. With the Abbe flap, it is very important to design the flap in the middle of the lower lip. In this fashion, the scar will be dead center, which prevents asymmetric distortion of the lower lip. Secondary scar revisions to get the scar in the center will only give limited success. The design of the Abbe flap should allow closure of the lower lip without pull on the vermilion to prevent distortion. Abbe flaps in men need special consideration with regard to hair growth. By turning the lower lip skin upside down, the direction of hair growth is incorrect. In addition, the hair growth on the lower lip skin is often less than that on the upper lip skin. In some cases, additional hair follicle transplants at a later date can be considered.

Step deformities, which are very visible after all wounds are healed, are caused by incorrect realignment of the white roll at initial surgery. Careful realignment after full wound healing will improve the white roll appearance. The lip vermilion can be touched up during the second operation if asymmetry resulting from bulkiness across a scar exists. Careful restoration of the continuity of the orbicularis oris muscle has to be performed to prevent a whistling deformity. The continuity of the orbicularis oris muscle can be restored secondarily, if required. In the case of persistent commissural deformity, two opposing mucosal rhomboid flaps, which are transposed laterally to reconstruct the angle, may be best used. Mucosal deficiency of the vermilion may be overcome by using an anterior-based tongue

flap, which is divided after 10 to 14 days,[12] or by using a facial artery musculomucosal flap.[13]

Microstomia can be particularly troublesome for patients who use dentures. They have to be instructed how to remove and insert these appliances, so that the least amount of strain is put on the lip. A splinting device may be used for several months to treat microstomia.

SUMMARY

Functional and aesthetic outcome enhancement of facial reconstruction is a very challenging discipline. It is important not only to have a thorough understanding of the functional anatomy of the area that requires reconstruction but also be aware of the aesthetic and anthropometric properties of the area involved. The surface anatomy as we visually perceive our fellow humans during social interaction needs to be recreated in a fashion so that asymmetry and scarring do not distract us. Only with a continuous quest for perfection and an open mind will we be able to improve our results.

REFERENCES

1. McDowell F. The classic reprint. Ancient ear-lobe and rhinoplastic operations in India. Plast Reconstr Surg 1969;43(5):515–22.
2. Esser JFS. Artery flaps. Reprint of 1932 book. Rotterdam, The Netherlands: Erasmus Publishing; 2003.
3. Menick FJ. Facial reconstruction with local and distant tissue: the interface of aesthetic and reconstructive surgery. Plast Reconstr Surg 1998;102(5): 1424–33.
4. Gottlieb LJ, Krieger LM. From the reconstructive ladder to the reconstructive elevator.[Editorial]. Plast Reconstr Surg 1994;93(7):1503–4.
5. Walton RL, Cohn AB, Beahm EK. Epidermal overgrafting improves coloration in remote flaps and grafts applied to the face for reconstruction. Plast Reconstr Surg 2008;121(5):1606–13.
6. Mureau MAM, Moolenburgh SE, Levendag PC, et al. Aesthetic and functional outcome following nasal reconstruction. Plast Reconstr Surg 2007;120(5): 1217–27.
7. Burget GC, Menick FJ. The subunit principle in nasal reconstruction. Plast Reconstr Surg 1985;76(2): 239–47.
8. Menick FJ. A 10-year experience in nasal reconstruction with the three-stage forehead flap. Plast Reconstr Surg 2002;109(6):1839–55.
9. Mureau MAM, Posch NAS, Meeuwis CA, et al. Anterolateral thigh flap reconstruction of large external facial skin defects: a follow-up study on functional

and aesthetic recipient- and donor-site outcome. Plast Reconstr Surg 2005;115(4):1077–86.

10. Carroll CM, Pathak I, Irish J, et al. Reconstruction of total lower lip and chin defects using the composite radial forearm–palmaris longus tendon free flap. Arch Facial Plast Surg 2000;2(1):53–6.

11. Ninkovic M, Spanio di Spilimbergo S, Ninkovic M. Lower lip reconstruction: introduction of a new procedure using a functioning gracilis muscle free flap. Plast Reconstr Surg 2007;119(5):1472–80.

12. Jackson IT. Local flaps in head and neck reconstruction. 2nd edition. St. Louis (MO): QMP Publishers; 2007.

13. Pribaz JJ, Meara JG, Wright S, et al. Lip and vermilion reconstruction with the facial artery musculomucosal flap. Plast Reconstr Surg 2000;105(3): 864–72.

Reconstruction of Scalp and Forehead Defects

Iris A. Seitz, MD, PhD, Lawrence J. Gottlieb, MD*

KEYWORDS

- Scalp • Forehead • Defects
- Facial reconstruction • Calvarial reconstruction

Reconstruction of scalp and forehead defects is a complex field with a broad variety of reconstructive options. Initially, one must ask: what are the goals and priorities? What is the easiest way to close the defect and what is the best way to close the defect? Is the goal to close the wound or to reconstruct the defect?

To define the initial goals of reconstruction, one considers size and location of the defect; etiology and depth of the defect or injury; surrounding tissue quality; exposure of vital structures such as bone, dura or brain parenchyma; age and health of the patient; and, in the case of malignancy, status of disease (control or palliation.) If the goal includes aesthetic reconstruction, then hair growth pattern, hairline and brow position, skin color, texture and composition, as well as aesthetic subunit principles have to be considered. Next, one determines the realistic expectations of the patient, family and surgeon as well as limitations that may preclude obtaining initial goals.

To successfully reconstruct any defect, a detailed knowledge of anatomy and the ability to perform a variety of different reconstructive options are necessary. The unique anatomy of the scalp tissue with its hirsute quality gives rise to the aesthetic principle of preserving and manipulating native scalp tissue to cover the defect whenever possible. Because of the relative inelasticity of the scalp tissue, primary closure is often not possible and healing by secondary intention, tissue expansion, skin graft coverage, local advancement/rotational flaps, regional pedicle flaps or free tissue transfer may be indicated to simply close the wound or reconstruct the defect. A detailed analysis of the preoperative (or anticipated) defect is essential to provide not only adequate wound coverage but also help tailor the method of reconstruction to achieve an optimal aesthetic result. Current techniques used for reconstruction of scalp and forehead defects are the subject of this article.

The scalp and forehead are the unique tissues that cover the cranium. When portions of the hirsute scalp are missing or deformed, donor sites for aesthetic reconstruction of the hair-bearing skin are by-in-large limited to the use of residual hirsute scalp. This limitation is a result of the fact that there is no other skin with the same quality, quantity, and density of hair on the human body. The quest to replace hair-bearing skin has led to clever manipulations of the residual hirsute scalp to resurface large areas of alopecia.[1,2] The advent of tissue expansion has revolutionized secondary reconstruction of large areas of alopecic scalp and is unrivaled in techniques for replacing "like with like". Transferring hair as grafts (strips, plugs or individual shafts) has become an art in itself to repopulate small or large surface areas with hair. When acute closure of a defect is required or when the surface area of residual hair bearing skin is not large enough to resurface large alopecic or full thickness scalp defects, then the reconstructive goals must be shifted to providing quality cutaneous coverage. Reconstruction of the bald head similarly requires stable coverage. Forehead skin is unique with its thick sebaceous skin spanning the space between the brows and the scalp. The primary challenge of reconstructing forehead

Section of Plastic and Reconstructive Surgery, The University of Chicago, 5841 S. Maryland Avenue, MC 6035, Chicago, IL 60637, USA
* Corresponding author.
E-mail address: lgottlie@surgery.bsd.uchicago.edu (L.J. Gottlieb).

Clin Plastic Surg 36 (2009) 355–377
doi:10.1016/j.cps.2009.02.001
0094-1298/09/$ – see front matter © 2009 Published by Elsevier Inc

defects is replacing skin of similar color and texture without distorting the brow or hairline.

ANATOMY OF THE SCALP AND FOREHEAD

Knowledge of the anatomy of the scalp and forehead will assist the reconstructive surgeon in the choice of local flap options as well as choosing a potential microsurgical recipient vessels site if needed. Furthermore, such knowledge is important for understanding, evaluating and adequately reconstructing complex full thickness calvarial defects.

The anatomy of the scalp and that of the forehead are very similar and, therefore, the two are often considered a single unit. The main difference between the scalp and the forehead is that the scalp is usually hirsute and has a fibrous aponeurosis (galea aponeurotica) connecting the occipital muscle posterior and the frontal muscle anterior whereas the forehead—instead of the aponeurotic layer—has the frontalis muscle. The different layers of the scalp and forehead may be remembered by using the mnemonic "SCALP" which stands for Skin, subCutaneous tissue, musculoAponeurotic layer, Loose areola tissue, and Pericranium.

The scalp has the thickest skin in the body, approximately 3–8 mm thick[3] and is connected to the deeper layers via vertical septae. The subcutaneous tissue underneath the skin contains fat and dense connective tissue including hair follicles, arteries, veins, lymphatics, and sensory nerves. The scalp is well vascularized; scalp injuries can lead to severe bleeding because to the high flow and the potential of the cut vessels to retract into the fat.

The occipitalis and frontalis muscles are thin, paired quadrilateral muscles joined in the midline by extensions of the galea. The frontalis muscles originate from the galeal aponeurosis and insert into the dermis at the level of the supraciliary arches where they join together with the procerus, corrugator supercilii and orbicularis oculi. The occipitalis muscles originate from the lateral two-thirds of the superior nuchal line and the mastoid part of the temporal bone and insert into the galea with a deep portion extending into the subgaleal fascia.[4] The galea aponeurotica covers the cranium between both muscles and is continuous with the temporoparietalis fascia (superficial temporal fascia) laterally, which is confluent with the subcutaneous musculoaponeurotic system (SMAS) of the face. The loose areaola (subgaleal) layer is a relative avascular plane, this layer enables the above layers to slide as a unit over the cranium and provides a safe plane for dissection.

The pericranium is the periosteum of the calvarium and is continuous with the deep temporal fascia (temporalis muscle fascia) laterally at the superior temporal line. Caudally, the deep temporal fascia divides into superficial and deep layers, with the temporal fat pad in between, inserting deep and superficial on the zygomatic arch respectively.[4]

Vascular Supply

The blood supply to the scalp is divided into four vascular territories: anterior, lateral, posterior, and posterolateral. The vessels travel in the subcutaneous tissue, which allows for large regional flaps to be safely elevated in the subgaleal plane.[5]

The supratrochlear and supraorbital vessels arise from the internal carotid system via the ophtalmic artery and enter vertical at the level of the supraorbital rim. They travel deep and pierce through the frontalis muscle above the brow, traveling superficial and anastomosing with each other as well as branches of the superficial temporal arteries, supplying the forehead and anterior scalp. The superficial temporal arteries are terminal branches of the external carotid artery, traveling through the superficial lobes of the parotid gland, becoming more superficial at the zygomatic arch. The superficial temporal artery supplies the lateral scalp including the skin, subcutaneous tissue, and superficial temporal (temporoparietalis) fascia. It lies within the superficial temporal fascia and divides into frontal (anterior) and parietal (posterior) branches. These branches connect via the galea to the posterior blood supply of the scalp and also connect to the pericranium at the superior temporal line contributing to perfusion of the outer cortex of the parietal cranium.[6] The temporalis muscle is supplied by the deep temporal branch of the maxillary artery. The deep temporal fascial (overlying the temporalis muscle) is supplied by the middle temporal artery and has no vascular connections to the temporoparietalis fascia or the superficial temporal artery.

The posterior scalp is primarily supplied by the occipital arteries, which are branches of the external carotid arteries. The occipital arteries travel along the vertebral muscles, becoming more superficial as they pierce through the cranial part of the trapezius muscle approximately 2 cm from the midline at the nuchal line. The posterolateral/mastoid area is supplied by the posterior auricular arteries.

The venous drainage follows the above named arteries and, in addition, there is an internal drainage system via the emissary veins of the diploe of the cranium to the dural sinuses. Those emissary veins have no valves and are a potential route for the spread of scalp infections intracranially.[7]

The lymphatic drainage system lies in the subdermal and subcutaneous tissue. No lymph nodes are found in the scalp tissue; the lymph from the scalp drains to the preauricular, postauricular, parotid, upper cervical and occipital nodes.

Nerves

Scalp and forehead sensory innervation is provided by the branches of the trigeminal nerve, cervical spinal nerves, and the cervical plexus. The supraorbital nerve, a branch of the first division of the trigeminal nerve, divides into a superficial branch and a deep branch. The superficial division pierces the frontalis muscle and supplies the skin of the forehead and anterior hairline region. The deep division runs along the periosteum and pierces the galea 0.5–1.5 cm medial to the superior temporal line at the level of the coronal suture to innervate the frontoparietal scalp.[8] The zygomaticotemporal nerve, which is a branch of the maxillary division of the trigeminal nerve, supplies a small region lateral to the brow up to the superficial temporal crest. The lateral scalp and preauricular area are innervated by the auriculotemporal nerve, which is a branch of the mandibular division of the trigeminal nerve. The occipital region is supplied by the greater occipital nerve from the dorsal rami of the cervical spinal nerves and the lesser occipital nerve from the cervical plexus. The greater occipital nerve emerges 3 cm below the occipital protruberance, next to the semispinalis muscle, approximately 1.5 cm lateral to the midline.[9] Another important structure is the temporal branch of the facial nerve, which travels within the temporoparietal fascia allowing for safe dissection in the deep plane of the loose areola tissue when raising a coronal flap.[10]

Aesthetic Units of the Scalp and Forehead

The hair-bearing scalp is its own aesthetic unit, with no further subunits but rather with anatomical areas like parietal, temporal, occipital and vertex.

The forehead is a separate aesthetic unit with its own subunits: paramedian, lateral, lateral temporal region and eyebrows.[11] It is important to understand and respect those aesthetic units in facial reconstruction and to be aware that contour is the primary determinant of normalcy,[12] followed by color and texture of the skin surface.

FOREHEAD AND SCALP RECONSTRUCTION PRINCIPLES AND TREATMENT GUIDELINES
Goals and Priorities

When considering a defect or deformity, the initial question is: what are the goals and priorities? Recognizing that the easiest way to close a defect may not be the best or ideal way, one must ask: is the goal to simply close a wound or to reconstruct the part to obtain the best aesthetic and functional outcome possible? (**Table 1**).

Considerations include: location and size of defect; depth of defect and surrounding tissue quality; age and health of patient; and status of disease (control or palliation) (**Table 2**). If wound closure is the primary goal, a sequential thought process following the steps of the "wound closure" ladder is appropriate. If the main goal is to reconstruct the defect, especially in aesthetic reconstruction, then the thought process should not be sequentially, but the best option should be used, even if a more straightforward procedure would work to close the wound.[13] The next consideration is determining the limitations that may preclude obtaining initial goals and being sure that the patient, family and surgeon have realistic expectations.

Principle Replace Like Tissue with Like Tissue

Scalp tissue is unique in its composition and its hair-bearing capacity. Therefore the ideal tissue for scalp defect coverage would be scalp tissue. If there is significant damage to surrounding tissue due to trauma, infection or radiation, defect coverage with local tissue may not be a good option to obtain reliable, stable wound closure. Medical and aesthetic considerations are involved in the decision-making about which reconstructive option to use. The goal of wound coverage from a functional and protective

Table 1
Goals and priorities: first step
After disease or injured tissue is removed, ask the question:
What are our goals & priorities?
To close the wound or to reconstruct the part
What is the *easiest* way to close and what is the *best* way to close the defect?

Table 2
Goals and priorities: considerations

Location, size, depth and etiology of defect
Quality of surrounding tissue
Previous or active infection
Pre- or postoperative radiation
Exposure of vital structures such as bone, dura or brain parenchyma
Age and health of patient
Status of disease (control or palliation)
Aesthetic considerations such as hair growth pattern, hairline and brow position and aesthetic subunits

standpoint has to be combined with the goal of achieving a cosmetically pleasing (or acceptable) result. Often, this goal requires a combination of different procedures and several surgical stages. In order to achieve an optimal aesthetic result, frequently the final revisions (using loco-regional flaps, tissue expansion or hair transplantation) must be delayed until stable wound coverage is obtained.

Etiology and Analysis of Defects

The magnitude of scalp and forehead defects is dependent on the underlying causative factors leading to the defect or injury. They may be full thickness or partial thickness and can be classified as congenital or acquired (**Table 3**). Congenital defects[14] may include: cutis aplastica, congenital nevus, congenital vascular malformations, and congenital tumors. Acquired scalp and forehead defects may be caused by: injuries such as burns; mechanical trauma such as blunt, penetrating injuries; avulsion injuries leading to "degloving" of the scalp; or from tumor invasion, infection, oncologic resection, radiation or wound-healing difficulties. Preoperative

anticipation of potential difficulty with direct closure when the scalp or forehead has been compromised by one of the above circumstances or conditions is crucial to success.

The initial evaluation of the defect is based on its size and location, tissue involved, and structures exposed like pericranium, cranium, devascularized bone flaps, prosthetic material, dura, brain parenchyma or vessels. In addition, the quality of the surrounding tissue (scarring, infection, radiation) and aesthetic concerns such as contour, skin color match, hairline, brow position and aesthetic subunits must be considered. A number of authors have established staging systems and treatment algorithms to be used at their institutions.[15,16]

After assessing the size and location of the defect (or anticipated defect), the structures involved, the surrounding tissue quality, and the patient's medical condition, the next step is to define the goals of the operation. Is the goal to close the wound or reconstruct the part? Sometimes these two goals are the same. If aesthetic reconstruction is the goal, then multiple operative procedures may be needed to obtain the best result. Frequently, wounds are initially closed in the most straightforward way, with

Table 3
Conditions leading to scalp, calvarian and forehead defects: congenital and acquired

Congenital	Acquired
Aplasia cutis congenita	Trauma: blunt, penetrating or avulsion injuries
Congenital nevus	Burns
Congenital vascular malformation	Tumor invasion
Congenital tumors	Oncologic resection
—	Radiation
—	Infection
—	Wound-healing difficulties

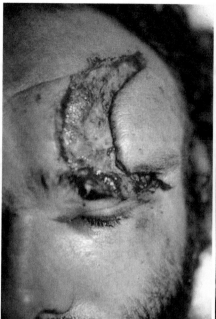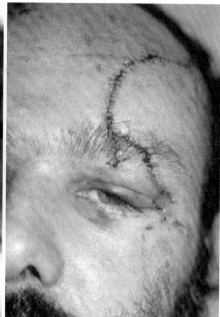

Fig. 1. Primary closure of traumatic avulsion injury.

the anticipation that secondary reconstruction with tissue expansion or other reconstructive technique will be performed secondarily. In the case of malignancies, one may adjust the reconstructive approach depending on whether the goal is cure or palliation. If tissue quality is poor due to scarring, radiation or infection and if local options are unavailable, then distant tissue is clearly indicated. Sometimes, even if local, less complicated options are technically feasible, distant tissue is safer and more reliable in ensuring uncomplicated healing. This approach is especially important if there is exposure of vital structures.

LOCAL AND REGIONAL RECONSTRUCTIVE OPTIONS SCALP AND FOREHEAD DEFECTS
Primary Closure

Frequently, post-traumatic wounds have the appearance of tissue loss but, on careful inspection, are found to not be missing any tissue. These wounds can usually be closed directly if minimal tissue needs to be debrided (**Fig 1**). If the defect is smaller then 3 cm in diameter, primary closure with undermining can usually be performed.[17] There may be limitations of that approach based on the surrounding tissue quality or exposure of vital structures. Local advancement flaps, undermining the tissue and scoring

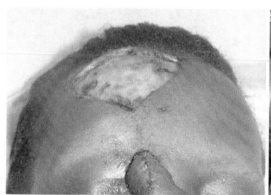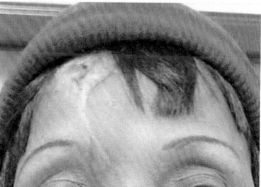

Fig. 2. Donor site of paramedian forehead flap left open to close by secondary intention (*top*). Same donor site 9 months later (*bottom*) with hypo and hyper pigmented scar.

of the galea,[18] helps in reducing tension and increases the chances of stable wound coverage. One needs to be careful to not score too deeply or close under too much tension, both of which will compromise the blood supply and lead to marginal necrosis or alopecia.

Secondary Intention Healing

Mohs initial approach of healing small forehead and scalp defects with secondary intention healing by granulation, contraction and re-epithelialisation, seems to have satisfactory results in the forehead area if the defect is not too close to the brow.[19] Experience with allowing paramedian forehead flap donor sites to heal secondarily leads credence to this approach, although the patient must be aware of the prolonged healing time required with this approach. Although healing by secondary intention frequently leads to acceptable results in Caucasians, patients with darker skin frequently heal with hypo- or hyperpigmented scars (**Fig 2**). In the scalp area, the healed defect will be alopecic but will also have reduced in size significantly because of the contraction component of secondary healing.[20]

Skin Grafting and Tissue Expansion

The main advantage of covering a defect with a skin graft is that it is a straightforward procedure achieving reliable wound closure. The downsides are: the difficulty in matching the color, texture and thickness; suboptimal restoration of the contour; and the lack of hair if used in scalp reconstruction. Patients with defects on bald heads are frequently best served with a skin graft, whereas, defects within the hair-bearing portion are frequently aesthetically unacceptable (**Fig. 3**). Split thickness skin grafts frequently do not tolerate radiation therapy very well, especially if a significant amount of desquamation occurs from the

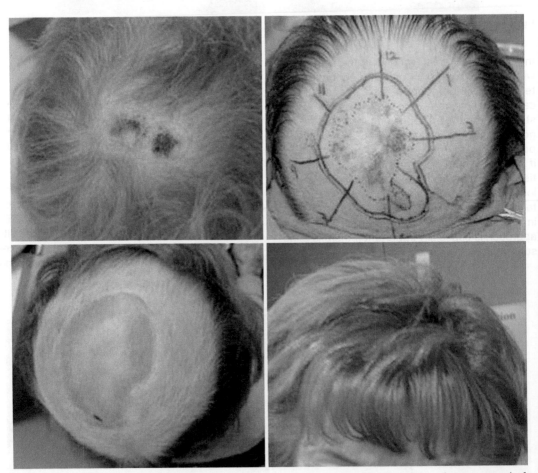

Fig. 3. 83-year-old female (*top left*) with recurrent squamous cell cancer of scalp. Extent of tumor noted after cutting hair (*top right*), proposed resection outlined. Wound closed with a STSG from lower abdomen with primary closure of donor site (*bottom left*). Camouflage of surgically created alopecia with hair piece (*bottom right*).

radiation. If postoperative radiation is anticipated, consideration should be given to using a fasciocutaneous flap that has the capacity to re-epthelialize rather than a skin graft or skin grafted tissue flap that have more limited capacity to re-epithelialize should desquamation occur (**Fig. 4**).

In 1908, Robinson was the first to describe that a skin graft can reliably be placed directly on pericranium rather than waiting for the wound to be covered by granulation tissue first.[21] Another method to be considered when the outer table of the cranium is exposed is to drill burr holes through the outer table into the diploe, await granulation tissue to cover the bone, then skin-grafting the granulation tissue. Alternatively, the outer table of the skull can be removed and a skin graft can be placed directly on the well-vascularizide diploe.[22]

More recently, artificial dermal substitute (Integra) has been used on burred outer table, and secondarily skin grafted after the acellular dermal matrix revascularizes.[23,24] Although grafts may take on burred bone, generally these grafts are not very stable and do not stand up to minor trauma.

For forehead defects, it is important to consider the subunits and avoid distorting brow and hairline. Frequently, resurfacing the entire aesthetic unit of the forehead with a skin graft or flap is preferable to a "patch" resurfacing. This can improve the cosmetic appearance if no significant contour deficit is present (**Fig. 5**). The main challenge with skin grafts on the forehead is achieving contour and color match, specifically if the defect in addition to missing skin involves loss of soft tissue with exposed bone. When pericranium is

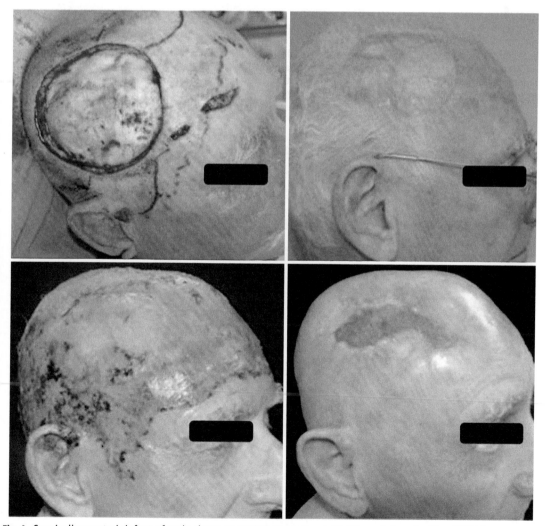

Fig. 4. Surgically created defect of scalp down to pericranium (*top left*). Wound closed with a STSG from contralateral scalp (*top right*). Desquamation from radiation therapy (*bottom left*). Native scalp spontaneously re-epithelialized but STSG site is healing slowly by contraction (*bottom right*).

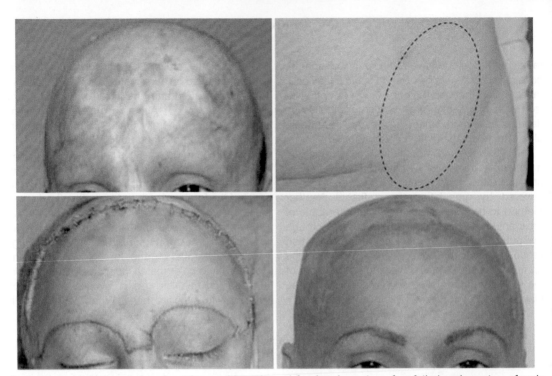

Fig. 5. 35-year-old Hispanic female with unstable scalp and forehead scarring after failed replantation of scalp and STSG coverage (*top left*). FTSG donor site from area of lower abdomen without stretch marks (*top right*). Immediately after surgery demonstrating entire aesthetic resurfacing (*bottom left*). Two years post-operative (*bottom right*). Eyebrows created with tattoo.

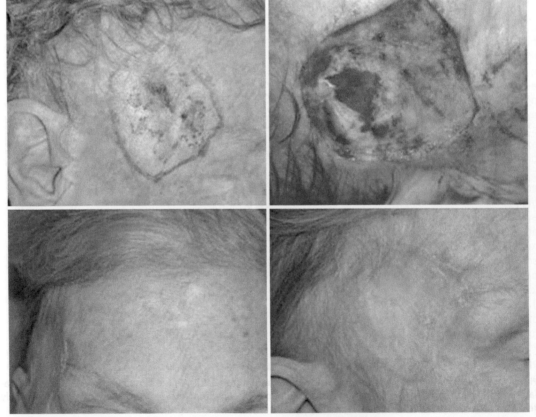

Fig. 6. 89-year-old female with extensive basal cell carcinoma (*top left*). Resection through deep temporal fascia (*top right*). 6 months post-operatively of STSG harvested from the scalp (*bottom*).

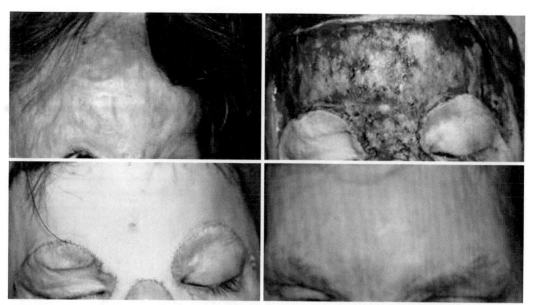

Fig. 7. 3-year-old male with severe forehead scarring from a 35% burn injury when he was 3 months old (*top left*). Aesthetic unit excision (*top right*). FTSG harvested from an expanded abdominal donor site (*bottom left*). Same patient, 18 years later (*bottom right*).

missing, local pericranial (periosteal) flaps can be raised to cover small to moderate size defects and allow for skin grafting over those pericranial flaps.[25] Ideally, if a split thickness graft is used to resurface the forehead, then, for better color match, a depilated split thickness graft harvested from the scalp should be considered (**Fig. 6**). Full thickness skin grafts (FTSG) are far superior to split grafts, which tend to contract more and have a shiny appearance. If there is a paucity of FTSG donor sites, then the FTSG donor site can be expanded to facilitate direct closure of the donor site. Unfortunately, even with preliminary tissue expansion, there is usually not enough available donor site skin above the clavicles to harvest a full thickness graft for the best color match of an entire forehead aesthetic unit.[9] Meticulous technique and hemostasis is essential, in that even a small loss of a graft used to reconstruct an entire subunit, will sully an otherwise aesthetic result. In addition, the inferior margin of the graft should be touching the eyebrows (if they are present) and the superior margin should be touching or just inside the scalp hairline (**Fig. 7**). If this is not done, a small amount of contraction or growth in children will lead to a rim of residual forehead skin above and below the graft.

Tissue expansion is clearly the reconstructive option of choice for both scalp and forehead defects, in that no other technique can provide "like tissue" for large defects.[26,27] Temporary skin grafting with the anticipation of subsequent

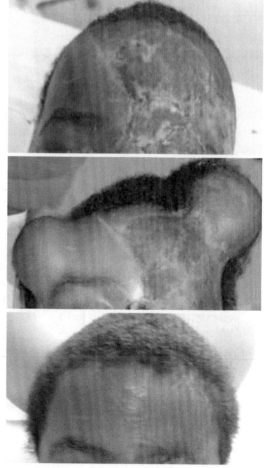

Fig. 8. Initial wound resurfaced with a STSG (*top*). Remnants of forehead expanded (*middle*). After transfer of expanded flaps, planning final scars to lie at borders of forehead subunits (*bottom*).

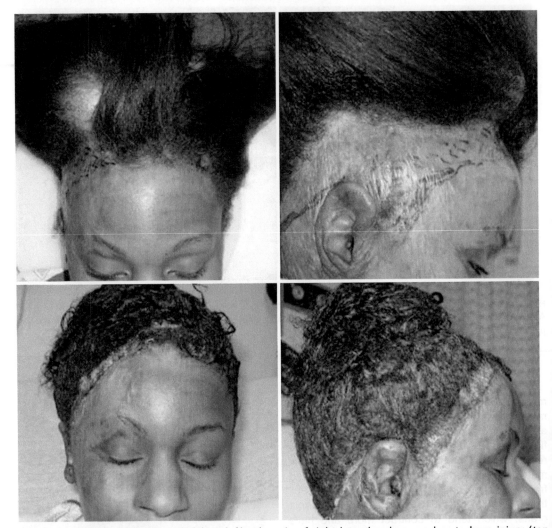

Fig. 9. Scalp expanders fully expanded (*top left*). Alopecia of right lateral scalp secondary to burn injury (*top right*). After recreation of natural hairline with expanded scalp flaps (*bottom*).

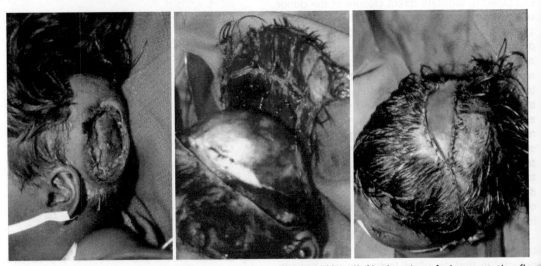

Fig.10. Asphalt "road rash" injury through pericranium in a 6-year-old boy (*left*). Elevation of a large rotation flap (*middle*). Despite galeal scoring incisions could not be closed without excess tension (*right*). Therefore, a STSG was used to relieve tension on the flap.

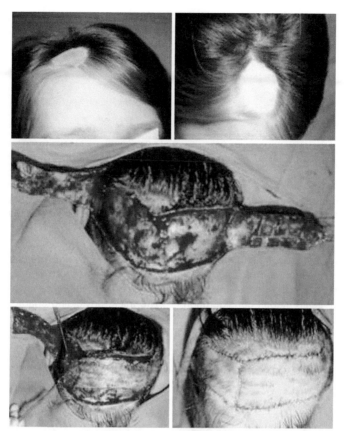

Fig. 11. 10-year-old female with aplasia cutis congenital (*top*). Ortichocha-type advancement flaps with galeal scoring (*middle*). De-epithelized alopecic area left attached to one of the flaps to anchor it to the deep tissue in attempt to minimize scar widening (*bottom light*). Scalp reconstructed with Ortichochea-type advancement flaps (*bottom right*).

removal after tissue expansion of adjacent local tissue from the same aesthetic unit provides a superior cosmetic outcome (**Figs 8** and **9**). The main disadvantages of tissue expansion are the need for multiple procedures, the temporary aesthetic deformity of having expanders, risks of extrusion, and the lengthy treatment period over several months.[26,28] Another consequence of tissue expansion is the molding/erosion of the skull from the pressure of the expander. Although this can potentially can lead to disastrous consequences,[29] bony contour irregularities caused by tissue expansion generally spontaneously improve with time.

LOCAL FLAP RECONSTRUCTION WITHIN THE SAME AESTHETIC UNIT

Tissue from the same aesthetic unit provides the best cosmetic results in reconstructing a defect.

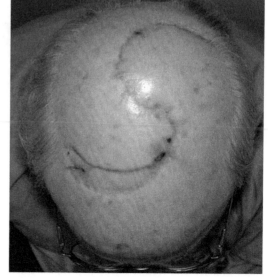

Fig. 12. Aesthetically unacceptable scar on bald head.

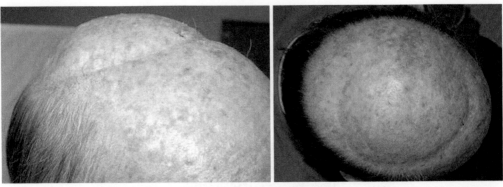

Fig. 13. Scars of large rotation flap on bald head. Although a STSG was not needed to supplement flap closure, wound contraction lead to unacceptable aesthetic from "biscuiting" of the curved incision.

There are no separate aesthetic units of the scalp, but there is a clear distinction between the hair-bearing scalp and the aesthetic unit of the fore-head. When utilizing scalp flaps, consideration needs to be given to the direction of hair growth. A swatch of hair growing in the wrong direction can mar an otherwise excellent reconstruction. The thick, unyielding characteristics of scalp and

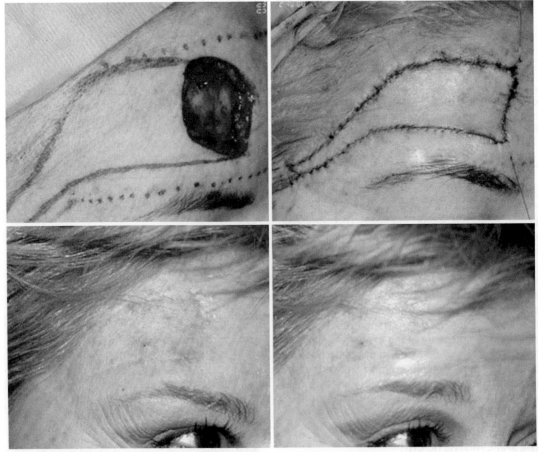

Fig. 14. Forehead defect with proposed v-y flap outlined to minimize any change in eyebrow position (*top left*). Flap Advanced and wound closed (*top right*). 6-month follow-up (*bottom left*). Patient raising her eyebrows (*bottom right*).

forehead skin frequently make local tissue rearrangements (with direct closure of the donor site) a challenge. Closure under tension will frequently lead to loss of hair in a widened scar or marginal necrosis. To avoid this, when large local flaps are performed, the donor sites frequently need to be skin grafted to minimize tension (**Fig. 10**).

Undermining and scoring of the galea can help closing a small to moderate size defect if the surrounding tissue is of good quality and has not been violated by severe trauma, scarring, infection or radiation. Rotation, transposition, or geometric flaps can provide acceptable cosmetic results if the defect is small to moderate size[30,31] (**Fig. 11**). Multiple techniques using loco-regional flaps have been described.[1,2] Rapasio described the use of three adjacent rhomboid flaps in the vertex area that can reconstruct the natural whorl pattern of the hair in that region.[32]

A combination of rotation and advancement is often utilized to cover larger defects requiring a long curvilinear incision, which incorporates at least one of the named scalp vessels allowing for maximal excursion while maintaining vascularity. The length of the rotation flap should exceed five times the diameter of the defect to get adequate tension free closure.[33] Galeal scoring, back cutting, and undermining of the scalp in the subgaleal plane can help minimize tension as well. The results of these flaps appear better in hirsute scalps as compared to the bald head; bald heads do not have hair or skin lines to hide the scars (**Figs. 12** and **13**).

Up to 40% of the forehead can be closed with a rotation-advancement flap based on the supratrochlear and supraorbital vessels providing a good aesthetic result.[33] Dependent on the defect location and skin laxity, as well as the presence or absence of facial lines, V-Y advancement flaps or H-flaps can provide good results as well (**Figs. 14** and **15**). Rocha described a frontalis-based V-Y musculocutaneous flap for forehead defects up to 5.5 cm in diameter.[34]

RECONSTRUCTIVE OPTIONS OUTSIDE OF THE AESTHETIC UNIT
Crane Principle and Island Pedicle Flaps

Reconstruction of defects with flaps from outside the aesthetic unit in which the defect is located is

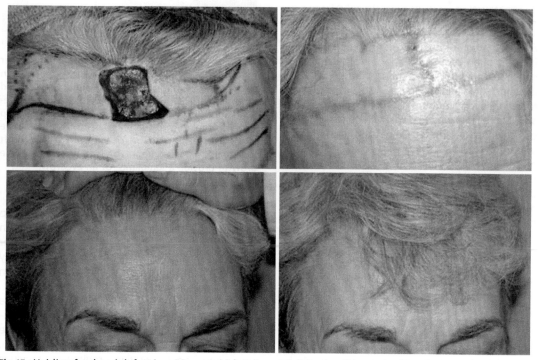

Fig. 15. Hairline forehead defect in a 58-year-old female executive who did not want to allow the wound to heal by secondary intention (*top left*). Forehead skin lines marked. Bilateral v-y advancement flaps placing incisions within or parallel to skin lines (*top right*). Acceptable scars 4 months postoperatively (*bottom left*). Further camouflage of scars with bangs (*bottom right*).

often required if there is not enough laxity of tissue within the same aesthetic unit. One of the techniques used crossing the aesthetic units of the scalp and the forehead is the crane principle. In 1969, Millard described the crane principle in which a flap is used as an engineering crane to lift and transport subcutaneous tissue from one area to deposit in another; the pedicle and overlying scalp skin can be returned to its bed later.[35] This principle was applied for forehead defects not amenable to closure with a skin graft. This two-stage method used a hair-bearing scalp flap to resurface the forehead. After waiting for the deep surface of the flap to get revascularized from the wound bed, the hair-bearing skin was returned to its original site leaving the subcutaneous flap tissue down, placing a split thickness skin graft over it (**Fig. 16**).[36]

Island fasciocutaneous scalp flaps based on the superficial temporal vessels also move tissue from one aesthetic unit into another. These flaps have been used for eyebrow reconstruction but generally have been found to transfer too much hair; free hair transplants achieve superior aesthetic results. The temporoprietalis fascial/subcutaneous flap, which is subsequently skin grafted, can be useful to augment forehead contour deficiencies.[37]

Reconstruction with Regional and Distant Pedicle Flaps

Reconstruction of defects with regional or distant flaps is often required if the surrounding tissue has poor quality due to prior trauma, scarring, infection or radiation changes. Also, if post-surgical radiation is required, the defect must be closed in a stable reliable way that will withstand the stress of radiation treatment. Defects in the occipital area can be reliably closed with a pedicle trapezius musculocutaneous flap based on the deep branch of the transverse cervical artery.[38] The latissimus dorsi pedicle flap can also be utilized to cover most areas of the scalp.[39] If regional or distant pedicle flaps are not adequate for wound coverage, free tissue transfer should be considered.

FREE TISSUE TRANSFER, MICROSURGICAL RECONSTRUCTION
Muscle, Musculocutaneous and Fasciocutaneous Flaps

Many reconstructive surgeons will choose to close large scalp and forehead wounds with a free-tissue transfer, even if one could technically be closed with a distant pedicle flap. Their reasoning is that free tissue transfers provides the most robust vascular supply of the flap to the wound,

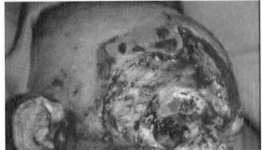

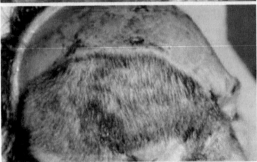

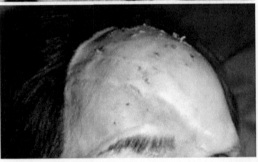

Fig. 16. After debridement of electrical injury, lower forehead and orbit wounds unable to support a skin graft (*top*). Transposition of a "scalping" flap based on the superficial temporal vessels to close right forehead and orbit (*middle*). After the hair bearing scalp skin was replaced to the scalp, deep tissue was able to be left behind to be closed with a skin graft (*bottom*). A small amount of hair was left on the brow to provide a semblance of an eyebrow.

compared to the distal portion of the pedicle flap (which frequently has less robust vascularity). In addition, it is usually easier to inset and tailor free-tissue transfers then pedicle flaps, thereby making the free flap option not only the best option but the easiest.

Although the general principle of "replacing like with like tissue" is an important concept, specifically in scalp and forehead reconstruction there are patients in whom the presence of infection, pre- and post-operative radiation, previous surgery, or simply the size of the defect precludes using "like" local or regional reconstructive options. In those cases, a more advanced

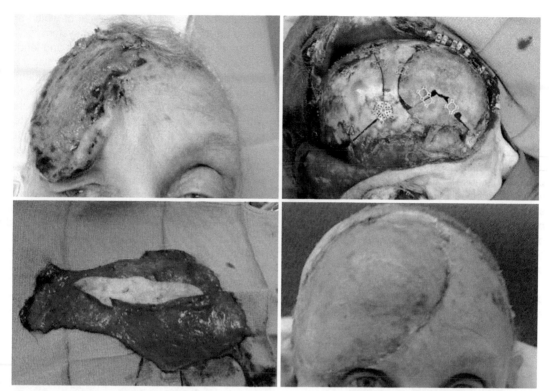

Fig. 17. 79-year-old female with a neglected basal cell carcinoma invading into the cranium (*top left*). After radical resection including frontal bone and performing a cranioplasty with autologous split calvarium from posterior lateral skull (*right*). Latissimus dorsi musculocutaneous flap (*bottom left*). Note that the skin paddle on this thin patient was able to be used as a monitor without a contour deformity. 2 weeks after placing STSG on flap (*bottom right*).

approach utilizing free tissue transfer with different tissue components—depending on the complexity of the defect—is indicated. This is frequently the case in the setting of aggressive malignancies when expedient wide excision, often down-to-bone or even including the calvarium leaving exposed dura or brain parenchyma, requires immediate reliable coverage.

The increasing use of pre- and post-operative radiation therapy not only creates a patient population presenting with increased scarring and radiation damage of the surrounding tissue but one that requires timely healing and a durable construct stable enough to withstand post-operative radiation therapy as well.[40]

Beasley and colleagues[15] developed a staging system based on defect size and surrounding tissue quality indicating free flap coverage for defects of the forehead and scalp with heavy trauma, infection, radiation damage and previous local flap failure, as well as for forehead defects greater than 50 cm^2 and scalp greater than 200 cm^2. Those numbers are guidelines; every case has to be carefully analyzed with an individualized

treatment plan. The decision about which type of free flap is indicated depends also on multiple factors, including defect size, location, wound condition, tissue availability, donor site morbidity,

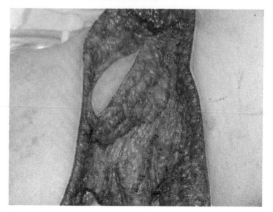

Fig. 18. Cutaneous portion of a latissimus dorsi musculocutaneous flap on an obese patient. The thickness of the subcutaneous tissue precludes using this on the scalp because of the significant contour deformity that would result.

as well as surgeon's and patient's preference. If there is previous or ongoing infection or osteomyelitis, then a free flap including a significant amount of muscle is thought to be to be beneficial.[41,42] The latissimus dorsi is a suitable muscle flap with a long vascular pedicle, adequate surface area, thickness and contourability to cover the convex surface of the scalp and forehead (**Fig. 17**). Although the latissimus dorsi flap has the option of including a skin paddle for postoperative monitoring, the skin is usually excluded in obese patients because of the significant deformity that would be caused by the skin with its underlying subcutaneous tissue (**Fig. 18**). If a bony defect is present, the latissimus dorsi flap may include the option of incorporating vascularized rib, based on the intercostal perforators of the thoracodorsal system, with the flap.[43–46]

If more tissue is required than the latissimus dorsi free flap can provide, it can be combined with the serratus muscle flap as well as with the scapular/parascapular free flap—all of which are based off the subscapular vascular system.[47]

Depending on the size of the defect and length of pedicle required, almost any muscle flap can be used. One of the most versatile flaps frequently used for small to moderate size defects is the rectus abdominis muscle flap. It is relatively thin with a long pedicle and can be rapidly harvested in the supine position thereby facilitating simultaneous harvest and tumor resection or recipient site preparation.[48] Although it can be raised as a musculocutaneous flap, because of excess abdominal fat in the western population, skin is usually not included in this flap when used for scalp or forehead coverage. It should be noted that muscle flaps will atrophy and thin with time; frequently, this adds to the aesthetic outcome, but if there is an underlying contour irregularity, it will be visible after the muscle atrophies (**Fig. 19**).

The omental flap was the first successful free flap used for scalp reconstruction.[49] The

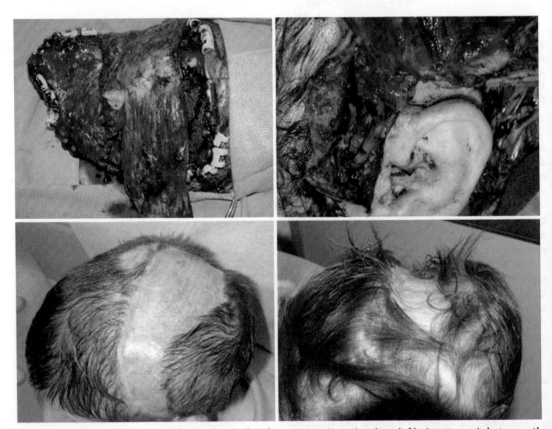

Fig. 19. Rectus abominis flap draped over the skull defect prior to insetting (*top left*). Anastomosis between the deep inferior epigastric vessels and the superficial temporal vessels (*top right*). Skin grafted muscle flap three months postoperatively (*bottom left*). 18 months postoperatively photo demonstrates the atrophy of the muscle flap (*bottom right*). Although scalp integrity is still intact, the original contour deformity from resection of bone is now visible.

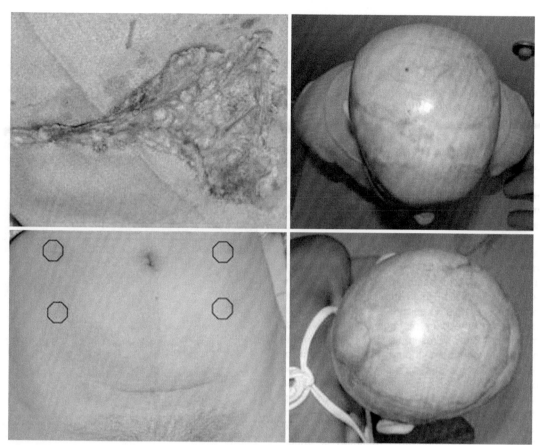

Fig. 20. Same patient as in **Fig. 5** who had an unstable scalp graft after scalp avulsion. Omental free flap (*top right*). Stable coverage with skin grafted omentum 2 years later (*top left and bottom right*). The Gastroepiploic vessels are visible through the graft. Four 1.5 cm incisions (*circles*) and previous Pfannenstiel incision were used for harvesting the omentum to limit donor site scars and morbidity (*bottom left*).

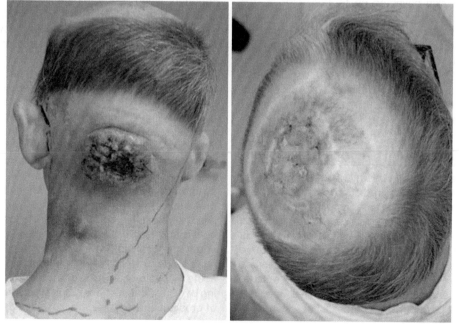

Fig. 21. 56-year-old male with previous squamous cell carcinoma on vertex of scalp, now with metastatic lesions of occiput.

advantage of the omental flap is its pliability, long vascular pedicle, thin contour and rich vascularity, which can be beneficial—specifically in areas of prior severe radiation damage, infection or cerebrospinal fluid leak. Although the vascular pedicle can be lengthened significantly up to over 90 cm,[50] when it is lengthened, the amount of surface area available for coverage is decreased. The main disadvantage is the need for laparotomy and potential associated complications,[51] although it may be harvested laparoscopically, which limits scars and donor site morbidity (**Fig. 20**).

Whereas fasciocutaneous flaps work well to reconstruct forehead defects, the paucity of hair makes them less optimal in scalp reconstruction. The scapular and parascapular, radial forearm and anterior lateral thigh free flap are common options. The radial forearm free flap has a thinner dermis than the back or thigh skin and by that may more closely resemble facial skin in forehead reconstruction although the color match of all these flaps is suboptimal. Until recently, the only flap with a large enough surface area (without pre-expansion) to cover extensive scalp defects has been the latissimus/serratus combined flap or the omentum. As mentioned above, when postoperative radiation is anticipated, fasciocutaneous flaps are superior to soft tissue flaps that require split thickness skin grafts. In near total scalp defects, the authors found the giant vascularized anterior lateral thigh (GVALT) fasciocutaneous (or musculocutaneous) free flap to be the best option for single-stage coverage.[52] This subtotal thigh free flap can reliably provide a large amount of soft tissue including skin coverage up to 1200 cm[2].[53] This option has been useful for patients undergoing resection of aggressive malignancies requiring immediate reconstruction of massive defects and early postoperative radiation therapy. This large skin territory can safely be transferred if medial and lateral perforators of the lateral femoral circumflex vascular pedicle are included in the flap (**Figs. 21–24**).[52,54]

The Complex Full-thickness Calvarial Defect

Combined-modality treatment of tumors with surgical resection and radiation can lead to tissue compromise resulting in combined scalp and cranial defects. Radiation, scar, dural violation and cerebrospinal fluid leak usually preclude local flap options[45] and, in fact, frequently require distant tissue from outside the zone of injury. Although controversial, the authors believe that it is important to evaluate the potential need for structural support in the initial stage of

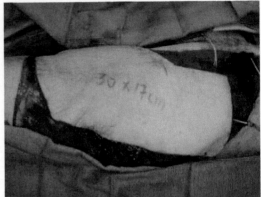

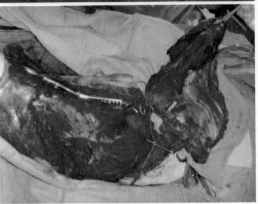

Fig. 22. 30 cm × 17 cm musculocutaneous thigh flap (*top*). Undersurface of the flap (*bottom*). Rectus femoris muscle included to help fill suboccipital dead space.

reconstruction. This consideration is particularly important when complex defects lie posterior or lateral to the vertex of the skull. In these situations, external pressure from a recumbent patient with a soft tissue-only reconstruction can theoretically transmit enough pressure to increase intracranial pressure, resulting in negative neurological sequelae, such as seizuriform activity. Neurological impairment has also been described from external compression from the flap weight itself, especially for bony defects over the frontal lobe,[55] as well as from compression of the cortex just from atmospheric pressure;[56] the neurologic sequelae from this entity is known as the syndrome of the trephined.[57] Although various prosthetics (titanium mesh, polymethylmethacrylate, polyethylene, or hydroxyapetite cement) or nonvascularized bone have been used to reconstruct the cranium, in the authors experience, more times than not, the clinical scenario requiring acute reconstruction is associated with a preexisting or history of infection, which precludes the use of prosthetics if possible. In these circumstances,

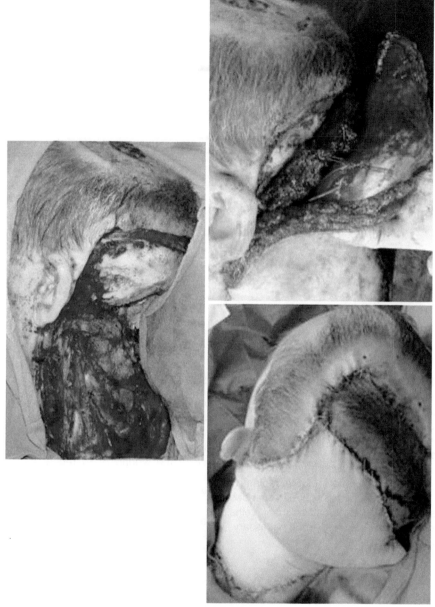

Fig. 23. Extensive surgical defect of posterior scalp and neck (*left*). Rectus femoris fascia anchored to the occiput to counteract gravity and pulling on the suture lines (*upper right*). Thigh flap was designed with a superior extension to allow the posterior hair-bearing scalp to be transposed to close the previous wound on the vertex with exposed cranium (*lower right*). The donor defect from the scalp transposition flap was then in continuity to the occipital defect & able to be closed with the extension of the thigh flap.

the authors prefer autologous vascularized bone. In the authors' experience, the latissimus dorsi composite free flap including vascularized rib can successfully cover those large complex cranial defects, provide skeletal support, restore contour, and significantly improve functional outcome with limited donor site morbidity

(**Fig. 25**).[46] Smaller defects can be reconstructed using the iliac or scapular plate.[58]

Replantation

The ultimate reconstruction utilizing the concept of reconstructing "like with like" is scalp replantation.

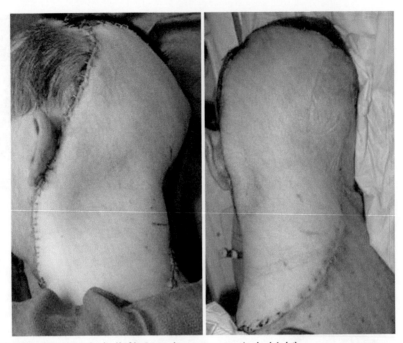

Fig. 24. Immediately post-operatively (*left*). 2 weeks post-operatively (*right*).

Successful replantation of scalp avulsion gives the best cosmetic result possible. The condition of the avulsed scalp has to be evaluated carefully, being sure that adequate donor and recipient vessels, preferably outside the zone of injury, are available for revascularization. Ideally, multiple vessels should be anastomosed to assure adequate arterial inflow and venous outflow of the replanted scalp. As with most replants, adequate venous drainage is crucial to success and as many veins as possible should be anastomosed. If necessary, vein grafts should be used.

FUTURE DIRECTIONS

The future directions of reconstruction are tissue engineering and composite tissue allograft transfer (CTA). Although genetically engineered growth of hair follicles has only been demonstrated in an animal model,[59] CTA of other facial parts have been clinically performed in humans.[60–64] Because the standard methods of scalp and forehead coverage and reconstruction are usually able to obtain an acceptable aesthetic result (albeit sometimes only with a wig), isolated scalp and forehead CTA in patients who are not otherwise immunosuppressed is not likely to become clinically relevant until a tolerance model is developed and substantiated.

SUMMARY

As mentioned, reconstruction of scalp and forehead defects is a complex field with a broad variety of reconstructive options. It is important to determine goals and priorities. Is the goal to close the wound or to reconstruct the defect? What is the easiest way to close the defect versus what is the best way to close the defect?

Defining those initial goals and choosing a reconstructive option is influenced by size and location of the defect, etiology and depth of the defect, surrounding tissue quality, exposure of vital structures like bone, dura or brain parenchyma, age and health of the patient and status of disease (control or palliation). A detailed preoperative defect analysis is essential to provide not only adequate wound coverage but also help tailor the method of reconstruction to achieve an optimal aesthetic result, taking in consideration hair growth pattern, hairline and brow position as well as aesthetic subunits.

ACKNOWLEDGMENTS

The authors want to acknowledge their Neurosurgery and Head and Neck Surgery colleagues as well as all the residents in Plastic and Reconstructive Surgery at the University of Chicago who were all crucial in the care of the patients presented in this manuscript.

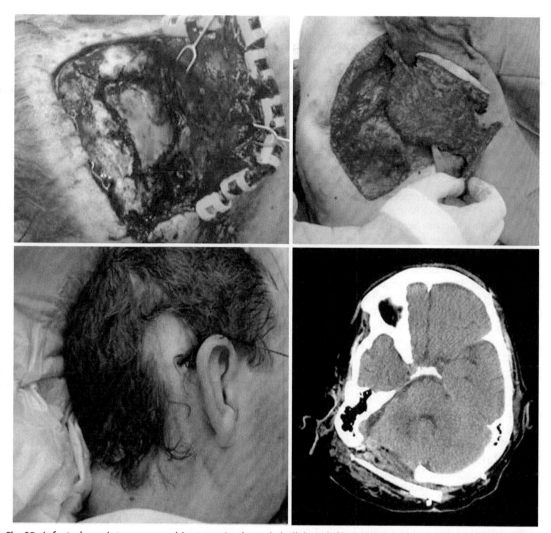

Fig. 25. Infected craniotomy wound in posterior lateral skull (*top left*). Latissimus dorsi osteomusculocutaneous flap with skin component to minimize tension on wound closure and the facilitate monitoring the microsurgical transfer (*top right*). The vascularized rib would provide a strut to protect the brain from pressure. Attachment of rib by intercostal perforators allowed for flexibility of insetting. Six months postoperatively (*bottom left*). Patient was allowed to lay on his flap immediately postoperatively. Follow-up CT scan showing vascularize rib spanning the cranial defect (*bottom right*).

REFERENCES

1. Orticochea M. Four flap scalp reconstruction technique. Br J Plast Surg 1967;20:159–71.
2. Lesavoy MA, Dubrow TJ, Schwartz RJ, et al. Management of large scalp defects with local pedicle flaps. Plast Reconstr Surg 1993;91:783–90.
3. Crawford BS. An unusual skin donor site. Br J Plast Surg 1964;17:311–3.
4. Tolhurst DE, Carstens MH, Greco RJ, et al. The surgical anatomy of the scalp. Plast Reconstr Surg 1991;87(4):603–12.
5. Seery GE. Surgical anatomy of the scalp. Dermatol Surg 2002;28(7):581–7.
6. Cutting CB, McCarthy JG, Berenstein A. Blood supply of the upper craniofacial skeleton: the search for composite calvarial bone flaps. Plast Reconstr Surg 1984;74(5):603–10.
7. McCarthy JG, Zide BM. The spectrum of calvarial bone grafting: introduction of the vascularized calvarial bone flap. Plast Reconstr Surg 1984;74(1):10–8.
8. Knize DM. Reassessment of the coronal incision and subgaleal dissection for foreheadplasty. Plast Reconstr Surg 1998;102:478–89.

9. Mosser SW, Guyuron B, Janis JE, et al. The anatomy of the greater occipital nerve: implications for the etiology of migraine headaches. Plast Reconstr Surg 2004;113:693–7.

10. Stuzin JM, Wagstrom L, Kawamoto HK, et al. Anatomy of the frontal branch of the facial nerve: the significance of the temporal fat pad. Plast Reconstr Surg 1989;83(2):265–71.

11. Siegle RJ. Reconstruction of the forehead. In: Baker SR, Swanson NA, editors. Local flaps in facial reconstruction. St. Louis (MO): Mosby–Year Book; 1995. p. 421–42.

12. Menick FJ. Facial reconstruction with local and distant tissue: the interface of aesthetic and reconstructive surgery. Plast Reconstr Surg 1998;102(5):1424–33.

13. Gottlieb LJ, Krieger LM. From the reconstructive ladder to the reconstructive elevator. Plast Reconstr Surg 1994;93(7):1503–4.

14. O'brien BM, Drake JE. Congenital defects of the skull and scalp. Br J Plast Surg 1960;13:102–9.

15. Beasley NJ, Gilbert RW, Gullane PJ, et al. Scalp and forehead reconstruction using free revascularized tissue transfer. Arch Facial Plast Surg 2004;6(1):16–20.

16. Lutz BS, Wei FC, Chen HC, et al. Reconstruction of scalp defects with free flaps in 30 cases. Br J Plast Surg 1998;51(3):186–90.

17. Terkonda RP, Sykes JM. Concepts in scalp and forehead reconstruction. Otolaryngol Clin North Am 1997;30:519–39.

18. Raposio E, Santi P, Nordstrom REA. Effects of galeotomies on scalp flaps. Ann Plast Surg 1998;41:17–21.

19. Bennett RG. Mohs' surgery: new concepts and applications. Dermatol Clin 1987;5(2):409–28.

20. Becker GD, Adams LA, Levin BC. Secondary intention healing of exposed scalp and forehead bone after Mohs surgery. Otolaryngol Head Neck Surg 1999;121:751–4.

21. Robinson EF. Total avulsion of the scalp. Surg Gynecol Obstet 1908;7:663.

22. Pitkanen JM, Al-Qattan MM, Russel NA. Immediate coverage of exposed, denuded cranial bone with split thickness skin grafts. Ann Plast Surg 2000;45:118–21.

23. Komorowska-Timek E, Gabriel A, Bennett D, et al. Artificial dermis as an alternative for coverage of complex scalp defects following excision of malignant tumors. Plast Reconstr Surg 2005;115(4):1010–7.

24. Koenen W, Goerdt G, Faulhaber J. Removal of the outer table of the skull for reconstruction of full-thickness scalp defects with a dermal regeneration template. Dermatol Surg 2008;34(3):357–63.

25. Terranova W. The use of periosteal flaps in scalp and forehead reconstruction. Ann Plast Surg 1990;25:450–6.

26. Gottlieb LJ, Parsons RW, Krizek TJ. The use of tissue expansion techniques in burn reconstruction. J Burn Care Rehabil 1986;7(3):234–7.

27. Iwahira Y, Maruyama Y. Expanded unilateral forehead flap (sail flap) for coverage of opposite forehead defect. Plast Reconstr Surg 1993;92:1052–6.

28. Gottlieb LJ, Dreyfuss DA. Tissue expander in head and neck reconstruction in local skin flaps and free skin grafts in head and neck reconstruction [chapter 9]. St. Louis: Mosby; 1992. p. 132–43.

29. Fudem GM, Orgel MG. Full-thickness erosion of the skull secondary to tissue expansion for scalp reconstruction. [letter]. Plast Reconstr Surg 1988;82:368–9.

30. Lida N, Ohsumi N, Tonegawa M, et al. Reconstruction of scalp defects using simple designed bilobed flap. Aesthetic Plast Surg 2000;24:137.

31. Vecchione TR. Multiple pinwheel scalp flaps. [chapter 2]. In: Strauch B, Vasconez LO, Hall-Findlay EJ, editors, Grabb's encyclopedia of flaps, vol. 1. Boston: Little, Brown; 1990. p. 10–2.

32. Raposio E, Nordstrom REA, Santi PL. Aesthetic reconstruction of the vertex area of the scalp. Case report. Scand J Plast Reconstr Surg 1998;32:339–41.

33. Yap LH, Langstein HN. Reconstruction of the scalp, calvarium, and forehead. In: Aston SJ, Beasley RW, Thorne CHM, et al, editors. Grabb and Smith's plastic surgery. 6th edition. Philadelphia: Lippincott Williams and Wilkins; 2007. p. 358–66.

34. Rocha LS, de Oliveira LC, Filho JV, et al. Frontal reconstruction with frontal musculocutaneous V-Y island flap. Plast Reconstr Surg 2007;120:631–7.

35. Millard DR. The crane principle for transport of subcutaneous tissue. Plast Reconstr Surg 1969;43:451–62.

36. Hamilton R, Royster HP. Reconstruction of extensive forehead defects. Plast Reconstr Surg 1971;47(5):421–4.

37. Borah GL, Chick LR. Island scalp flap for superior forehead reconstruction. Plast Reconstr Surg 1990;85(4):606–10.

38. Lynch JR, Hansen JE, Chaffoo R, et al. The lower trapezius musculocutaneous flap revisited: versatile coverage for complicated wounds to the posterior cervical and occipital regions based on the deep branch of the transverse cervical artery. Plast Reconstr Surg 2002;109(2):444–50.

39. Har-El G, Bhaya M, Sundaram K. Latissimus dorsi myocutaneous flap for secondary head and neck reconstruction. Am J Otol 1999;20(5):287–93.

40. Hussussian CJ, Reece GP. Microsurgical scalp reconstruction in the patient with cancer. Plast Reconstr Surg 2002;109(6):1828–34.

41. Mathes SJ, Alpert BS, Chang N. Use of the muscle flap in chronic osteomyelitis: experimental and clinical correlation. Plast Reconstr Surg 1982;69:815–28.

42. Eshima I, Mathes SJ, Paty P. Comparison of the intracellular bacterial killing activity of leukocytes in musculocutaneous and random-pattern flaps. Plast Reconstr Surg 1990;86:541.

43. Schlenker JD, Indresano AT, Raine T, et al. A new flap in the dog containing a vascularized rib

graft–the latissimus dorsi myoosteocutaneous flap. J Surg Res 1980;29(2):172–83.

44. Schmidt DR, Robson MC. One-stage composite reconstruction using the latissimus myoosteocutaneous free flap. Am J Surg 1982;144(4):470–2.

45. Robson MC, Zachary LS, Schmidt DR, et al. Reconstruction of large cranial defects in the presence of heavy radiation damage and infection utilizing tissue transferred by microvascular anastomoses. Plast Reconstr Surg 1989;83(3):438–42.

46. Seitz IA, Adler N, Odessey E, et al. Latissimus dorsi chimeric free flap reconstruction in complicated scalp and calvarial defects. Plast Reconstr Surg 2008;vol. 122(Suppl 4):116–7.

47. Aviv JE, Urken ML, Vickery C, et al. The combined latissimus dorsi-scapular free flap in head and neck reconstruction. Arch Otolaryngol Head Neck Surg 1991;117(11):1242–50.

48. Mehrara BJ, Disa JJ, Pusic A. Scalp reconstruction. J Surg Oncol 2006;94(6):504–8.

49. McLean DH, Buncke HJ. Autotransplant of omentum to a large scalp defect with microsurgical revascularization. Plast Reconstr Surg 1972;49:268–74.

50. Alday ES, Goldsmith HS. Surgical technique for omental lengthening based on arterial anatomy. Surg Gynecol Obstet 1972;135(1).103–7.

51. Hultman CS, Carlson GW, Losken A, et al. Utility of the omentum in the reconstruction of complex extraperitoneal wounds and defects donor-site complications in 135 patients from 1975 to 2000. Ann surg 2002;235(6):782–95.

52. Adler N, Cohn AB, Villa MT, et al. Subtotal thigh perforator free flap for coverage of large soft tissue defects. [abstract]. Proceedings of The American Society of Reconstructive Microsurgery, Maui, Hawaii 2009.

53. Cohn AB, Wu LG, Lohman R, et al. Near-circumferential musculocutaneous/perforator thigh flap on a single arterial pedicle: a novel option for large soft-tissue defects [abstract]. Proceedings of The American Society of Reconstructive Microsurgery, Tucson, AZ, 2006.

54. Villa MT, Cohn AB, Gottlieb LJ. The versatility of free-style thigh perforator flaps for reconstruction of the head neck and upper extremity. Plast Reconstr Surg 2006;118(Suppl 4):167.

55. Nahabedian MY, Chevray P, Olivi A, et al. Clinically manifested frontal lobe compression after anterior craniectomy and deep inferior epigastric perforator flap reconstruction. Plast Reconstr Surg 2003; 112(4):1040–5.

56. Richaud J, Boetto S, Guell A, et al. Effects of cranioplasty on neurological function and cerebral blood flow. Neurochirurgie 1985;31:183–8.

57. Grant FC, Norcross NC. Repair of cranial defect by cranioplasty. Ann Surg 1939;110:488–512.

58. Agarwal JP, Agarwal BS, Adler N, et al. Intrinsic chimera flaps: a review. Ann Plast Surg, in press.

59. Ito M, Yang Z, Andl T, et al. Wnt-dependent de novo hair follicle regeneration in adult mouse skin after wounding. Nature 2007;447:316–20.

60. Devauchelle B, Badet L, Lengelé B, et al. First human face allograft: early report. Lancet 2006; 368(9531):203–9.

61. Guo S, Han Y, Zhang X, et al. Human facial allotransplantation: a 2-year follow-up study. Lancet 2008; 372(9639):631–8.

62. Lantieri L, Meningaud JP, Grimbert P, et al. Repair of the lower and middle parts of the face by composite tissue allotransplantation in a patient with massive plexiform neurofibroma: a 1-year follow-up study. Lancet 2008;372(9639):639–45.

63. First near total face transplantation in the US. New York Times. December 16, 2008.

64. Cleveland clinic surgeons perform nations first near-total face transplant. Surgery largest, most complex of its kind; 80 percent of trauma patient's face transplanted; Press conference. Cleveland Clinic, Cleveland, OH; December 17, 2008.

Aesthetic Eyelid Reconstruction

John D. Stein, MD, FRCSC[a], Oleh M. Antonyshyn, MD, FRCSC[b],*

KEYWORDS

- Eyelid morphology • Eyelid reconstruction
- Upper eyelid • Lower eyelid • Lateral canthus
- Medial canthus

The eyelids are critical in the protection of the conjunctiva and sclera of the globe and in the preservation of vision. Aesthetically, the position and shape of the eyelids defines a distinctive frame for the eyes. Although periorbital morphology varies by age, gender, and ethnicity, minor asymmetries or disproportions in any given individual are immediately obvious. Reconstruction of the eyelids must address both functional and aesthetic requirements.

PERIORBITAL MORPHOLOGY

The aesthetics of the periorbital region are dictated primarily by the shape, position, and inclination of the palpebral fissure. Although the size and inclination of the eyelid aperture change with age in any given individual, a remarkable degree of symmetry is maintained. Previous anthropometric studies have demonstrated that paired eyelid dimensions differ by less than 1 mm, and inclinations by less than 1 degree.[1] Minor degrees of asymmetry are immediately obvious and readily perceived. Aesthetic reconstruction of the eyelids generally relies on analysis of morphology in the contralateral unaltered periorbital region, and aims to achieve a symmetric reconstruction.

The palpebral fissure is generally inclined upward at an angle of three to four degrees towards the lateral canthus, relative to a horizontal plane between the medial canthi (**Fig. 1**).[2] The eyelid aperture measures 33 mm in width and 10 mm in height in an average man[1] and is slightly smaller in women.

The ciliary margin of each eyelid traces a three-dimensional curve. The lower lid follows a gentle curve that just touches or covers the lower limbus. Generally, there is no scleral show below the limbus, but this is variable. Scleral show is more prevalent with age, and in individuals with negative axis (downward sloping) palpebral inclination. The upper lid similarly traverses a curve that covers the superior limbus and apexes at a point between the medial and superior limbus before it descends toward the lateral canthus. Normal mean upper eyelid position is 3.5 ± 1 mm above the center of the cornea, covering the top 2 mm of the superior limbus (see **Fig. 1**).[3] The normal position of the upper lid is important to reference in assessing lagophthalmos or ptosis.

The lateral canthal region is renowned for its crisp v-shape and notorious for rounding if the tendon's attachments are disturbed or the junction of the upper and lower lids scarred. The medial canthal has a slightly rounder transition between the upper and lower lids and possesses a complex relationship with the canalicular system and the concavity of the nasal-orbital-ethmoid region, easily becoming blunted or webbed with scarring.

The morphology of the lids is further defined by the lid folds (see **Fig. 1**). The supratarsal fold corresponds to the skin insertion of the levator superioris, and is located 8 to 11 mm above the ciliary margin in the mid pupillary line. The infratarsal fold corresponds to the skin insertion of the capsulopalpebral fascia, and is generally 5 mm below the ciliary margin in the midpupillary line.

[a] Craniofacial Surgery, University of Toronto, M1 520, Sunnybrook Health Sciences Centre, 2075 Bayview Avenue, Toronto, Ontario, Canada M9A 3GB
[b] Adult Craniofacial Program, University of Toronto, M1 520, Sunnybrook Health Sciences Centre, 2075 Bayview Avenue, Toronto, Ontario, Canada M9A 3GB
* Corresponding author.
E-mail address: oleh.antonyshyn@sunnybrook.ca (O.M. Antonyshyn).

Clin Plastic Surg 36 (2009) 379–397
doi:10.1016/j.cps.2009.02.011
0094-1298/09/$ – see front matter © 2009 Elsevier Inc. All rights reserved.

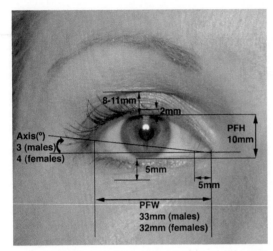

Fig. 1. Anthropometric norms of the eyelid. PFH, palpebral fissure height; PFW, palpebral fissure width.

FUNCTIONAL ANATOMY

Eyelid reconstruction aims to restore the structural integrity and function of the eyelids. Specific anatomic features are of particular importance to reconstructive surgeons, because they dictate optimal reconstructive requirements.

Eyelids

The eyelid is a bilamellar structure. The anterior lamella consists of the skin and orbicularis oculi muscle. The skin is extremely thin and adherent over the tarsus to the level of the supratarsal fold in the upper lid and infratarsal fold in the lower. More peripherally, over the preseptal and preorbital portions of the orbicularis muscle, the skin becomes thicker and more mobile. The posterior lamella is made up of the conjunctiva and tarsal plate (Fig. 2). The tarsal plates are composed of a dense connective tissue spanning the width of the lid for a distance of 25 mm. The tarsal plates are very thin and pliable, measuring only 1 mm in thickness. Although supportive, they conform easily to the contour of the globe.

Medial Canthus

The medial canthal region is a mere 5 mm wide in most cases but represents a unique and complex area of anatomy (Fig. 3). Considering the skin alone, it is the thinnest of the body with little to no subcutaneous tissue visible, even when viewed histologically. Immediately deep to the skin lies the medial canthal tendon, a tripartite structure derived from dense connective tissue attachments of the tarsus and the pretarsal and preseptal orbicularis oculi. Embedded within this structure are the upper, lower, and common canalicular ducts en route to the lacrimal sac. The sac lies in the lacrimal fossa of the lacrimal bone and is bounded by periosteum medially and a leaf of fascia that spans the fossa arising from the posterior and anterior lacrimal crests. Both the pretarsal and the preseptal orbicularis have a superficial and deep head. The horizontal tendon arises from the superficial heads of the pretarsal and preseptal orbicularis muscles and inserts broadly onto the anterior lacrimal crest creating the first of the three parts. The second part is a superior branch of the horizontal tendon that inserts onto the frontal bone just cephalad to the anterior crest. The deep heads of the pretarsal (Horner's muscle) and preseptal orbicularis comprise the third (and weakest[4]) part, which runs from the medial tarsus posteriorly. Although authors agree that Horner's muscle connects the tarsus to the posterior

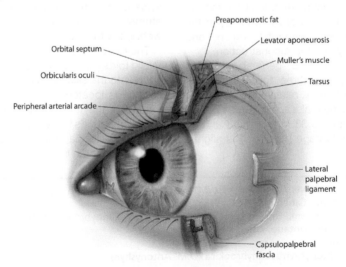

Fig. 2. Cross-sectional anatomy of the upper and lower eyelid in perspective.

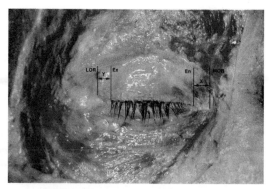

Fig. 3. Right orbit dissection, revealing pretarsal, preseptal, and preorbital portions of the orbicularis muscle. Note that the medial canthus (En) is separated from its bony insertion into the medial orbit (MOR) by the medial canthal tendon length X (approximately 5 mm). Similarly, the lateral canthus surface landmark (Ex) is separated from its insertion into bone (LOR) by the tendon Y (mean length = 7.52 mm[10]). Note that this lateral canthal tendon length varies with age, trauma, and scar contracture. It can attenuate and lengthen, predisposing to ectropion and lateral canthal dystopia.

lacrimal crest, there is renewed debate in the literature about the exact arrangement of the deep head of the preseptal orbicularis' attachments around the lacrimal sac and whether or not they insert directly onto the sac or just above its fornix.[5–7] In any event, the tripartite arrangement of the medial canthal tendon creates a net force vector that with every blink brings the eyelid medially and posteriorly into tight approximation with the globe and provides a "pump" action for the lacrimal apparatus.

Lateral Canthus

The lateral canthal tendon is a band of dense connective tissue rigidly anchoring the lateral edge of the tarsus to the lateral orbit (see **Fig. 3**). At the tarsus, the lateral canthal tendon is intimately associated with the septum orbitale, which lies immediately superficial to it. It is also associated here with the pretarsal orbicularis oculi fascia because histologic examinations of the tendon have revealed interwoven muscle fibers.[8] As it progresses laterally, the tendon diverges to become the deep and superficial canthal tendons.[9] The deep tendon has an average height of 10.2 mm at its insertion onto the orbit[8] and an average length of 7.52 mm but ranges from 2 to 12 mm in cadaveric dissections.[10] The deep tendon inserts onto the orbit at Whitnall's tubercle, which lies 1.5 to 4 mm posterior to the orbital rim and, on average, is 10.24 mm below the frontozygomatic suture.[10] Clinically, the position can be determined to be 3 to 4 mm below the center of the pupil. The superficial lateral canthal tendon continues on toward the anterior edge of the lateral orbital rim. Here, it is part of a greater superficial fascia that is continuous with the superficial temporal fascia, pretarsal, and preseptal orbicularis oculi fascia.[11] Between these two leafs of the canthal tendon lies Eisler's fat pad.

Vasculature

The upper and lower lids are each supplied by a network of anastomosing vessels. In the upper lid, four arterial arcades have been described: (1) the marginal, (2) the peripheral, (3) the superficial orbital, and (4) the deep orbital.[12,13] The marginal and peripheral arcades are derived from the medial and lateral palpebral arteries, branches of the ophthalmic and lacrimal arteries, respectively. The medial palpebral artery divides into superior and inferior branches before entering the eyelid along a line directly below the trochlea[13] and superior to the medial canthus. Once in the eyelid, the superior branch of the medial palpebral artery branches to form the marginal and peripheral arcades. The marginal arcade runs parallel and anterior to the lower border of the tarsus (deep to the orbicularis) and the peripheral arcade runs within Muller's muscle at the superior tarsal border. The superficial and deep orbital arcades course parallel to the orbital rim on their respective surfaces of the orbicularis oculi. Dedicated arteries running within the orbicularis oculi have not been observed, leading Kawai and colleagues[12] to suggest that cutaneous flaps of the upper lid skin could be raised without including muscle. The superficial and deep orbital arcades are essentially anastomotic connections between three lateral arteries: (1) the frontal branch of the superficial temporal artery; (2) the zygomatico-orbital artery; and (3) the transverse facial artery and branches of the supratrochlear, medial palpebral,[12,13] and occasionally the ophthalmic arteries. Contributions by the superior orbital artery to this system of arcades have not been observed.[12]

The lower lid similarly receives its blood supply from an inferior palpebral arcade derived from the lateral and medial palpebral arteries, which runs parallel and anterior to the lower border of the tarsus. Anastomosing vessels from the transverse facial, angular, and infraorbital arteries similarly contribute to lower lid perfusion.

Venous drainage for the lids is less well defined in the literature. In general, venules coalesce in the fornices draining into the supraorbital and supratrochlear veins superiorly and the facial and infraorbital veins inferiorly.

Lymphatic Drainage

The lymphatic drainage of the upper and lower lids has been historically described as involving two major basins for the anterior lamella. The upper lid, lateral canthus, and lateral region of the lower lid typically drain into the preparotid lymph nodes. The supratrochlear region, medial canthus, and medial two thirds of the lower lid drain into the submandibular glands. The continued publication of sentinel lymph node studies for the treatment of periorbital tumors will further refine the understanding of this topic.[14–16]

Orbicularis Muscle Innervation

The orbicularis oculi muscle is innervated on its deep surface by branches of the facial nerve. A more detailed understanding of the innervation to the upper and lower orbicularis oculi has been achieved with several recent anatomic investigations.[17–20] In most cases the upper orbicularis is innervated by three to six temporal and zygomatic branches[19] of the facial nerve that enter the muscle at close to 90 degrees, lateral and superior to the lateral canthus but inferior to the superior orbital rim.[17,19] The pattern of innervation to the lower orbicularis consists of several contributions of the zygomatic and buccal branches that enter the muscle in its lateral and medial substance.[18,20] Laterally, the branches enter the muscle near the origin of the zygomaticus major[18,19] and medially the branches enter medial to the lateral limbus.[18,20]

Lid Support and Dynamics

The upper eyelid provides 90% of the dynamic protection of the globe with a normal excursion of approximately 12 mm from complete downgaze to complete upgaze. Facilitating this is the levator palpebrae superioris muscle originating from the lesser wing of the sphenoid and extending anteriorly approximately 40 mm to Whitnall's ligament. Here the levator tendon spreads to become the aponeurosis and its direction of pull changes from horizontal to vertical. The levator aponeurosis inserts onto the tarsus along its superior border and blends into the canthal ligaments laterally. Following its merger with the orbital septum, the aponeurosis sends fibrous projections into the overlying skin. The position of the merger of the septum and the levator determines the position of the supratarsal fold. In the occidental eyelid, the merger lies at or near to the superior border of the tarsus approximately 8 to 10 mm from the lid margin centrally. In the Asian eyelid, the merger occurs below the superior border of the tarsus,[21,22] approximately 1 to 3 mm above the lid margin. A soft, mobile eyelid is essential for both closing and opening the palpebral fissure. As a basic principle of reconstruction, all efforts are focused on maintaining both the dimensions and the mobility of the upper lid.

The lower eyelid is far less mobile. A static, stable reconstruction of sufficient height is generally adequate in ensuring good apposition of the upper to the lower lid during closure. The primary objective of lower lid reconstruction is to restore the integrity of the tarsoligamentous sling (**Fig. 4**).

EYELID RECONSTRUCTION
Etiology of Eyelid Defects

Defects of the eyelid can be broadly classified by etiology into congenital and acquired defects. Congenital defects, such as coloboma, may be idiosyncratic or can arise as part of a syndrome, such as Treacher Collins syndrome. Acquired defects arise either traumatically or following surgical resection. Traditionally, defects have been further subcategorized based on the thickness of the loss (partial or full) and the percentage missing from the lid.

Defects of the Anterior Lamella

Defects of the anterior lamella involve the skin and potentially the underlying orbicularis oculi muscle. The reconstructive principles are as follows: (1) resurface the cutaneous defect using thin pliable skin with optimal color and texture match, (2) place incisions in natural lid crease lines, and (3) minimize any vertically oriented tension on the lid margin.

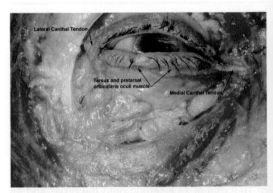

Fig. 4. Right orbit dissection. Septum orbitale and preseptal orbicularis muscle resected. Note the medial canthal tendon presenting as a clearly defined white structure immediately beneath the skin. Note the role of the tarsal-ligamentous sling (tarsus, pretarsal orbicularis muscle, medial and lateral canthal tendons) in supporting lower eyelid position.

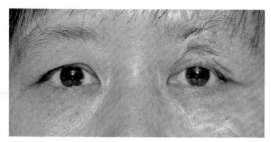

Fig. 5. Hyperpigmented contracted skin graft left upper eyelid retracts the ciliary margin and distorts the normal fullness of the supratarsal region.

Full-thickness skin grafts, harvested from contralateral upper eyelid, postauricular, or neck donor sites, can be used for this purpose. They are certainly the first choice in the primary treatment of traumatic defects. Skin grafts, however, can become depressed and pigmented. Graft scar contracture can obliterate normal eyelid contours and can potentially cause ectropion or lagophthalmos (**Fig. 5**).

Local skin flaps and myocutaneous flaps incorporating the orbicularis oculi muscle provide a far superior aesthetic result in most cases (**Fig. 6**).

Colour and texture match are more predictable. Scars can be placed within normal periorbital creases, minimizing visible scarring.

Defects of the Posterior Lamella

Defects of the posterior lamella may involve the conjunctiva, the tarsus, or both. Defects limited to the conjunctiva alone are very rare. When they represent a small (<25%) surface area of the lid, epithelialization from surrounding conjunctiva is expected. Larger defects do require resurfacing with a nonkeratinizing graft material. Large conjunctival defects are encountered most commonly during fornix reconstruction in enucleated orbits. Effective restoration of conjunctival integrity relies on precise resurfacing of the defect with a thick mucosal graft and appropriate mechanical stenting of the graft. Palatal mucosa provides the most appropriate donor site, yielding a relatively large amount of thick mucosal graft with minimal tendency to contract (**Fig. 7**).

Defects of the posterior lamella more commonly involve the tarsus. Loss of support to the eyelid, ectropion, and loss of infratarsal volume are commonly associated. These are generally

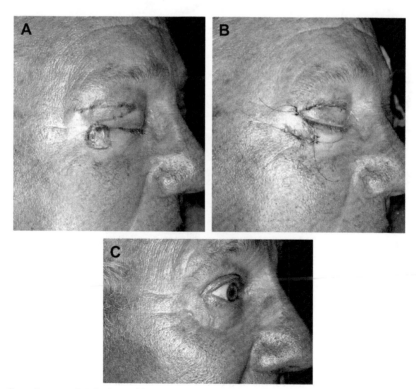

Fig. 6. Basal cell carcinoma of right lateral lower eyelid. (*A*) Planned reconstruction involves a laterally based myocutaneous flap (hemi-Triper) comprising supratarsal skin and orbicularis muscle. (*B*) Transposition of the flap leaves a donor scar in the supratarsal fold, and slings the lower lid superolaterally to provide mechanical support to the lower eyelid. (*C*) Final result at 3 months.

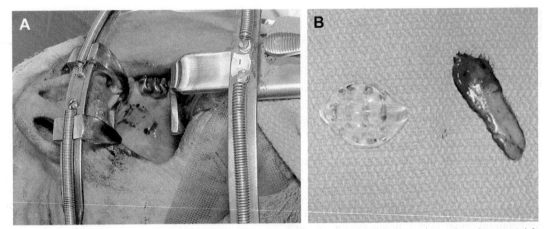

Fig. 7. Mucosa harvested from the paramedian aspect of the hard palate (*A*) provides optimal graft material for reconstruction of isolated conjunctival defects. The donor site is allowed to heal secondarily. Particular care is required to ensure the mucosa is harvested over the hard palate only, and that the bone is not denuded of periosteum. (*B*) When mucosal grafts are used in the relining of curved surfaces, such as the fornices, some form of mechanical stenting is required.

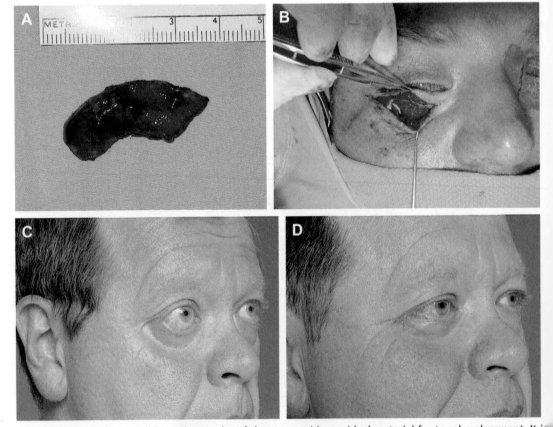

Fig. 8. (*A*) Cartilage harvested from the concha of the ear provides an ideal material for tarsal replacement. It is slightly thicker than tarsus, but has similar mechanical properties. (*B*) When used as a support for the lower eyelid, it must span the full height of the lower eyelid, and be fixed with sutures to the lower margin of the tarsus superiorly, and the infraorbital rim inferiorly. In circumstances where the internal lamella is deficient, but skin and lining are adequate (*C*), the conchal graft provides satisfactory support and volume augmentation (*D*).

complex postablative or posttraumatic eyelid deformities where the tarsus is deficient and restoration of the integrity of the tarsoligamentous sling necessitates stable support. Fascial and tendon slings are frequently used for this purpose. Where there is an associated retraction or volume deficiency in the infratarsal area, the authors prefer to use conchal cartilage graft (**Fig. 8**).

Deficiencies in Periorbital Volume

Periorbital volume deficiencies are frequently overlooked. These represent contour defects in the upper or lower eyelids, which can occur following traumatic fat atrophy, enucleation, or scar adhesion. Both the anterior and posterior lamellae are generally intact, and the contour depression occurs as a consequence of fat atrophy and adhesion of the anterior lamella to deeper structures.

Smaller defects are amenable to grafting. Both fat autograft injection and dermis fat grafting have been very effectively used for this purpose. More substantial volume deficiencies, however, particularly in a scarred recipient site, benefit from vascularized soft tissue augmentation. The authors prefer to use temporoparietal fascia for this purpose because it provides soft, pliable, well-perfused permanent volume replacement (**Fig. 9**).[23]

Full-Thickness Defects of the Lower Eyelid

Full-thickness defects of the lower lid and its margin may be repaired primarily when they represent less than 25% to 33% of the lid width (**Fig. 10**). Closure is performed in layers (conjunctiva with tarsus, orbicularis, and skin) to avoid a fistula. Small (7-0) absorbable sutures are used for the conjunctiva and the tails for the skin sutures are left long and become incorporated under the next knot away from the margin.

Faced with a subtotal defect that is not easily repaired primarily, many authors have suggested a lateral cantholysis to gain the necessary extra length. The canthal regions are aesthetically sensitive areas, however, possessing attributes that are very difficult reliably to reproduce. In addition, they are vital to proper lid closure. Faced with the option of performing a lateral cantholysis to assist with lid closure, the authors instead prefer flap reconstruction. Although this method is more involved, the benefit of maintaining the natural canthal appearance outweighs the additional effort.

In considering full-thickness lid reconstruction, options to reconstruct the posterior lamella can be categorized into either grafts or flaps. Among the more frequent graft choices are hard palate mucosa, a composite tissue graft of septal cartilage and mucoperichondrium, and tarsoconjunctival grafts. Hard palate mucosa is relatively abundant; however, it lacks the necessary strength to restore

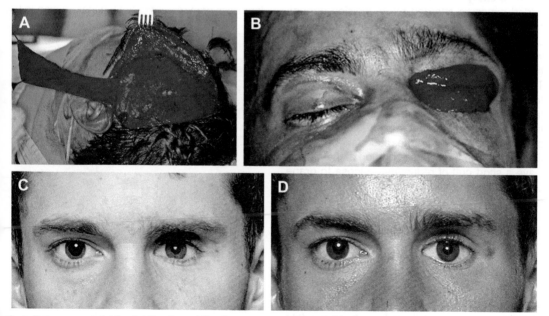

Fig. 9. Temporoparietal fascial flap for orbit volume augmentation following enucleation. (*A*) Elevation of flap by hemicoronal incision for exposure. (*B*) Preliminary inset of flap delivered by subcutaneous tunnel. Sizing and shaping of the flap can be easily accomplished and compared with contralateral volume. (*C*) Preoperative appearance ocular prosthesis in situ. (*D*) Postoperative result at 4 months shows improvement in supratarsal hollow.

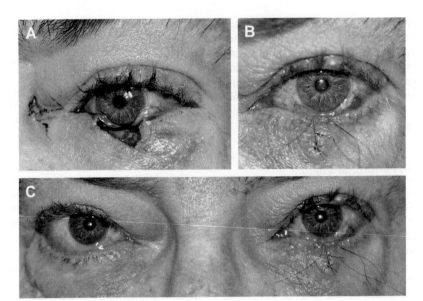

Fig. 10. (*A*) A full-thickness defect is converted to a pentagon-type shape. Note that the taper occurs inferior to the tarsus. (*B*) The skin suture tails are left long enough to permit their inclusion in the next knot away from the margin (not yet incorporated). (*C*) Although the postoperative result suggests increased scleral show at the lower limbus, a comparison is made with the right side demonstrating equivalence.

the tarsoligamentous sling. It is best reserved for central, intermediate length defects. It also generally requires that the donor defect be left to heal secondarily leading to a prolonged period of intraoral discomfort for patients postoperatively.

Composite chondromucosal septal grafts can be more easily harvested from the nose with the added exposure afforded by an incision through the nasal-alar groove. Reflecting the ala, a composite graft of suitable width and height with its attached mucosa can be harvested and the donor defect left to heal secondarily (**Fig. 11**). The graft is then fixed to the remaining medial canthal ligament and to the free border of the lateral tarsus (**Fig. 12**). If there is no suitable point of fixation one has to be reconstructed (see later). The conjunctiva is sutured to the mucoperichondrium. Care is taken in the cephalic portion of the graft to leave a short cuff of redundant mucosa to drape over the free margin of the graft once the anterior lamella is reconstructed. The graft spans the entire vertical height of the reconstructed lid and rests on the infraorbital rim. This ensures the lid margin is maintained at an appropriate level.

These grafts are advantageous because the septal cartilage is strong enough to maintain its shape and contour and resist contractile forces generated at the lid. In addition, there is a relative abundance of tissue available for even a complete lid reconstruction. Disadvantages include the additional incision in the nasal alar groove for access and the risk of creating a septal

perforation. Furthermore, the stiffness of the cartilage may be excessive in some cases preventing the lid from adequately conforming to the globe. Under these circumstances, it may be advantageous to shave the cartilage to a thickness that approaches a normal tarsal plate (ie, 1 mm).

Vascularized flap reconstruction of the posterior lamella is primarily indicated when perfusion to the

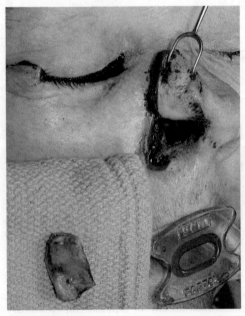

Fig. 11. Septal composite chondromucosal graft. Alar releasing incision for ease of exposure.

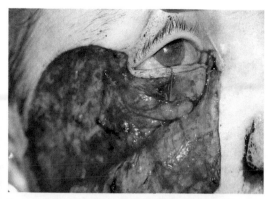

Fig. 12. Reconstruction of the posterior lamella. The lateral canthal tendon and remaining lateral aspect of the tarsoligamentous sling are not disturbed. The chondromucosal graft is sewn under tension to restore the integrity of the sling right out to the medial canthal tendon. Particular care is taken in ensuring the limbus is covered by the graft, leaving no scleral show.

periorbital region is compromised by previous scar, infection, or radiation. When local cheek skin does not provide reliable cover, vascularized lining and support is provided by the modified Hughes tarsoconjunctival flap. The flap, pedicled at the superior fornix, provides a well-perfused internal lamella that can support a full-thickness skin graft for anterior lamellar reconstruction. Limitations to the modified Hughes flap include a temporary obstruction of vision, requirement for a pseudosecond stage, and insufficient support for taller defects. The available tarsus is insufficient adequately to support the lower lid in the vertical dimension because it does not reach the inferior orbital rim as easily as a larger cartilage graft. Although a Hughes tarsoconjunctival flap can be the primary means of lower lid reconstruction, the authors prefer to leave the upper lid untouched except in the specific circumstances listed previously, where revascularization of a posterior lamellar graft may be compromised.

Reconstruction of the anterior lamella of the lower lid must accomplish several goals. Apart from providing a reliable skin layer, the reconstructed lower eyelid should appear to blend seamlessly with the cheek in both contour and color. Furthermore, the anterior lamella reconstruction should ideally be designed to counteract significant contractile forces that overcome either the native or reconstructed posterior lamella and create an ectropion. A standard principle for achieving this has been to avoid using split-thickness skin grafts or inferiorly based flaps, choosing instead flaps that are based either horizontally, or better still oblique-superiorly. The final

appearance of the reconstructed lower lid margin is determined by the width of the lid, provision of adequate lid support, and the relative position of the medial and lateral canthi. Unlike the upper lid, it is this collection of variables and not the shape of the globe that significantly affects the contour of the lower eyelid.[24]

For most full-thickness lower lid defects, the authors prefer to reconstruct the anterior lamella with the Mustardé cheek rotation flap (**Fig. 13**). The flap provides sufficient tissue to reconstruct the entire anterior lamella while satisfying the major criteria: oblique-superior flap orientation, resistance to contracture, color and texture approximation, and seamless transition into the malar region. The flap can be designed to avoid distortion in the lateral canthal region, using a subciliary incision that courses around the lateral canthus (see **Fig. 12**). From here, the incision arcs superiorly into the temporal skin (see **Figs. 12 and 13**), then inferiorly toward the root of the helix and continues in the preauricular skin to the lobule. Here a decision can be made to perform either a bilobed cheek flap or extend the flap down toward the neck posterior to the angle of the jaw. The bilobed cheek flap is indicated for cases where insufficient skin is available in the cheek to close both the lid and donor defects. In general, this arises when one third to one half of the skin between the lateral canthus and the ear has been resected (**Fig. 14**). The incision for the bilobed flap continues around the lobule, courses superiorly in the postauricular sulcus, and apexes near the hairline. It then turns to run inferiorly off of the posterior hairline and into the neck skin.

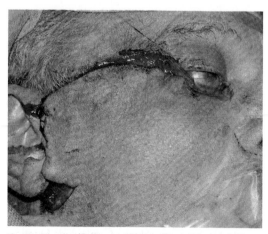

Fig.13. Mustardé cheek rotation flap with a "back-cut" below the earlobe to enhance ease of rotation. Note the arc of the flap extending superior to the lateral canthus.

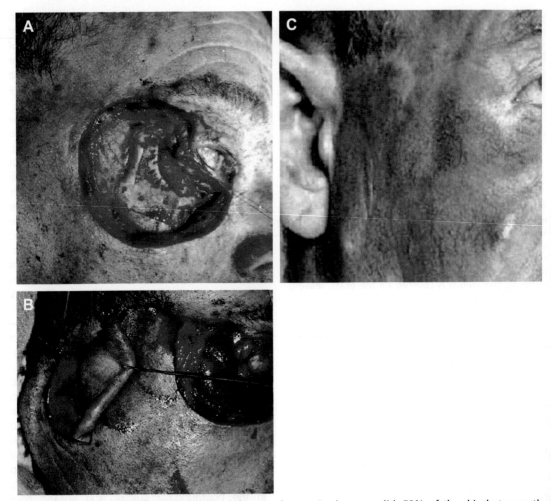

Fig. 14. Bilobed cheek flap. (*A*) Postablative defect involves entire lower eyelid, 50% of the skin between the lateral canthus and ear. (*B*) Bilobed cheek flap elevated to provide anterior lamella and cheek coverage. Retroauricular defect is closed primarily. (*C*) Final result at 4 months.

At this point, the dissection for the bilobed and an extended cheek flaps are equivalent. In the neck, the incision is propagated inferiorly as necessary to achieve adequate coverage. Additional ease of rotation can be realized with a back-cut at the terminus of the incision (see **Fig. 13**). The flap is elevated superficial to the SMAS and care is taken to ensure the malar fat pad is not distorted by avoiding its inclusion on the undersurface of the flap. A vacuum drain is placed under the flap. The greatest risk following Mustardé lower lid reconstruction is downward sagging resulting in retraction and ectropion. Contributing factors include loss of integrity of the tarsoligamentous sling, atonicity of the reconstructed lid because of loss of orbicularis function, postoperative swelling, and gravitational pull. As noted by Callahan and Callahan,[25] the surgeon must actively counteract postoperative sagging

using the following steps: (1) reconstruct the posterior lamella under sufficient tension, fixing the posterior lamellar graft to medial and lateral canthi or lid remnants; (2) design the cheek rotation flap such that it arcs superiorly, above the lateral canthus; and (3) anchor the deep surface of the cheek flap to the lateral orbital rim periosteum and the deep temporal fascia laterally. Finally, the medial standing cone is excised within the tear trough and all incisions repaired (**Fig. 15**).

The clinical course of a lower eyelid defect, which also partially involves the skin of the medial canthal region, tear trough, and nasal side wall, appears in **Fig. 16**. Reconstruction of this defect required two cutaneous flaps to avoid blunting the nasal-cheek junction. The anterior lamella and medial canthus were resurfaced with a Mustardé cheek rotation flap. A glabellar flap resurfaced the nasal side wall.

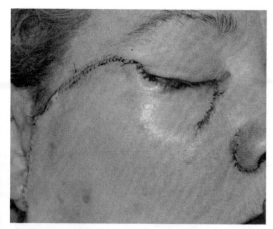

Fig. 15. Mustardé cheek rotation flap. Medial standing cone excised in tear trough.

The Mustardé cheek flap is versatile. It is well vascularized and in the older patient, with skin laxity in the cheek and upper neck, the flap can be rotated to the medial canthus with relative ease especially if a back-cut at the inferior terminus of the incision is made. In a young person, or in subacute cases where there are larger defects, an expanded cheek flap is another option considering the aesthetic results that can

be accomplished (**Fig. 17**). Again, the plane of dissection for insertion of the tissue expander is immediately superficial to the SMAS.

Full-Thickness Defects of the Upper Eyelid

Reconstruction of the upper lid shares similar principles with the lower lid: providing a conjunctival or mucous membrane for lining, a tarsal equivalent, and an anterior lamella. Avoidance of contracture leading to lagophthalmos with subsequent corneal exposure is the primary goal. Athough the shape of the reconstructed lid is more dependent on the protrusion of the globe than the shape of the underlying cartilage (unlike the lower lid),[24] the ability of the reconstruction to resist contraction can be limited without a tarsal equivalent imbedded. For this reason, the authors recommend including a cartilage framework in upper lid defects that involve significant resection of the tarsus. A further feature of the upper lid to be considered is providing both eyelid opening and closure. Wide, full-thickness lid defects not involving significant proportions of the levator aponeurosis generally remain animated. Tarsal reconstruction also permits any remaining levator aponeurosis to be secured to the construct. Modest lid opening is possible provided the

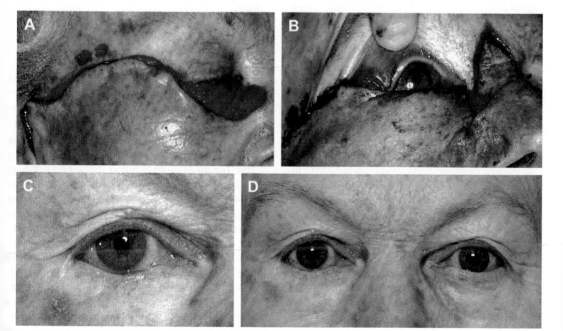

Fig. 16. Lower eyelid defect partially involving the medial canthal skin, tear trough, and nasal side wall. (*A*) The Mustardé flap has been incised; however, two excisional biopsies constrained the height of the flap's apex. (*B*) The lower lid and medial canthus are resurfaced with the Mustardé cheek flap; the tear trough is closed in a V-Y fashion and the remaining nasal side wall defect will be covered with a glabellar flap to avoid blunting this convex border region. (*C*) The result at 6 months shows the lid margin is stable, positioned only slightly below the lower limbus. (*D*) The result is acceptable both functionally and, compared with the left eyelid, aesthetically.

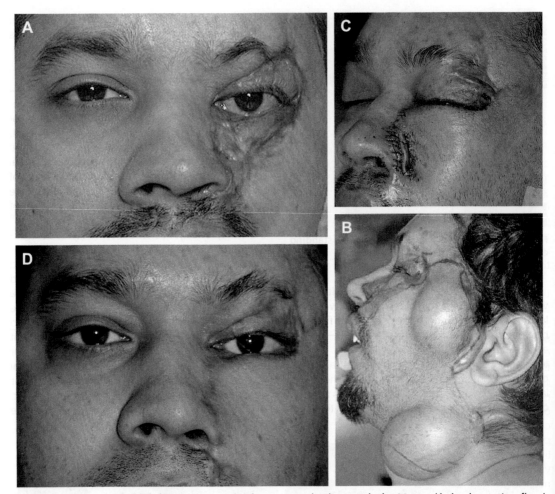

Fig. 17. (*A*) Posttraumatic lid deformity. For optimal texture and color match the Mustardé cheek rotation flap is chosen. (*B*) Inadequate tissue is present to reconstruct entire lid so an expanded cheek flap is chosen. The immediate postoperative result is shown in (*C*) and the final appearance at 15 months is shown (*D*).

anterior lamella remains supple enough to telescope within the upper sulcus. Lid closure can remain voluntary if sufficient innervated orbicularis oculi muscle remains, particularly medially.[26,27] In the absence of orbicularis oculi, however, lid closure can be achieved passively with gold weight implants, as in cases of facial nerve palsy, or reanimated with a temporalis muscle transposition. Free-functioning muscle transfer to achieve lid closure has also been reported.[28]

Reconstructing upper lid animation can be challenging if the defect involves significant portions of the levator aponeurosis. A fascial graft between the remaining levator palpebrae superioris muscle and the reconstructed tarsus may achieve some lid elevation. Care must be taken to ensure the balance of lid opening and closure does not compromise corneal protection.

Established local flap options for the reconstruction of full-thickness upper lid defects not

amenable to primary repair include the Tenzel-Stewart rotation-advancement, Mustardé lid switch, Tripier flaps, and the Cutler-Beard flap.

The Tenzel-Stewart rotation advancement flap is indicated for defects representing 40% to 60% of the width of the upper lid. This option does hold certain advantages in that it is a single-stage procedure and provides an uninterrupted lash line, albeit medially situated. The technique relies on a selective lateral canthotomy of the upper limb of the canthus to achieve the requisite mobility of the remaining lid and a semicircular suborbicularis oculi myocutaneous flap in temporal region. Similar to the lower lid the authors hold reservations against performing a canthotomy because reproducing the lateral canthal angle can be unpredictable even when the flap is sutured to the orbital rim periosteum. Over time, under the influence of the orbicularis, dermal-periosteal scar stretches and the canthus becomes rounded.

The Mustardé lid switch flap seems to be less often practiced, although there are some contemporary advocates for its use[29] in narrow full-thickness defects. The horizontal limb of the incision is placed below the tarsus of the lower lid to ensure the inferior palpebral artery is included. The repair to the upper lid remnant is made in layers with the tails of the caudal skin sutures included in the knots of the adjacent cephalic stitches. Benefits include the transfer of exact tissue matches in the reconstruction and the provision of a lash line for the upper lid. The donor site morbidity includes a loss of tarsal support and predisposition to either ectropion or entropion as the wound contracts when left to heal secondarily. During the 3-week attached pedicle phase there is a risk of corneal ulceration where the flap and the lashes cross the visual axis.

For tall and wide (up to complete width) full-thickness defects of the upper lid, the Cutler-Beard composite flap from the lower lid provides an exact tissue match for the conjunctiva and skin. The lack of tarsal support predisposing to entropion in wide defects can be overcome with the inclusion of an auricular cartilage graft imbedded in the flap.[30,31] The flap is pedicled on the inferior conjunctival fornix, preorbital orbicularis, and cheek skin. The superior margin of the flap is created with a full-thickness incision running parallel to the inferior tarsal border of the lower lid, preserving the inferior palpebral artery. Two vertical incisions are made corresponding to the medial and lateral borders of the upper lid defect. These incisions are carried inferiorly to the fornix, and the flap is then advanced under the remaining rim of the lower lid into the upper lid defect. If a cartilage graft is to be used to restore tarsal integrity, the flap can be filleted at its superior edge deep to the orbicularis. The graft is placed over the repaired conjunctiva and secured to the remaining medial and lateral tarsus. The free border of the levator aponeurosis can be secured either to the cartilage or, if a graft is not used, the free edge of orbicularis or the capsulopalpebral fascia. The remaining myocutaneous flap is inset and closed in layers.

Most authors leave the flap pedicled for longer than is required for revascularization alone, with the extra time intended to allow for some tissue expansion. The small increase in flap length gained assists in establishing a tension-free closure of the lower lid to avoid ectropion and ensures that the reconstructed upper lid margin lies flush with the remaining lid.

After at least 4 weeks, and up to 8,[31,32] the flap is divided at the upper margin of the lower lid. In this way, there is sufficient skin to establish the ideal margin for the upper lid. A small cuff of conjunctiva is retained on the upper lid by stepping the full-thickness incision. This cuff is then rolled anteriorly to the skin incision to help prevent keratinizing epithelium from contacting the globe. The remaining donor half of the flap is inset into the lower lid. Care is taken when freshening up the inferior margin of the lower lid not to injure the inferior palpebral artery, which lies just deep to the secondarily healed wound edge. Repair is performed in three layers.

The Cutler-Beard flap (**Fig. 18**) is a good option for reconstructing large upper lid defects because it provides a supple anterior lamella to permit lid opening and a true conjunctival surface. It is easily modified to provide tarsal support by imbedding any number of grafts options (contralateral tarsus, auricular or nasal cartilage, fascia, donor sclera). The major criticisms of this method are the lack of inherent support and the prolonged period of visual obstruction. A minor criticism over the lid switch flap is the inability to provide upper lid eyelashes. Another feature to consider is the fact that the transferred orbicularis muscle is inanimate. This may not be critical in most central and lateral defects, but it may become an issue when the reconstruction involves a significant amount of the medial upper lid, the region most responsible for blinking. Furthermore, anatomic studies cited previously suggest full-width defects repaired by this method may denervate the pretarsal orbicularis of the lower lid because of the breadth and depth of dissection such a reconstruction demands. In those cases, a lateral canthopexy of the lower lid may be indicated to avoid or treat an established ectropion. Nevertheless, the reconstruction does provide very good tissue texture and color match for most upper lid reconstructions enabling the surgeon to deliver a result capable of meeting most if not all functional and aesthetic goals.

More extensive defects of the upper lid can be reconstructed with regional flaps; however, the Fricke and forehead flaps are quite thick and require multiple flap thinning procedures to achieve a pliability that permits lid opening. Furthermore, these flaps lack a conjunctival lining, which necessitates a mucosal graft given that the defects' size precludes use of adjacent or contralateral conjunctiva. Flap pedicles can be divided at 3 weeks, at which point staged flap thinning procedures can be undertaken.

RECONSTRUCTION OF THE LATERAL CANTHUS

The functional goal of lateral canthal reconstruction is to provide a rigid point of attachment for

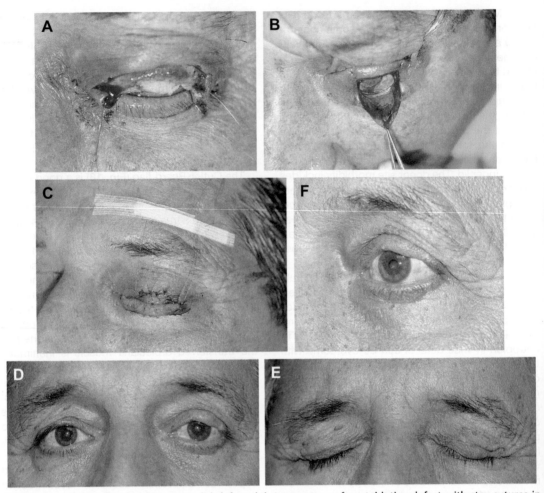

Fig. 18. Cutler-Beard flap for 40% upper lid defect. (*A*) Appearance of postablative defect with stay sutures in tarsus. (*B*) Full-thickness flap from the lower lid dissected to the inferior fornix with preservation of a 4-mm lower lid margin. (*C*) Flap inset into upper lid, passing under the lower lid margin; Frost stitch supporting lower lid to reduce flap tension. Postoperative photos at 6 months with eyes open (*D*), closed (*E*), and oblique view to demonstrate flap thickness (*F*).

both lids to maximize the efficiency of the orbicularis oculi to complete lid closure.[33] Aesthetically, the goals are to achieve an acute angle between the upper and lower lid, control the shape of the palpebral fissure, and position the lower lid at the lower limbus. In general, this is only possible provided the functional goal is met and the tarsal-tendon junction is secure. The reconstructed tendon is subject to constant tension from the action of the orbicularis oculi muscle. Over time, a failure to achieve rigid stabilization eventually results in rounding and medial displacement of the canthus.

To achieve a rigid point of attachment for the canthal tendon, the skeletal structure must first be reconstructed if it is deficient (ie, following ablation of any tumor also involving the lateral orbital rim). Options for this include bone graft (**Fig. 19**)

or bridging implants (eg, titanium mesh, high-density polyethylene). Consider using a temporalis muscle flap to cover any skeletal reconstruction for additional soft tissue coverage if radiation therapy is also planned.

Options for reconstructing the lateral canthal tendon can be categorized into either local flaps, fascial, or tendon grafts. The available local flaps include a tarsal strip if the defect is not very wide and there is sufficient pre-existing laxity in the lid. In this way, the tarsus can be advanced and secured to the desired position on the lateral orbital rim. This can be accomplished most reliably with two 1.1-mm drill holes in the lateral orbit corresponding in position to Whitnall's tubercle. McCord and colleagues[34] suggest the upper canthal sutures should traverse the lower hole with the lower canthal sutures passing through the upper drill hole. The

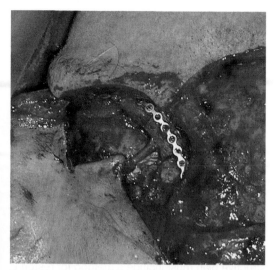

Fig. 19. Squamous cell carcinoma of combined upper and lower lids, temple, and lateral canthus. Lateral orbitotomy repaired; however, bone grafting would be identical. Superficial temporal fascia graft used to reconstruct the lateral canthal tendon.

sutures are then tied to one another over the lateral rim. Although this method is more elaborate, the alternative of simply suturing the tarsus to the periosteum of the lateral orbital wall in this setting carries a risk of long-term dehiscence.

If tarsal advancement is not suitable, a turn-over periosteal-temporal fascia flap is a reasonable option. The flap is elevated and pedicled on the inner surface of the lateral orbital wall. It is then split into upper and lower leaflets and secured to their respective tarsal plates (**Fig. 20**). Leone[35]

further suggested that the two leafs of the reconstructed canthal tendon be crossed over to assist in creating the acute angle between the upper and lower lids. If the periosteum of the lateral orbit is not available a graft of temporal fascia (see **Fig. 19**), tendon, or fascia from a remote site (eg, palmaris, plantaris, tensor fascia lata) can be secured to the lateral orbit and the tarsus. Finally, in cases where the lid defect necessitates a posterior lamellar reconstruction the tissue used to reconstruct the tarsus can be secured with stainless steel suture directly to the lateral orbit through drill holes in the orbital rim.

To reconstruct the acute angle between the upper and lower lids, the best results are most often realized by overlapping the upper lid's lateral raw deep surface over the lower lid's surface and allowing the wound to heal secondarily. Suturing the free edge of the upper lid to the corresponding wound on the lower lid often introduces an unnaturally blunted appearance to the canthus.

MEDIAL CANTHUS RECONSTRUCTION

Compared with the intricate anatomy and function of the medial canthus, the reconstructive goals for defects involving the medial canthal tendon are relatively modest: to fixate rigidly the medial tarsus at the superior junction of the anterior and posterior lacrimal crests,[4] ensure lid apposition to the globe with proper anteroposterior placement of the bony insertion, and avoid a telecanthic appearance. Damage to the lacrimal apparatus and its subsequent reconstruction is not covered in this article except to mention dacryocystorhinostomy

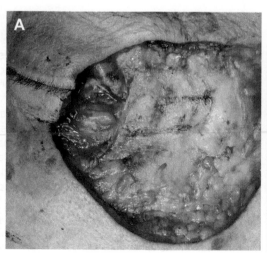
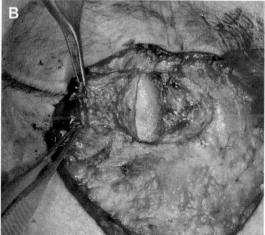

Fig. 20. Periosteal-fascial flap for lateral canthal tendon reconstruction. (*A*) Design of flap pedicled at lateral orbital rim. (*B*) Flap elevated turned toward tarsus and attachment to lateral orbital rim preserved. Note: division of the flap into superior and inferior halves not yet completed.

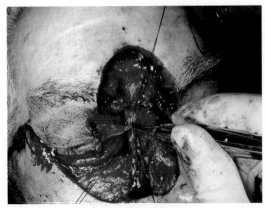

Fig. 21. Superficial temporal fascia used to reconstruct the medial canthal tendon. Fascia secured to upper and lower tarsus. Three SherLock bone anchors placed. Superior anchor obscured by graft. It is positioned superior and posterior to the original tendon insertion and just anterior to the lacrimal sac. Forceps are holding fascia to tension the lids appropriately and indicate where, specifically, the facia should be fixed to the anchor. The lower two anchors will be used to provide points of fixation for Mustardé cheek rotation flap.

or analogous procedures are typically performed once the lid reconstruction has been completed.[36]

The authors prefer to reconstruct all medial canthus defects, regardless of size, with local flaps. Despite published reports of satisfactory results for healing by secondary intention,[37] the risks of epiphora, epicanthal folds, and medial ectropion are minimized by flap rotation. To that end, local flaps elevated to cover the medial canthus should be designed with a horizontal or superior oblique line of tension to aid in supporting the medial lids. Jelks and colleagues[36] expand on the use of a medially based, upper lid myocutaneous flap to cover defects in the medial canthal region. The flap is a good option in these cases because it provides thin, supple skin and has a superiorly directed tension vector. Another option for larger partial-thickness defects in the medial canthus is the partially thinned glabellar flap in the method described by Onishi and colleagues.[38] A caudally based glabellar flap is transposed 90 degrees into the defect and the donor site is closed with a Rintala flap. The thinned portion of the flap is used to cover the canthal tendon and provides a reasonable approximation of the original skin texture of this region.

In cases where the medial canthal tendon is resected, the authors reconstruct this structure with a regionally available fascia graft, such as superficial temporal fascia or galea. The graft is secured to the medial tarsus and the nasal end

of the graft is secured to the lacrimal bone with appropriate tension. The method of fixation can include transnasal wiring in the method of Zide and McCarthy[4] or with bone anchors placed in the ideal position: posterior to the anterior lacrimal crest and superior to the point of the original medial canthal tendon insertion (**Figs. 21** and **22**).

COMBINED UPPER AND LOWER EYELID DEFECTS

Confronted with large defects involving significant portions of both the upper and lower eyelids (**Fig. 23**) the same reconstructive principles as isolated eyelid reconstruction apply. By their nature, full-thickness defects involving both lids often involve one of the canthal tendons and the reconstructive plan must include a method for restoring their integrity. There is no single local flap that can resurface both eyelids, so in most instances at least two flaps,[39] and subsequent flap thinning procedures, particularly for the upper lid, are required.

In many cases, the cheek rotation flap remains available to provide cover for much of the medial canthus and the entire lower lid. The same methods of reconstructing the posterior lamella, discussed previously, still apply. In reconstructing

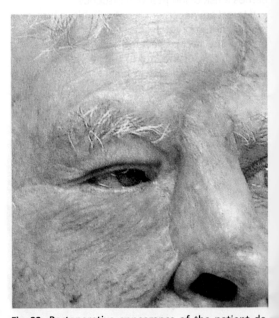

Fig. 22. Postoperative appearance of the patient depicted in **Fig. 21.** Mustardé cheek rotation flap used to cover the lower lid and medial canthal region. Medial edge of the cheek flap has been secured to Sherlock bone anchors to reconstruct nasojugal groove. A contralateral forehead flap has provided coverage for the nasal and glabellar defects.

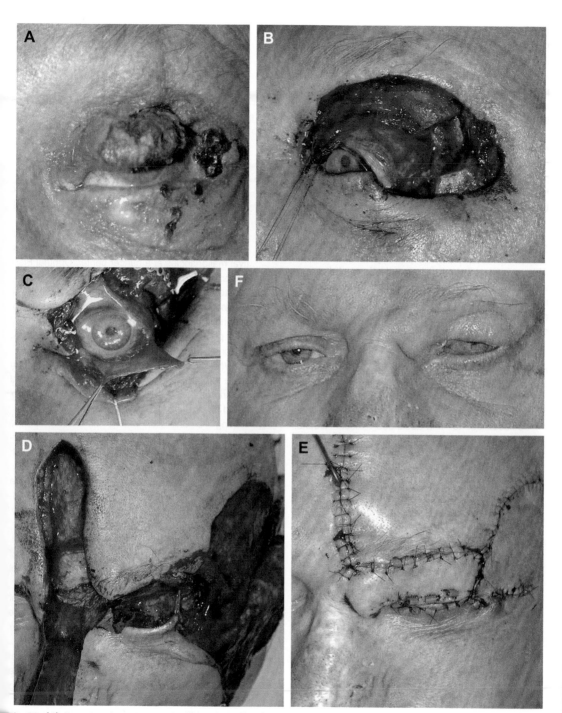

Fig. 23. (*A*) An extensive squamous cell carcinoma involving three quarters of upper lid, lateral canthus, and one third of the lower lid. (*B*) Postablative defect with lateral orbitotomy to facilitate excision of involved lacrimal gland and lateral rectus. (*C*) Remaining conjunctiva of lower lateral eyelid will be approximated to upper lid conjunctiva. Forehead flap elevated for upper lid reconstruction and Mustardé cheek flap for lower lid. (*D*) Temporal fascial graft to reconstruct lateral canthus of lower lid. (*E*) Flaps rotated into place and lids secured with temporary medial and central tarsorrhaphy. (*F*) Final result at 6 months. There has been an interval release of temporary tarsorrhaphy and division of conjunctival flap at 6 weeks.

the upper lid, the favored options for reconstruction based on the lower lid are unavailable. The Fricke or forehead flaps, despite their bulk, possess the required length and reliability to provide coverage for the entire upper lid. Their stiffness in these situations often makes cartilage support unnecessary. Secondary procedures to address the pedicle and flap thickness may permit some degree of upper lid animation. In the short to medium term, these flaps and a tarsorrhaphy provide static corneal protection. With the use of lubricants and artificial tears, patients can go on to experience useful vision.

SUMMARY

Although there is an art to aesthetic eyelid reconstruction, fundamentally it is based on an appreciation of the anatomy and morphology of the eyelid and an understanding of the reconstructive goals and principles summarized in this article.

REFERENCES

1. Ferrario VF, Sforza C, Colombo A, et al. Morphometry of the orbital region: a soft-tissue study from adolescence to mid-adulthood. Plast Reconstr Surg 2001;108(2):285–92 [discussion: 293].
2. Kunjur J, Sabesan T, Ilankovan V. Anthropometric analysis of eyebrows and eyelids: an inter-racial study. Br J Oral Maxillofac Surg 2006;44(2):89–93.
3. Small RG, Meyer DR. Eyelid metrics. Ophthal Plast Reconstr Surg 2004;20(4):266–7.
4. Zide BM, McCarthy JG. The medial canthus revisited: an anatomical basis for canthopexy. Ann Plast Surg 1983;11(1):1–9.
5. Kakizaki H, Zako M, Miyaishi O, et al. The lacrimal canaliculus and sac bordered by the Horner's muscle form the functional lacrimal drainage system. Ophthalmology 2005;112(4):710–6.
6. Yamamoto H, Morikawa K, Uchinuma E, et al. An anatomical study of the medial canthus using a three-dimensional model. Aesthetic Plast Surg 2001;25(3):189–93.
7. Kakizaki H, Zako M, Mito H, et al. The medial canthal tendon is composed of anterior and posterior lobes in Japanese eyes and fixes the eyelid complementarily with Horner's muscle. Jpn J Ophthalmol 2004;48(5):493–6.
8. Gioia VM, Linberg JV, McCormick SA. The anatomy of the lateral canthal tendon. Arch Ophthalmol 1987;105(4):529–32.
9. Knize DM. The superficial lateral canthal tendon: anatomic study and clinical application to lateral canthopexy. Plast Reconstr Surg 2002;109(3):1149–57 [discussion: 1158–63].
10. Rosenstein T, Talebzadeh N, Pogrel MA. Anatomy of the lateral canthal tendon. Oral Surg Oral Med Oral Pathol Oral Radiol Endod 2000;89(1):24–8.
11. Muzaffar AR, Mendelson BC, Adams WP Jr. Surgical anatomy of the ligamentous attachments of the lower lid and lateral canthus. Plast Reconstr Surg 2002;110(3):873–84 [discussion: 897–911].
12. Kawai K, Imanishi N, Nakajima H, et al. Arterial anatomical features of the upper palpebra. Plast Reconstr Surg 2004;113(2):479–84.
13. Erdogmus S, Govsa F. The arterial anatomy of the eyelid: importance for reconstructive and aesthetic surgery. J Plast Reconstr Aesthet Surg 2007;60(3):241–5.
14. Nijhawan N, Ross MI, Diba R, et al. Experience with sentinel lymph node biopsy for eyelid and conjunctival malignancies at a cancer center. Ophthal Plast Reconstr Surg 2004;20(4):291–5.
15. Amato M, Esmaeli B, Ahmadi MA, et al. Feasibility of preoperative lymphoscintigraphy for identification of sentinel lymph nodes in patients with conjunctival and periocular skin malignancies. Ophthal Plast Reconstr Surg 2003;19(2):102–6.
16. Ho VH, Ross MI, Prieto VG, et al. Sentinel lymph node biopsy for sebaceous cell carcinoma and melanoma of the ocular adnexa. Arch Otolaryngol Head Neck Surg 2007;133(8):820–6.
17. Hwang K, Cho HJ, Chung IH. Pattern of the temporal branch of the facial nerve in the upper orbicularis oculi muscle. J Craniofac Surg 2004;15(3):373–6.
18. Hwang K, Lee DK, Lee EJ, et al. Innervation of the lower eyelid in relation to blepharoplasty and midface lift: clinical observation and cadaveric study. Ann Plast Surg 2001;47(1):1–5 [discussion: 5–7].
19. Ouattara D, Vacher C, de Vasconcellos JJ, et al. Anatomical study of the variations in innervation of the orbicularis oculi by the facial nerve. Surg Radiol Anat 2004;26(1):51–3.
20. Lowe JB III, Cohen M, Hunter DA, et al. Analysis of the nerve branches to the orbicularis oculi muscle of the lower eyelid in fresh cadavers. Plast Reconstr Surg 2005;116(6):1743–9 [discussion: 1750–1].
21. Hwang K, Kim DJ, Chung RS, et al. An anatomical study of the junction of the orbital septum and the levator aponeurosis in Orientals. Br J Plast Surg 1998;51(8):594–8.
22. Doxanas MT, Anderson RL. Oriental eyelids: an anatomic study. Arch Ophthalmol 1984;102(8):1232–5.
23. Cowen DE, Antonyshyn O. The vascularized temporoparietal fascial flap for correction of the deep superior sulcus. Ophthal Plast Reconstr Surg 1995;11(2)100–7 [discussion: 107–8].
24. Malbouisson JM, Baccega A, Cruz AA. The geometrical basis of the eyelid contour. Ophthal Plast Reconstr Surg 2000;16(6):427–31.

25. Callahan MA, Callahan A. Mustarde flap lower lid reconstruction after malignancy. Ophthalmology 1980;87(4):279–86.

26. McCord CD Jr, Coles WH, Shore JW, et al. Treatment of essential blepharospasm. I. Comparison of facial nerve avulsion and eyebrow-eyelid muscle stripping procedure. Arch Ophthalmol 1984;102(2): 266–8.

27. McCord CD Jr, Shore J, Putnam JR. Treatment of essential blepharospasm. II. A modification of exposure for the muscle stripping technique. Arch Ophthalmol 1984;102(2):269–73.

28. Frey M, Giovanoli P, Tzou CH, et al. Dynamic reconstruction of eye closure by muscle transposition or functional muscle transplantation in facial palsy. Plast Reconstr Surg 2004;114(4):865–75.

29. Stafanous SN. The switch flap in eyelid reconstruction. Orbit 2007;26(4):255–62.

30. Carroll RP. Entropion following the Cutler-Beard procedure. Ophthalmology 1983;90(9):1052–5.

31. Fischer T, Noever G, Langer M, et al. Experience in upper eyelid reconstruction with the Cutler-Beard technique. Ann Plast Surg 2001;47(3): 338–42.

32. Colour Atlas of Pthalmic Plastic Surgery, 3rd edition. Tyers AG, Collin JRO, editors. Philiadelphia: Butterworth Heinemann Elsevier 2008. p. 422–69.

33. McCord CD, Boswell CB, Hester TR. Lateral canthal anchoring. Plast Reconstr Surg 2003;112(1):222–37 [discussion: 238–9].

34. McCord CD, Ford DT, Hanna K, et al. Lateral canthal anchoring: special situations. Plast Reconstr Surg 2005;116(4):1149–57.

35. Leone CR Jr. Lateral canthal reconstruction. Ophthalmology 1987;94(3):238–41.

36. Jelks GW, Glat PM, Jelks EB, et al. Medial canthal reconstruction using a medially based upper eyelid myocutaneous flap. Plast Reconstr Surg 2002; 110(7):1636–43.

37. Moy RL, Ashjian AA. Periorbital reconstruction. J Dermatol Surg Oncol 1991;17(2):153–9.

38. Onishi K, Maruyama Y, Okada E, et al. Medial canthal reconstruction with glabellar combined Rintala flaps. Plast Reconstr Surg 2007;119(2):537–41.

39. Motomura H, Taniguchi T, Harada T, et al. A combined flap reconstruction for full-thickness defects of the medial canthal region. J Plast Reconstr Aesthet Surg 2006;59(7):747–51.

Endoscopic-Assisted Reconstructive Surgery of the Lacrimal Duct

René M.L. Poublon, MD, PhD[a],*, K. de Roon Hertoge, MD[b]

KEYWORDS

- Lacrimal duct stenosis
- Endoscopic management • Dacryocystorhinostomy

Tearing eyes, or epiphora, is a complaint that can occur in early childhood and in adulthood, especially in the elderly. It is caused mostly by stenosis of the lacrimal duct system but not seldom is associated with hypersecretion due to atopic disease. It also can occur when the pump function of the lacrimal duct system is lacking as a result of paralysis of the orbicularis muscle. Dacryocystorhinostomy (DCR) has been the treatment of choice in cases of blocked lacrimal duct for the past 100 years. The approach can be performed externally and endonasally. Toti[1] was the first to describe the external approach, in 1904. A skin incision in the medial corner of the eye and an osteotomy in the lacrimal bone were made. Dupuy-Dutemps and Bouguet[2] modified this technique with the introduction of mucosal flaps to enhance a better functional result. The external approach became the gold standard treatment of lacrimal duct stenosis, with a success rate of more than 90%.

Caldwell[3] reported the endonasal approach in 1893, although the technique using an electric burr was not widely advocated because the success rates were low owing to problems with visualization. This changed in the 1980s and 1990s with the introduction of nasal endoscopes. Visualization of intranasal structures with modern endoscopes is excellent, and surgery, combined with the use of fine rhinology instruments, has become more controlled. McDonogh and Meiring[4] described the first modern endonasal procedure in 1989. Currently, endoscopic DCR can be

performed with punches, chisels, or powered instrumentation and laser assistance. The success rates vary from 60% to 90%.

ANATOMY

Tears are produced and secreted in the lacrimal glands located in the upper orbital margins deep to orbicularis and levator muscles, anterior to the orbital septum. Tears moisten the front of the eye and migrate to the puncta in the medial margins of the lids, where they enter the upper and lower canaliculus (**Fig. 1**). Both canaliculi are 10 to 12 mm long and run between fibers of the orbicularis muscle (deep head of the preseptal and pretarsal orbicularis) posterior to the medial canthal ligament. They fuse as the common canaliculus and drain into the lacrimal sac. Contraction of the orbicularis muscle gives rise to a negative pressure in the lacrimal sac ("tear pump"). A valve system in the lacrimal sac and nasolacrimal duct prevents backflow (valves of Rosenmüller, Krause, and Hasner). The lacrimal sac can be found in the medial aspect of the orbit between the anterior and posterior lacrimal crest (lacrimal fossa), where lacrimal bone and frontal process of the maxilla are fused together. The suture line between both runs exactly halfway the lacrimal fossa in the craniocaudal direction. The ventrodorsal distance of the lacrimal fossa is 7.2 to 8.6 mm. The craniocaudal length of the lacrimal sac is approximately 12 to 15 mm and runs into the nasolacrimal duct, which

a Department of Otorhinolaryngology and Head and Neck Surgery, Erasmus MC Center Location, Erasmus University Rotterdam, 's Gravendijkwal 230, 3015 CE Rotterdam, The Netherlands
b Department of Ophthalmology, Erasmus MC Center Location, Erasmus University Rotterdam, 's Gravendijkwal 230, 3015 CE Rotterdam, The Netherlands
* Corresponding author.
E-mail address: r.poublon@erasmusmc.nl (R.M.L. Poublon).

Clin Plastic Surg 36 (2009) 399–405
doi:10.1016/j.cps.2009.02.002
0094-1298/09/$ – see front matter © 2009 Elsevier Inc. All rights reserved.

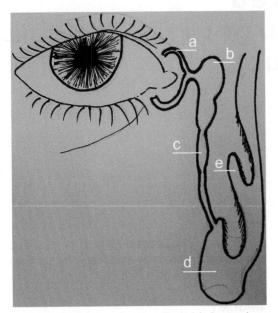

Fig. 1. Lacrimal apparatus: canaliculi (a), lacrimal sac (b), lacrimal duct (c), inferior nasal meatus (d), and middle nasal meatus (e).

opens onto the inferior meatus of the nose, just behind the head of the inferior turbinate.

The region of the nasolacrimal sac endonasally is approximately 5 mm anterior to the attachment and head of the inferior turbinate and runs in craniocaudal direction for approximately 10 mm (**Figs. 2** and **3**). The attachment of the uncinate process corresponds with the posterior part of the lacrimal fossa and the anterior part of the medial orbital wall or papyraceous plate.

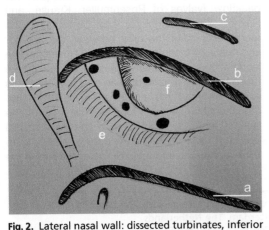

Fig. 2. Lateral nasal wall: dissected turbinates, inferior turbinate (a), middle turbinate (b), superior turbinate (c), uncinate process (e), and ethmoidal bulla (f). The region anterior to the middle turbinate shows the outlines of the lacrimal sac (d) and part of the nasolacrimal duct.

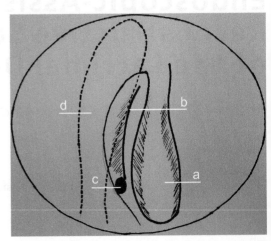

Fig. 3. Frontal view with projection of the lacrimal sac on the lateral nasal wall and relation to the middle turbinate. Middle turbinate (a), uncinate process (b), and natural ostium of maxillary sinus (c). The dotted line represents the outline of the lacrimal sac (d).

PATIENT SELECTION

A history of excessive tearing is mostly due to an obstruction of the lacrimal duct system but must be excluded from hypersecretion resulting from atopic disease, foreign body, or dry eye syndrome, frequently seen in postmenopausal women. Also, disturbance of the tear pump function can give rise to hypersecretion in cases of laxity of the lower lid (after facial motor paralysis) or ectropion and a history of recurrent dacryocystitis with dilation of the lacrimal sac. Munk and colleagues[5] advocated a classification of hypersecretion from grade 1 (only two times a day cleaning of the eyes is necessary) to grade 4 (continuous tearing during the day). Secondary acquired nasolacrimal duct obstruction can be observed after chronic dacryocystitis, autoimmune disease (Wegener's granulomatosis or sarcoidosis), trauma (Le Fort 2 skull fracture), paranasal sinus surgical procedures, tumors, and radiotherapy. A causative factor is lacking in primary acquired nasolacrimal duct stenosis. Congenital nasolacrimal duct stenosis can give rise to excessive tearing in early childhood as seen in some facial anomalies or syndromes.

Preoperative Evaluation

Schirmer's test
It is possible to exclude a dry eye syndrome with Schirmer's test. A test strip is placed in the lateral conjunctival fornix of both lower eyelids. After 5 minutes the strips are removed and the amount of moisture measured. Young persons normally moisten 15 mm of the paper strip. In the elderly

only 10 mm is moistened. In patients who have sicca syndrome, less than 5 mm is moistened in 5 minutes.

Dye disappearance test

The simplest and most reliable technique for assessing the function of the lacrimal apparatus is the dye disappearance test. It is performed by instilling a drop of 2% fluorescein in the conjunctival fornix of the lower lids. The fluorescein has to disappear and be transported into the lacrimal apparatus within 15 minutes. This test can be combined with Schirmer's test. The color dilution on the paper strip can be compared with a scale of known standards and the most closely comparable color dilution chosen or recorded on visual analog scale.

Anel test

Patency of the lacrimal apparatus can be tested mechanically. Therefore a Bowman's probe is introduced in the puncta of the lower lid to dilate the lower canaliculus. Irrigation is performed by introducing an Anel needle, which is connected to a syringe filled with saline (**Table 1**). The nasolacrimal duct is patent if the patient tastes the saline. Reflux of saline through the upper and lower canaliculus occurs if the distal part of the lacrimal apparatus is completely blocked. If reflux occurs through only the irrigated canaliculus, a proximal stenosis is obvious.

Dacryocystography

Imaging is indicated when neoplasms in the lacrimal sac or immediate surrounding tissue are suspected (less than 5% of all cases of nasolacrimal duct obstruction) or dacryoliths. A contrast medium (Lipiodol) is injected after dilating the inferior canaliculus to visualize the total nasolacrimal system. The image quality in plain radiography can be enhanced with subtraction techniques. CT and MRI can provide more insight in the skeletal and soft tissues in combination with intraluminal contrast. These adjunct techniques, however, are not necessary in the majority of patients.

Nasal endoscopy

Patency of the nose is a prerequisite for an endonasal approach to the lacrimal duct and sac. Septal deviation, nasal polyps, or nasal tumors have to be excluded. Surgery to the lacrimal duct is difficult or not possible if the middle turbinate is not visible with a 30° endoscope owing to a vomerian crest and spur, septal spine, or nasal polyps. Simultaneous septal correction, therefore, sometimes is needed with a DCR.

TREATMENT

DCR is indicated when the nasolacrimal duct is relatively or totally obstructed and the common canaliculus is patent. A fistula is made between the lacrimal sac and the nasal cavity. A permanent fistula between the medial conjunctival fornix and the nasal cavity has to be made if the upper and lower canaliculus or the common canaliculus is stenotic. Glass or Pyrex tubes (Jones tubes) have to be placed to prevent recurrent stenosis.

Surgical Technique

Surgery is performed under general anesthesia. The mucosa of the lateral nasal wall anterosuperior to the middle turbinate is infiltrated with 2 mL epinephrine (1:100,000) after decongestion of the nasal mucosa with cocaine (3% solution) with 0.5 mL epinephrine (1 mg/mL). The mucosal lining of the lateral nasal wall has to be incised and elevated under endoscopic control with a rigid 4-mm wide endoscope (30°) for endonasal exposure of the medial aspect of the lacrimal fossa. The incision for this mucosal flap begins 5 to 8 mm above the insertion of the head of the middle turbinate and runs forward approximately 8 mm anterior to the middle turbinate and ends just above the insertion of the inferior turbinate. Information as to the localization of the lacrimal sac can be provided by transillumination with an optical fiber introduced into the inferior canaliculus, which is connected to a xenon light source. The maximal brightness corresponds to the posterior end of the lacrimal fossa where the overlying

Table 1 Anel test (lacrimal irrigation)	
Patent	No Anatomic Obstruction
Patent with reflux	Partial obstruction
Not patent with reflux	Total obstruction
Not patent without reflux	Proximal total obstruction

Patients in whom reflux occurs with total obstruction can benefit from DCR.

bone is thinnest. The suture line, or maxillary line, between the frontal process of the maxilla and lacrimal bone is exposed after elevating the mucosal flap. A chisel (4 mm) is used to mobilize the firm bone of the posterior part of the frontal process, which is anterosuperior to the lacrimal sac. This mobilized bone and the thinner lacrimal bone are removed with forceps. All the bone of the lacrimal fossa has to be removed to allow the mucosal medial wall of the lacrimal sac to be flatter on the lateral nasal wall. This is ensured by tenting the medial wall of the sac with an illuminated optical fiber. The sac is incised in a C shape to create a large posterior-based mucosal flap. The mucosal flap can be excised or reflected onto the lateral nasal wall.

The lacrimal system is intubated with a bicanalicular silicon stent, which is stabilized in the nose with a small silicon button. Gauze soaked in antibiotic ointment is left behind in the middle nasal meatus for the initial postoperative healing period. No oral antibiotics are given. The nasal packing is removed on the fourth postoperative day. Saline nasal douches are advised to moisten the mucosa for 6 weeks at minimum. Also topical nasal steroids (fluticasone diproprionate) are given twice a day for 6 weeks. Intubation with silicon tubes lasts for 3 months.

RESULTS

Successful functional result can be defined as relief of symptoms or marked improvement in tearing. Munk's score can be used for this purpose (**Table 2**). Success also can be defined as normal passage of fluorescein at the dye disappearance test and a patent lacrimal ostium with nasal endoscopy.

Rotterdam Experience

The authors conducted a retrospective case review of 48 consecutive patients (34 women and 14 men; mean age 62 years, range 25–86 years) in a tertiary referral center who underwent 57 operations between 2004 and 2007. All underwent an endoscopic procedure. Twenty-one patients (30 operations) had no previous surgery. Twelve patients had some other surgical procedures (13) in the past, including extended paranasal sinus surgery for inverted papilloma (7), schwannoma (1), neuresthesioblastoma (2), squamous cell carcinoma (1), orbital reconstruction after trauma (1), and frontomaxillar dysplasia (1). Seventeen patients had previous lacrimal surgery in their history—external DCR (10) and endonasal DCR (7). Postoperative improvement or subjective resolution of epiphora was assessed with Munk's score.[5] Grades 0, 1, and 2 were classified as successful. All patients were classified preoperatively as grade 4.

All patients completed a telephone questionnaire to evaluate the long-term postoperative improvement after an average follow-up of 26 months. The overall success rate was 88% (50/57 patients). Patients who had no previous surgery had more successful outcomes (93%; 28/30 operations) (**Figs. 4** and **5**). The success rate of those patients who underwent other surgical procedures in the past was less (85%; 11/13 operations), whereas the success rate after lacrimal surgery in the past was 82% (14/17). No statistical difference was found because of small numbers.

COMPLICATIONS

Endoscopic nasal procedures can lead to major or minor complication. Damage to the extraocular muscle results in double vision, whereas optic nerve damage results in blindness. Thus far, double vision has not been reported in the literature.

Trauma to the medial orbital wall always has to be prevented. This can occur if the dissection is taken too far posterior. The first sign of entering the orbit during surgery is exposure of the yellow colored orbital fat. Damage to small postseptal vessels that retract in the orbital fat during the surgical procedure results in a retrobulbar hematoma, which may lead to blindness.

Table 2	
Munk's score: a classification system for the severity of tearing	
Grade 0	No Epiphora
Grade 1	Occasional epiphora requiring dabbing with a handkerchief less than twice a day
Grade 2	Epiphora requiring dabbing 2 to 4 times a day
Grade 3	Epiphora requiring dabbing 5 to 10 times a day
Grade 4	Epiphora requiring dabbing more than 10 times a day or constant tearing

Patients who have grade 3 or 4 can benefit from DCR.

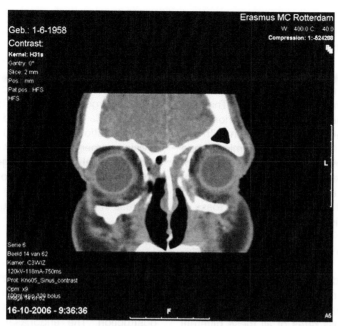

Fig. 4. Postoperative section of a coronal CT in which the surgincalle made ostium can be observed of the lacrimal fossa on the right side.

Laceration of the lacrimal puncta can occur after traumatic dilatation of the canaliculus with a Bowman's probe or too tight fixation of the silicon tubing during the postoperative period. A minor complication is a hematoma in the lower lid resulting from damage of the preseptal orbital vessels. Postoperative nose bleeding can be treated easily with nasal packing. The authors observed two major complications in the data (laceration of the puncta): no loss of vision, double vision, orbital fat exposure, or orbital hematomas occurred. There were no cases of postoperative nasal bleeding.

DISCUSSION

Surgery for epiphora changed during the last decades of the twentieth century, from an external approach (external DCR)[1] to an endonasal approach (endoscopic DCR).[4]

The reported success rates for the external DCR was 80% to 99% and became the gold standard for nasolacrimal duct obstruction.[6–10] The main disadvantage of this procedure, however, is the required dissection of the orbicularis muscle and damage to the medial palpebral ligament, which is likely to interfere with the pump function. Also, the visible scar in the medial corner of the eyelid and the possible effect of the surgical procedure on the nasal mucosa (mucosal adhesions; nasal bleeding) can be a problem.

The improved visualization with nasal endoscopes, however, allows easy identification of

the lacrimal sac and, therefore, there no longer is a need for a skin incision. The success rates are between 75% and 97% for primary cases,[11–16] which makes the endonasal approach more favorable than the external approach. Endoscopic DCR allows rhinologists to correct the concomitant intranasal pathology, such as septal deviation, enlarged bullous middle turbinate, and nasal polyps,[17,18] at the same time. Meticulous surgery is needed to prevent major and minor[19] intraorbital complications. Endoscopic DCR also is a safe and

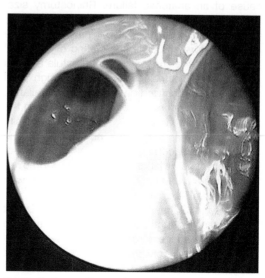

Fig. 5. Postoperative endoscopic view of the lateral nasal wall with a patent lacrimal ostium.

effective means of treating nasolacrimal duct obstruction in infants and young children.[20–22]

Different methods are advocated for endoscopic localization of the medial wall of the lacrimal fossa. The simplest is the technique of transillumination of the lacrimal sac with a sterile optical fiber, used in retinal surgery.[23,24] The fiber is preferably introduced through the inferior canaliculus and the light then can be seen with the endoscope. Some prefer to use a microscope instead of an endoscope.[25] In cases of loss of anatomic landmarks or extensive scar tissue, image guidance recently has been advocated.[26]

The bony medial wall of the lacrimal fossa is mobilized after incising the mucoperiosteum of the region, anterior to the middle turbinate. The mucoperiosteal flap can be preserved as a posterior-based flap.[14,27] Fixation with sutures is never necessary. The window in the bony lacrimal fossa can be performed mechanically with a chisel or with powered instrumentation, such as a burr.[16] The reported success rates of all these different methods vary from 80% to 97%.

Results of endonasal KTP-laser DCR compared with external DCR are poor, 64% versus 94%,[9] whereas endolacrimal KTP laser is more successful, 83%.[28] Other laser equipment, such as holmium-YAG,[29,30] can be used safely and has similar results in relieving symptoms of distal lacrimal duct obstruction. The argon-HGM laser has shown excellent outcomes (97%).[31]

Failure of function after surgery to the nasolacrimal duct is most common because of lack of tear pump function as can been seen after muscular weakness due to facial palsy and ectropion.[32] Scar contracture of the rhinostomy can be the cause of an anatomic failure. Rhinostomy size, however, seems not to effect success rate after the external approach.[33] The original fistula initially is wider before gradually contracting over time.[34] Intubation of the surgically formed fistula aims to prevent the cicatrizing closure, although until recently no randomized data have been available.

Most investigators use bicanicular stents in the postoperative period.[13,14,16,18,22] Insertion of silicone tubes seems to have no benefit on the success rate according to a small randomized, prospective, parallel-group study.[35] Moreover, failures were found only in the group treated with silicon tubes (5 out of 23 patients).

Mitomycin C has been advocated to inhibit fibrosis as an antiproliferative agent and to increase the success rate of endonasal surgery in adults and in children.[36–38] No randomized study, however, has yet been performed.

The success rate for primary endonasal, endoscopic surgery of nasolacrimal duct obstruction in the authors' series was 93% and is in concordance with the literature. Success in primary surgery depends on creating a wide osteotomy and preservation of as much mucosal tissue as possible to reduce scarring.

The authors' data from endonasal, endoscopic revision surgery were 82%. These data are better than the 45% to 77% reported in the literature.[39,40] Scar formation around the nasolacrimal sac in revision surgery limits proper identification of the sac. Lacrimal revision surgery reported from a tertiary referral center accounted for 12.5% in the series of Ben Simon and colleagues,[39] whereas in this series it accounted for 29.8%.

SUMMARY

Reconstructive surgery of the nasolacrimal duct or DCR can be performed via an external or endonasal approach. For almost a century external DCR was the gold standard for correction of lacrimal duct obstruction. The endonasal approach became a safe surgical procedure using endoscopes and has the same anatomic and functional success rate as the external approach. It can be performed in adults and in children with close collaboration between a rhinologist and an ophthalmologist. An overview is given of the literature together with the authors' experience in this field.

REFERENCES

1. Toti A. Nuovo metodo conservatore dicura delle suppurazione croniche del sacco lacrimale (dacriocistorhinostomia). Clin Moderna (Firenza) 1904;10:385.
2. Dupuy-Dutemps L, Bouguet M. Note preliminaire sur en procede de dacryocystorhinostomie. Ann Oncol 1921;158:241.
3. Caldwell GW. Two new operations for obstruction of the nasal duct with preservation of the canaliculi and with an incidental description of a new lachrymal probe. Am J Ophthalmol 1893;10:189–93.
4. McDonogh M, Meiring JHJ. Endoscopic transnasal dacryocystorhinostomy. J Laryngol Otol 1989;103: 585–7.
5. Munk PL, Lin DT, Morris DC. Epiphora: treatment by means of dacryocystoplasty with balloon dilation of the nasolacrimal drainage apparatus. Radiology 1990;177(3):687–90.
6. Tarbet KJ, Custer PL. External dacryocystorhinostomy. Surgical success, patient satisfaction, and economic cost. Ophthalmology 1995;102:1065–70.
7. Shun-Shin GA, Thurairajan G. External dacryocystorhinostomy—an end of an era? Br J Ophthalmol 1997;81:716–7.
8. Delaney YM, Khooshabeh R. External dacryocystorhinostomy for the treatment of acquired partial

nasolacrimal obstruction in adults. Br J Ophthalmol 2002;86:533–5.

9. Mirza S, Al-Barmani A, Douglas SA, et al. A retrospective comparison of endonasal KTP laser dacryocystorhinostomy versus external dacryocystorhinostomy. Clin Otolaryngol Allied Sci 2002; 27(5):347–51.

10. Dolman PJ. Comparison of external dacryocystorhinostomy with nonlaser endonasal dacrycystorhinostomy. Ophthalmology 2003;110:78–84.

11. Metson R. Endoscopic surgery for lacrimal obstruction. (9 of 12 cases 75%). Otolaryngol Head Neck Surg 1991;104(4):473–9.

12. Hartikainen J, Jukka A, Matti V, et al. Prospective randomised comparison of endonasal endoscopic dacrycystorhinostomy and external dacryocystorhinostomy. Laryngoscope 1998;108:1861–6.

13. Woog JJ, Kennedy RH, Custer PL, et al. Endonasal dacryocystorhinostomy: a report by the American Society of Ophthalmology. Ophthalmology 2001; 108(12):2369–77.

14. Tsirbas A, Wormold PJ. Mechanical endonasal dacryocystorhinostomy with mucosal flaps. Br J Orthod 2003;87(1):43–7.

15. Tsirbas A, Davis G, Wormold PJ. Mechanical endonasal dacryocystorhinostomy versus external dacryocystorhinostomy. Ophthal Plast Reconstr Surg 2004;20(1):50–6.

16. Saratziotis A, Emanuelli E, Gouveris H, et al. Endoscopic dacryocystorhinostomy for acquired nasolacrimal duct obstruction: creating a window with a drill without use of mucosal flaps. Acta Otolaryngol 2008;31:1–4.

17. Nussbaumer MJ. Concomitant nasal procedures in endoscopic dacryocystorhinostomy. J Laryngol Otol 2004;118(4):267–9.

18. Onerci M. Dacryocystorhinostomy. Diagnosis and treatment of nasolacrimal canal obstructions. Rhinology 2004;40:49–65.

19. Fayet B, Racy E, Assouline M. Complications of standardized endonasal dacryocystorhinostomy with unciformectomy. Ophthalmology 2004;111(4):837–45.

20. Vander Veen DK, Jones DT, Tan H, et al. Endoscopic dacryocystorhinostomy in children. J AAPOS 2001; 5(3):143–7.

21. Barnes EA, Abou-Rayyah Y, Rose GE. Pediatric dacryocystostomy for nasolacrimal duct obstruction. Ophthalmology 2001;108(9):1562–4.

22. Jones DT, Fajardo NF, Petersen RA, et al. Pediatric endoscopic dacryocystorhinostomy failures: who and why? Laryngoscope 2007;117(2):323–7.

23. Siegert R, Weerda H. Die diaphonoskopische Lokalisation der Tränenwege bei der endonasalen Dakryozystorhinostomie. Laryngorhinootologie 1996;75:309–10.

24. May A, Fries U, Zubcov-Ivantscheff A, et al. Endoillumination-guided intranasal microscopic

dacryocystorhinostomy for difficult cases. ORL J Otorhinolaryngol Relat Spec 2002;64:11–5.

25. Weber R, Draf W, Kolb P. Die endonasale mikrochirurgische Behandlung von Tränenwegsstenosen. HNO 1993;41:11–8.

26. Day S, Hwang TN, Pletcher SD, et al. Interactive image-guided endoscopic dacryocystorhinostomy. Ophthal Plast Reconstr Surg 2008;24(4):338–40.

27. Sonkhya N, Mishra P. Endoscopic transnasal dacryocystorhinostomy with nasal mucosal and posterior lacrimal sac flap. J Laryngol Otol 2008;28:1–7.

28. Hofmann T, Lackner A, Muellner K, et al. Endolacrimal KTP Laser-assisted dacryocystorhinostomy. Arch Otolaryngol Head Neck Surg 2003;129(3):329–32.

29. Woog JJ, Metson R, Puliafito CA. Holmium:YAG endonasal laser dacryocystorhinostomy. Am J Orthop 1993;116(1):1–10.

30. Hehar SS, Jones NS, Sadiq SA, et al. Endoscopic holmium:YAG laser dacryocystorhinostomy—safe and effective as a day-case procedure. J Laryngol Otol 1997;111(11):1056–9.

31. Szubin L, Papageorge A, Sacks E. Endonasal laser-assisted dacryocystorhinostomy. Am J Rhinol 1999; 13(5):371–4.

32. Wormold PJ, Tsirbas A. Investigation and endoscopic treatment for functional and anatomical obstruction of the nasolacrimal duct system. Clin Otolaryngol Allied Sci 2004;29(4):352–6.

33. Linberg JV, Anderson RL, Bumsted RM, et al. Study of intranasal ostium external dacrycystorhinostomy. Arch Ophthalmol 1982;100(11):1758–62.

34. Mann BS, Wormold PJ. Endoscopic assessment of the dacryocystorhinostomy ostium after endoscopic surgery. Laryngoscope 2006;116(7):1172–4.

35. Smirnov G, Tuomilehto H, Teräsvirta M, et al. Silicon tubing is not necessary after primary endoscopic dacryocystorhinostomy: a prospective randomised study. Am J Rhinol 2008;22(2):214–7.

36. Camara JG, Bengzon AU, Henson RD. The safety and efficacy of mitomycin C in endonasal endoscopic laser assisted dacryocystorhinostomy. Ophthal Plast Reconstr Surg 2000;16:114–8.

37. Deka A, Bhattacharjee K, Bhuyan SK, et al. Effect of mitomycin C on ostium in dacrycystorhinostomy. Clin Experiment Ophthalmol 2006;34(6):557–61.

38. Dolmetsch AM, Gallon MA, Holds JB. Nonlaser endoscopic endonasal dacryocystorhinostomy with adjunctive mitomycin C in children. Ophthal Plast Reconstr Surg 2008;24(5):390–3.

39. Ben Simon GJ, Joseph J, Lee S, et al. External versus endoscopic dacryocystorhinostomy for acquired lacrimal duct obstruction in a tertiary referral center. Ophthalmology 2005;112(8):1463–8.

40. Tsirbas A, Davis G, Wormold PJ. Revision dacrycystorhinostomy: a comparison of external and external techniques. Am J Rhinol 2005;19(3):322–5.

An Algorithm for Treatment of Nasal Defects

Brian M. Parrett, MD, Julian J. Pribaz, MD*

KEYWORDS

- Nasal defects • Nasal reconstruction • Forehead flap
- Nasolabial flap • Nasal lining • Cartilage graft

The nose maintains the central position on the face and may be the most difficult facial feature to reconstruct well. Defects of the nose are common after cancer resection and trauma and, fortunately, there are many options available for reconstruction. The goal is to select the most appropriate option for a given defect. In this article, the authors' have sought to simplify the complex topic of nasal reconstruction with an algorithm for treatment of nasal defects based on their location, concentrating on local flap reconstruction of small to medium-sized defects. The more complex reconstruction of defects involving multiple layers and multiple subunits of the nose are discussed.

ANATOMY

The nose is a three-layered structure covered by skin, supported by a middle layer of bone and cartilage, and lined by mucoperichondrium. The skin has differing qualities in the various nasal regions. The skin of dorsum and sidewall is thin, smooth, and mobile; the skin of the tip and ala is thick and stiff with sebaceous glands. The nasal bones, septum, and upper and lower lateral cartilages provide structural integrity and projection, create contour and definition, and buttress the soft tissues. Nasal lining consists of specialized tissue that is thin and well vascularized with dry, hair-bearing skin at the vestibule and moist mucosa in the nasal vault.

Historically, Burget and Menick[1] divided the nose into aesthetic subunits, which are adjacent areas of characteristic skin quality, contour, and border outline. These subunits are the dorsum, tip, columella, and paired sidewalls, alae, and soft triangles. According to the subunit principle, if greater than 50% of a subunit is involved, excision of the entire subunit before reconstruction is recommended. However, this is not universally applicable, as enlarging small defects may result in increased use of the forehead flap for defects where smaller local flaps may suffice.[2–4] The subunit principle is a tool, not a rigid rule, and should be modified to fit the individual needs of the patient.

PLANNING

Preoperative planning is the most important aspect of a successful reconstruction. Although small defects may only require a single procedure, typically multiple procedures are needed to reconstruct a more extensive defect to obtain a functional and aesthetic nose. Poor planning leads to complications that result in nasal distortion or collapse, especially in multistage procedures.

Define the Defect

Define the defect in terms of size, depth, orientation, and location on the nose. In delayed reconstructions, this requires recreation of the original defect by releasing contractures and excising scars, returning structures to their normal positions. To simplify defining the defect, we arbitrarily divide the nose into thirds transversely (**Fig. 1**), and this will be the basis for our algorithm.

Division of Plastic Surgery, Harvard Medical School, Brigham & Women's Hospital, 75 Francis Street, Boston, MA 02115, USA
* Corresponding author.
E-mail address: jpribaz@partners.org (J.J. Pribaz).

Clin Plastic Surg 36 (2009) 407–420
doi:10.1016/j.cps.2009.02.004
0094-1298/09/$ – see front matter © 2009 Elsevier Inc. All rights reserved.

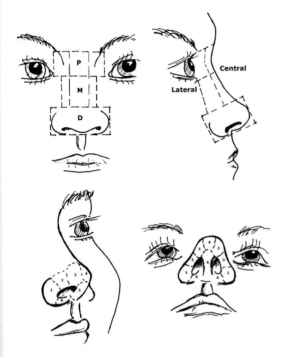

Fig. 1. (*Above*) Drawings demonstrate the three zones of the nose: P, proximal third zone; M, middle third zone; D, distal third zone. (*Below*) Distal zone subunits: 1, ala; 2, domal-alar groove; 3, dome; 4, central; 5, columella; 6, sill.

Next, understand the defect in terms of layers, as complex nasal defects are often multilayered with loss of lining, support, and skin cover. The goal is to replace like with like and the importance of an accurate diagnosis here cannot be overemphasized. After defining location and missing layers, the reconstruction can be broken down into component parts, with each part addressed in turn.

Identify Donor Sites

Donor sites for lining, support, and skin cover should be determined. Missing tissue should be replaced in the exact amount that has been removed or lost. Making flaps too small is a common mistake that should be avoided. Also, when designing a flap, avoid distorting adjacent structures including the eyelid, ala, and oral commissure.

ASSEMBLING THE NASAL LAYERS

The reestablishment of all deficient layers of the nose is the foundation of a successful reconstruction. The goal should be the reestablishment of a normal nasal contour; scarring will occur as part of the reconstruction but is much more tolerable than contour abnormalities in the nose.

External Skin

Nasal reconstructions usually rely on skin flap coverage from local or regional sources and this is the focus of the algorithm below. The reconstructive ladder provides a framework for analyzing the various coverage options. Direct repair may be considered in only very small defects. Skin grafts may be of some use, especially in elderly, multi-morbid patients that cannot or do not wish to undergo a more complex reconstruction. Skin grafts are often performed according to the subunit principle[1] but often do not provide the best cosmetic results. Composite grafts can be useful in the reconstruction of smaller defects of the alar rim. Local and regional flaps are the mainstay of nasal reconstruction as they use nearby tissue that provides an excellent color and texture match.[5,6] Finally, distant tissues in the form of free flaps may be needed if the forehead donor site is unavailable or if the defect is too large and complex. However, distant tissues often have a less desirable color and texture match.

Local and regional flaps give the best results and are the first choice for reconstruction. Flap tissue is generally recruited from either a vertical or a transverse direction. After defining defect geometry, determine from which direction skin will be donated. This depends on tissue laxity, vascularity, and resulting donor site distortion. Although many flaps are described for nasal reconstruction, most defects can be best closed with the miter flap, glabella flap, bilobed flap, V-Y advancement flap, nasolabial flap, or the forehead flap (**Fig. 2, Table 1**).

The forehead flap is the mainstay of reconstruction for larger nasal defects, including subtotal or total nasal defects.[8–10] Forehead flap reconstruction requires at least two stages: 3 weeks after flap elevation and inset, the pedicle is divided and the proximal portion of the flap is thinned. Since forehead skin is thicker than nasal skin, thinning of the flap is required. However, for larger and more complex defects, especially involving the nasal tip complex, Menick[9,10] describes a three-stage procedure to provide a better cosmetic result. During the first stage, a full-thickness forehead flap is harvested and inset atop reconstructed lining and support. The distal portion of the flap (the columellar inset) is thinned. Three weeks later, an intermediate stage entails reelevating the cutaneous part of the flap with a 4-mm tissue thickness, leaving the pedicle intact and with direct removal of distal hair follicles if present. The excess frontalis muscle and subcutaneous fat that have healed onto the underlying support structures can be appropriately thinned, sculpted

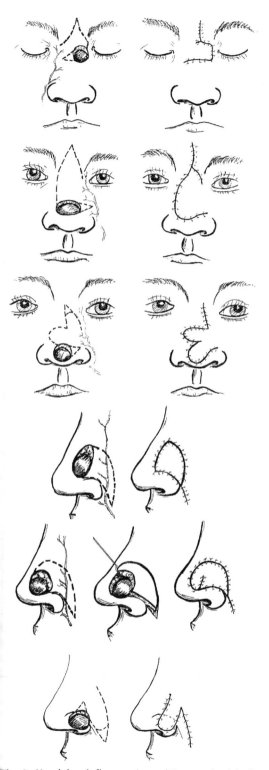

Fig. 2. Nasal local flap options. (*First row*) glabella flap; (*second row*) miter flap; (*third row*) bilobed flap; (*fourth row*) V-Y advancement flap; (*fifth row*) extended V-Y advancement flap; (*sixth row*) nasolabial flap.

and recovered with the thin forehead flap. At the final stage 3 weeks later, the pedicle is divided, thinned, and inset. Laser hair removal may be needed if the flap has residual hair growth after intermediate stage hair follicle removal.

Nasal Lining

Failure in nasal reconstruction is often due to a shortage of lining, as the unlined nose will distort because of scar contraction. Reestablishment of thin, supple, and well-vascularized lining is difficult. Full-thickness grafts can be used for lining when placed on the undersurface of a flap such as on the frontalis muscle of a forehead flap.[8,11] Skin grafts cannot sustain primary cartilage grafts or cover exposed cartilage or bone. However, delayed cartilage grafts can be placed at a second stage approximately 3 weeks later to ensure graft survival. Alternatively, the distal portion of a forehead or nasolabial flap can be folded over for lining. This will need to be thinned approximately 3 weeks later by an incision along the planned alar rim. At this stage, cartilage grafts may be placed.

Intranasal donor tissue provides thin, flexible, and vascularized lining to nourish primary structural grafts while conforming to the neoarchitecture of the nose and without obstructing the airway.[8] Designing these flaps requires a working knowledge of septal blood supply.[8] A flap of septal mucoperichondrium with or without cartilage can be based on a septal branch of the superior labial artery that enters the nasal septum lateral to the nasal spine. This axial flap is versatile because it can be long, with a 1.3 mm pedicle. Ipsilateral mucoperichondrial flaps can be transposed to replacing lining for the vestibule, alar margin, or lateral sidewall. This flap can be used in combination with a bipedicle flap to line an alar rim defect. In such cases, residual vestibular skin superior to the defect is transferred to the proposed alar rim as a bipedicle flap based medially on the septum and laterally on the nasal floor.[8] The donor defect is then closed with the ipsilateral mucoperichondrial flap or by a full-thickness skin graft (FTSG). In addition, an ipsilateral mucoperichondrial flap for lining the lower vestibule can be combined with a contralateral mucoperichondrial flap to line the middle and upper vaults. The contralateral design is based on the dorsum of the septum by way of the anterior ethmoidal vessels and is hinged laterally.[8] This was originally described by DeQuervain[12] as a composite chondromucosal hinge flap. A sufficient amount of dorsal septal support has to be left in place, thus limiting the flap's lateral reach.

When local flaps are unavailable, lining can be reconstructed using regional or distant tissue,

Table 1
Most common local and regional flaps for nasal defects

Flap Name	Flap Type	Characteristics
Miter flap	Advancement	Recruits tissue vertically; also referred to as the dorsal nasal advancement flap
Glabella flap	Transposition	Recruits tissue vertically from glabella region to cover the superior portion of nose
Bilobed flap	Transposition	Careful design important; Zitelli modification[6,7]; ideal for dome or central tip defects
Nasolabial flap	Transposition	Superiorly or inferiorly based; most require second stage for pedicle division, flap debulking, or to define alar facial groove
V-Y or extended V-Y flap	Advancement	Based on blood supply from flap base; useful for lateral defects of proximal or middle one third of the nose, and certain alar defects
Forehead flap	Transposition	Axial blood supply; excellent color–texture match; most commonly designed as paramedian flap based on supratrochlear pedicle; can have gull-wing extensions to cover heminasal or total nasal defects

such as intraoral flaps, free flaps, or prelaminated flaps as summarized in **Table 2**.[13,14]

Skeletal Support

The osteocartilaginous framework reestablishes support and shape, resists scar contraction, and buttresses the soft tissues. It is critical for soft-tissue dimensions to be maintained early in reconstruction because restoring contour is difficult once the soft tissues collapse.[15] To achieve this,

grafts must be used to mold the external skin into the desired nasal shape as early as possible.[16] For nasal support, the surgeon must address the central nasal skeleton, the nasal sidewalls, the alar arches, and the lateral alar elements.

Grafts for nasal reconstruction are summarized in **Table 3**.[8,15] These grafts must be placed in a well-vascularized bed to ensure survival. In addition to central support, tip and lateral alar structural grafts are often needed.[8,15,16] Alar batten grafts from the auricular concha or nasal septum

Table 2
Options for reconstruction of nasal lining

Options	Characteristics
Nasal turnover flap	Poor vascularity; thick and stiff
Nasolabial lining flap	Bulky; requires multiple stages
Forehead flap (turn-in)	Bulky; requires multiple stages
FTSG	Needs vascular bed; cannot support primary grafts
Chondromucosal–cutaneous graft	Needs vascular bed; unpredictable; incomplete take
Vestibular or mucosal bipedicle flap	Little available; since lined by dry skin, it is ideal for alar rim lining; may crust and bleed if used for alar rim
Septal mucoperichondrial flap	May incorporate cartilage; ipsilateral or contralateral; well vascularized; supports primary cartilage grafts; mostly used for the midvault
FAMM flap[13]	Superiorly based axial blood supply; provides moist mucosal lining
Prelaminated flap	Multistaged; can place skin or mucosa graft on undersurface of a forehead or radial forearm flap 3 weeks before transfer
Radial forearm flap[14]	Needs thinning; may be used solely for lining; can reconstruct surrounding tissues

Abbreviation: FAMM, facial artery musculomucosal flap.

Table 3
Cartilage and bone donor tissue options

Donor Tissue	Characteristics
Septal cartilage	Strong; straight; limited in quantity
Conchal cartilage	Weaker; intrinsic curve useful for alar batten or cartilage reconstruction
Costal cartilage	Stronger; from sixth to ninth ribs ideally; serve as central support elements; can form an L-strut that sits on nasal radix and bends sharply at proposed nasal tip to rest on anterior nasal spine
Cranial bone graft	From parietal skull; useful for reconstructing bony pyramid, nasal sidewall; provides strong central support; shaped and secured to maxilla and frontal bone with microplates
Iliac or costal bone grafts	Alternative for nasal pyramid and dorsum reconstruction

are often necessary to stiffen alar reconstructions to prevent retraction and to tent the airway open during inspiration. Tip anatomy is redefined by replacing missing alar cartilages.[8] If further tip definition and support is necessary, shield-type cartilage grafts and columellar strut grafts may be required.

Composite Grafts and Laminated Flaps

Small yet complex full-thickness nasal defects can be achieved using composite grafts or flaps. Composite grafts are most often taken from the ear and used for smaller full-thickness defects, especially involving the alar rim. They are most reliably and best performed secondarily, when the defect is recreated with local turndown flaps which increases the raw surface contact to maximize revascularization of the graft. Composite grafts used acutely, especially in Mohs defects that have been extensively cauterized, will likely not be revascularized adequately.

Composite flaps may be local or distant and may occur naturally in the body or be prelaminated at a separate site before transfer to the defect. For instance, the auricular ascending helical flap is similar in appearance and structure to the ala of the nose, providing excellent color and contour match.[17] It is a laminated structure available as a free flap based on the branches of the superficial temporal vessels and has been used to aesthetically reconstruct the ala, columella, and nasal sill.

Prelaminated flaps can be formed by introducing tissues into a flap without disturbing its blood supply.[18,19] The volar forearm is the most common site for prelamination in nasal reconstruction as it provides abundant and thin skin with reliable vascularity. Typically, in the first stage, the outline of the nose and surrounding involved tissues is made on the forearm, and skin and cartilage grafts are inserted for lining

and support, respectively.[18–20] Once these tissues have healed together, the composite three-dimensional flap is transferred to the defect by means of microvascular anastomosis.

ALGORITHM

After reviewing our experience, we have devised a treatment algorithm (**Table 4**), focusing on small- to medium-sized (1–2 cm) defects that can be best treated with local flaps. These are the most common defects encountered in clinical practice and often occur in patients who present for immediate reconstruction after Mohs micrographic excision of skin cancer. The algorithm is based on defect location and orientation, with the nose divided transversely into three zones (see **Fig. 1**).[6] This algorithm should narrow choices to allow for a quicker and simpler treatment selection, realizing that there is always more than one method of reconstruction. Most of these reconstructions can be performed under local anesthesia in an outpatient setting. Once defects exceed the 2-cm mark, it becomes difficult to rotate local tissue. The more complex management of multi-layered and larger defects will also be described.

Proximal Third of Nose

Defects in the proximal third of the nose can be centrally located on the dorsum or radix area or laterally on the upper sidewalls. They often have exposed periosteum or bone and rarely extend through the bone so that external skin reconstruction is the primary goal.

Central defects

Central defects can be horizontal, round, or vertical in orientation. A horizontal defect is best reconstructed with miter flap advanced from the

Table 4
Algorithm for nasal reconstruction with local and regional flaps

Nasal Divisions	Subdivision or Subunit	Orientation	Flap Choice
Proximal third	Central	Horizontal	Miter flap
		Round	Glabella flap
		Vertical	V-Y flap
	Lateral	Horizontal	Glabella flap, first choice; miter flap, second choice
		Vertical	V-Y flap
	Combined	—	Forehead flap
Middle third	Central	Horizontal, round	Miter flap
		Vertical	V-Y flap
	Lateral	Horizontal	Miter flap
		Vertical	V-Y flap, first choice; nasolabial flap second choice
	Combined	—	Forehead flap
Distal third	Alar	—	Nasolabial flap, first choice; V-Y flap, second choice
	Domal-alar groove	—	Nasolabial flap, first choice; V-Y flap, second choice
	Dome	—	Bilobed flap
	Central tip	—	Bilobed flap
	Columella	—	Composite graft, skin graft, ascending helical free flap
	Nasal sill	—	Nasolabial flap
	Combined	—	Forehead flap, first choice; nasolabial or extended V-Y flap, second choice
Combined[a]	—	—	Forehead flap

[a] Combination of the proximal, middle, and distal third divisions.

glabella region. A round defect is best reconstructed with a glabella flap transposed from the midforehead or glabella region. A vertical defect is best reconstructed with a V-Y advancement flap from the nasal sidewall.

Lateral defects

Lateral defects can be divided into horizontally or vertically oriented defects. Horizontal or round defects can be reconstructed most often with a glabella flap but also may be closed with a miter flap (**Fig. 3**). Vertical defects can be reconstructed with a V-Y flap from the dorsum of the nose extending onto contralateral sidewall if necessary. Other options for lateral sidewall defects include a FTSG from the lateral defects preauricular area; this is an area on the nose that a skin graft can give an acceptable result.

Combined lateral and central defects

Combined lateral and central defects are most commonly best reconstructed with a forehead flap, but occasionally can be closed with an extended glabella flap. In these proximal defects, a single-stage forehead flap may suffice.

Full-thickness defects

Full-thickness defects in this area are uncommon. Reconstruction of support using bone or cartilage is less important here, especially for smaller bone defects as nasal collapse is not a concern. Nasal lining in the upper vault does not require reconstruction with moist, intranasal tissues as most of the airflow in the nose is straight back in a horizontal direction.[21] For a full-thickness defect, the simplest reconstruction in this region is a local or forehead flap with a skin graft on its undersurface.

Middle Third of Nose

The middle third of the nose is divided into central and lateral zones, and includes the nasal bones and upper lateral cartilages.

Central defects

Central defects, if horizontal or round, are best reconstructed with a miter flap. Occasionally, a small vertical defect (<0.5 cm) can be directly closed; this must not distort nasal anatomy. A larger vertical defect can be closed with a V-Y advancement flap (**Fig. 4**A–C).

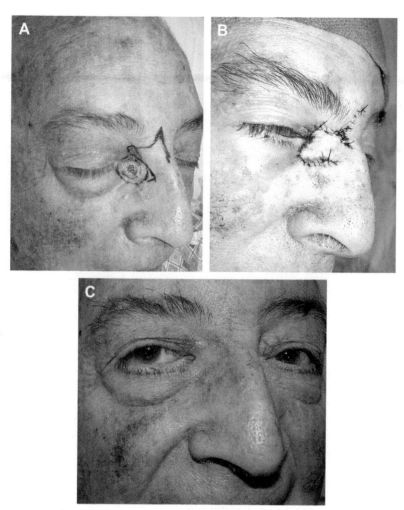

Fig. 3. (*A, B*) Horizontal defect of lateral proximal third of the nose is closed with a glabella flap. (*C*) Patient is shown 3-months postoperatively.

Lateral defects

Lateral defects are the most common middle third nasal defects and can be closed with either a V-Y flap, nasolabial flap, or a miter flap. Vertical defects are most amenable to closure with a V-Y advancement flap from the remaining sidewall and extending onto the medial cheek (**Fig. 4**D–F). We have isolated the VY flap on angular artery perforators at the lateral nasal region, allowing greater mobility. A nasolabial flap may also be used for vertically oriented defects in this region. For horizontal or transverse defects, a miter flap from the superior nose onto the dorsum is a reliable solution (**Fig. 5**).

Combined central and lateral defects

Combined central and lateral defects in the middle third of the nose will require forehead flap coverage. If the medial cheek is involved, a cheek advancement flap should be used to reconstruct the cheek defect and a forehead flap for the nasal defect.

Full-thickness defects

Full-thickness defects will need reconstruction of lining and, often, osteocartilaginous support (see **Tables 2** and **3**). As described earlier, a septal hinge flap or a contralateral mucoperichondrial flap with septal cartilage can provide support and lining for midvault full-thickness defects. Alternatively, a nasolabial flap or forehead flap can have a skin graft placed on the undersurface for lining with a cartilage graft placed at a second stage, 3 weeks later. Small cartilage defects often do not need reconstruction of support, and a flap with a skin graft on its undersurface will suffice.

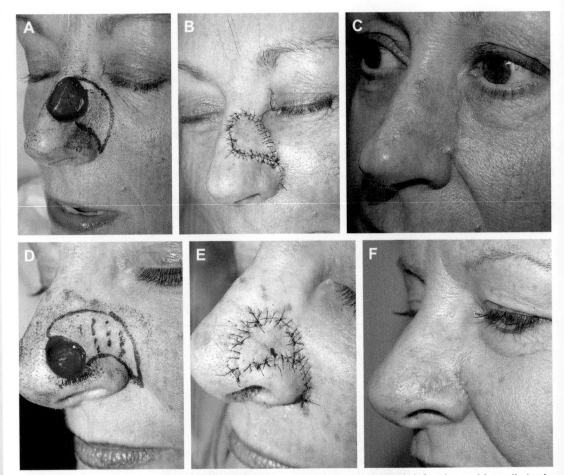

Fig. 4. The versatility of the V-Y advancement flap is shown. (*A, B, C*) A vertical defect located laterally in the middle third of the nose is closed with a V-Y flap. (*D, E, F*) A domal-alar groove defect is closed with an extended V-Y advancement flap based on angular artery perforators.

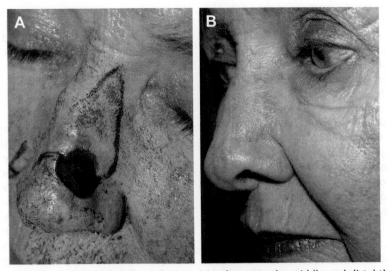

Fig. 5. (*A*) Horizontal defect located laterally at the transition between the middle and distal third of the nose, a miter flap is designed for closure. (*B*) Patient shown 3-months postoperatively.

Distal Third of Nose

The distal third zone of the nose is the most common location in our practice for nasal defects after cancer excision. This region can be divided into alar, domal-alar groove, dome, center (tip), columella, and sill subunits (see **Fig. 1**).

Alar defects

Alar defects are the most common in our practice and are most often reconstructed with a nasolabial flap (**Fig. 6**). For alar defects sparing the rim, a V-Y advancement flap may also be used with success. Any remaining alar rim will need a cartilage graft for support to prevent collapse of the rim. Small alar rim defects (up to 8 mm high) can be reconstructed with a composite graft of skin and cartilage from the root of the ear helix. Whenever a nasolabial flap is used, additional procedures to divide, inset the flap, and refine the reconstruction are generally required.

Full-thickness alar defects

Full-thickness alar defects will require a nasolabial flap, reconstruction of lining, and support. Lining can be provided with turnover flaps from local scar tissue or with a FTSG on the flap undersurface followed by a secondary cartilage graft from the septum or concha. We often take the FTSG from the dog-ear resection at the distal end of

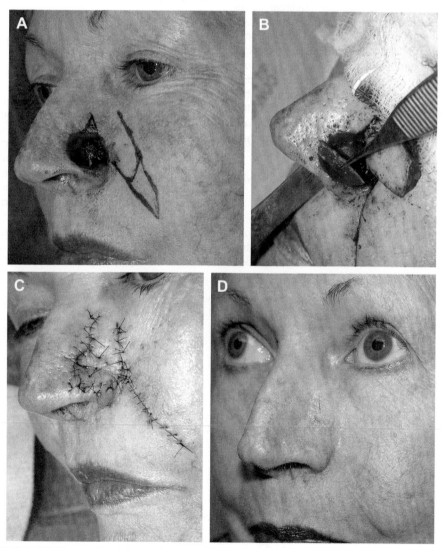

Fig. 6. (*A, B, C*) Full-thickness alar defect is shown with a small portion of alar rim intact. This was reconstructed with a superiorly based nasolabial flap with the distal portion of the flap used as a skin graft placed on the flap undersurface for lining. A septal cartilage graft was inserted into the remaining rim for support. (*D*) Patient is shown 3-months postoperatively.

the nasolabial flap. Other lining options (see **Table 2**) include a mucosal bipedicle flap or an ipsilateral mucoperichondrial flap with or without a bipedicle flap from the residual vestibular skin[8]; these can support primary cartilage grafts. When alar cartilages have been weakened or removed, they must be replaced or rebuilt.[8] If the alar rim is to be reconstructed, a cartilage graft should be placed along the new nostril margin to maintain projection and shape.

Domal-alar groove defects

Domal-alar groove defects are also common and are most often reconstructed with a nasolabial flap. A V-Y flap can be advanced from laterally to cover the defect and may be designed in an extended fashion for larger defects (see **Fig. 4**D–F). Less commonly, defects that are horizontal in orientation may be closed with a miter flap. For lining in full-thickness defects, a bipedicle lining flap or a turnover flap can be fashioned from local tissue, an ipsilateral mucoperichondrial flap can be used, or a skin graft can be placed on the flap undersurface. Cartilage grafts from the septum or concha may be needed depending on defect size and the amount of deficient cartilage.

Dome defects

Dome defects are best reconstructed with a bilobed flap.

Central defects

Central defects of the nasal tip are best reconstructed with a bilobed flap. Even large central defects are amenable to closure with extended bilobed flaps (**Fig. 7**). Cartilage tip grafts may need to be placed if there is deficient or weakened cartilage. Lining can be reconstructed with a mucoperichondrial flap or other options from **Table 2**.

Columella defects

Columella defects, if small, can be reconstructed with a composite graft from the antihelix of the ear. If no cartilage is deficient and there is intact periosteum, a FTSG may be placed. If the columella defect is large or encompasses the entire columella, a multistaged nasolabial flap or a single-staged ascending helical free flap from the ear may be the best option but is much more complex (**Fig. 8**).

Nasal sill defects

Nasal sill defects can be well reconstructed with a tunneled nasolabial flap.

Combined defects

Combined defects involving multiple subunits in the distal third of the nose will most often require a forehead flap for external skin cover. In such situations, the nasal subunit where the defect is located should be excised completely and then reconstructed with the forehead flap. If the combined defect is small, satisfactory reconstruction may still be accomplished with the previous described local flaps, especially if the defect is more lateral on the nose. In such cases, the extended V-Y or nasolabial flap are most often used. In select cases, an ascending helical free flap may provide excellent aesthetic

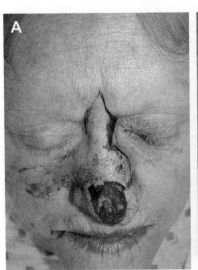
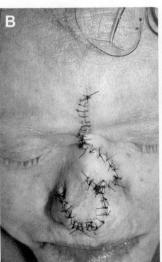
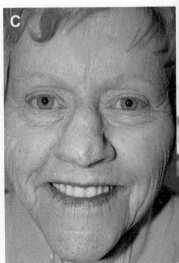

Fig. 7. (*A, B*) A bilobed flap is designed to close a central tip defect. It is important to design the dog-ear excision between the defect and flap pivot point, make the diameter of first lobe equal to the defect, and then reduce the width of the second lobe. (*C*) Patient is shown 4-months postoperatively.

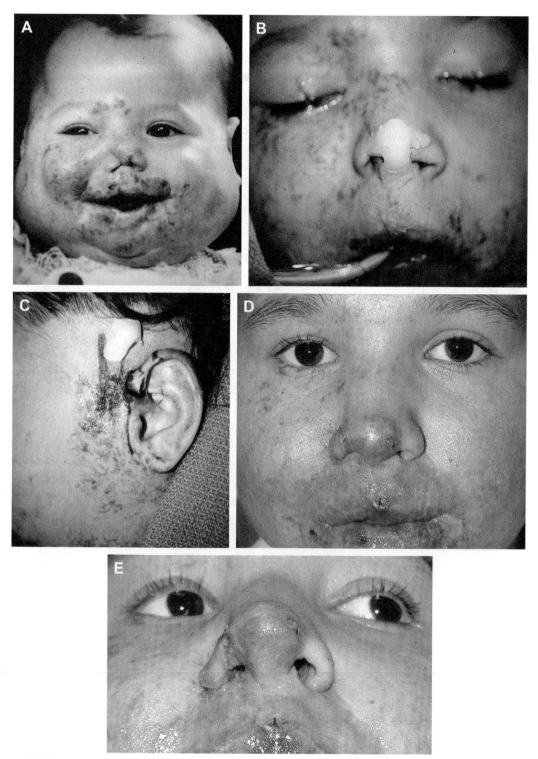

Fig. 8. (A) Shows a one-year-old baby with an aggressive hemangioma, leading to tissue necrosis and loss of the nasal columella. (B, C) At the age of 5 years, a free ascending helical flap was used for columella reconstruction. (D, E) The patient is shown 10-years postoperatively after scar revision, dermis fat grafting to the nasal tip, and dermabrasion.

results in these combined, larger defects involving the entire ala and alar rim.

Combined, full-thickness defects

Combined, full-thickness defects involving multiple zones in the distal third of the nose can be approached in various ways regarding timing and choices for lining and support. The options for nasal lining and support were discussed earlier. Commonly, a forehead flap can simultaneously be performed with a mucoperichondrial-lining flap (with or without a bipedicle flap) and cartilage grafts (**Fig. 9**). Also, a forehead flap can have a skin graft placed on its undersurface and 3 weeks later have a cartilage graft placed. Alternatively, especially for a larger lining and support defect, a well planned multistep reconstruction can be embarked on as is described for subtotal nasal loss in the next section.[22]

Combined Proximal-Middle-Distal Defects Including Subtotal or Total Nasal Loss

Defects that encompass a combination of the proximal, middle, and distal thirds of the nose will often require multistage reconstructions under general anesthesia (see **Fig. 9**). In these cases, external skin defects should be enlarged to excise

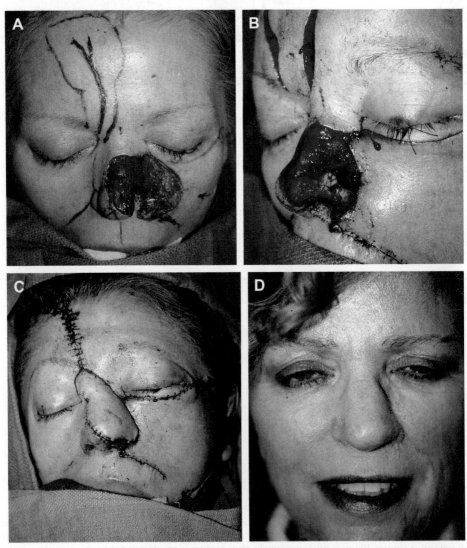

Fig. 9. (A) Shows a large nasal defect spanning multiple zones that is full-thickness in the left ala. (B) A mucoperichondrial-lining flap was raised and inset. Cartilage grafts are placed to provide support and to recreate the ala cartilage. (C) A forehead flap and cheek advancement flap were performed. (D) Patient is shown after two revisions including forehead flap thinning.

completely the aesthetic subunits involved, according to the principles by Burget and Menick.[1] This allows reconstruction of the entire subunit for maximal aesthetic benefit. If only skin is deficient, the initial procedure is most often the paramedian forehead flap. Flap thinning will need to be performed in a two- to three-staged procedure as described earlier.[9,10]

For subtotal or total nasal reconstruction with multiple layers involved, careful preoperative planning is required as this entails major multistep reconstructions with many pitfalls along the way. Large, complex central facial defects that involve the nose and surrounding structures usually require more tissue than is locally or regionally available. Conventional free tissue transfers that result in a blob reconstruction should be avoided.[15] The same principles as described above should guide reconstruction with focus on lining, support, and external skin coverage.

Burget and Walton have detailed their work in the difficult area of subtotal or total nasal reconstruction, and this should be reviewed before embarking on such complex reconstructions.[22] Their multistep procedure begins with a radial forearm flap for nasal lining with multiple paddles. This is followed in a second stage with an assembled framework of carved costal cartilage grafts and a forehead flap for external cover. The radial forearm flap provides a foundation onto which the construction of an osteocartilaginous framework and a forehead flap for external cover can be applied. Additionally, the radial forearm flap can be designed to fill cheek or upper lip defects. In a third stage, refinements including forehead flap thinning and subcutaneous sculpting are then performed before division of the forehead flap pedicle. In the final stage, the pedicle is excised and the nasal radix is sculpted and detailed. Secondary refinements may be needed in the future.

Prelaminated free flaps are also important options for total nasal reconstruction and provide well-vascularized tissue with lining and a cartilage framework that is eventually covered by a forehead flap.[18,19] Prelamination at a distant site allows recruitment of additional tissue for adjacent defects of the cheeks or lips and allows scar contracture and healing of the lining-framework construct to occur at a distant site before forehead flap placement.

SUMMARY

The treatment of nasal defects is challenging. This article and the references below have highlighted the complexity of nasal reconstruction. The authors hope that our algorithm has provided a simplified approach to this complex topic.

REFERENCES

1. Burget GC, Menick FJ. The subunit principle in nasal reconstruction. Plast Reconstr Surg 1985;76(2): 239–47.
2. Singh DJ, Bartlett SP. Aesthetic considerations in nasal reconstruction and the role of modified nasal subunits. Plast Reconstr Surg 2003;111(2): 639–48.
3. Rohrich RJ, Griffin JR, Ansari M, et al. Nasal reconstruction—beyond aesthetic subunits: a 15-year review of 1334 cases. Plast Reconstr Surg 2004; 114(6):1405–16.
4. Menick FJ. Aesthetic considerations in nasal reconstruction and the role of modified nasal subunits. Plast Reconstr Surg 2003;111(2):649–51.
5. Jackson IT. Nose reconstruction. In: Jackson IT, editor. Local flaps in head and neck reconstruction. 2nd edition. St. Louis (MO): Quality Medical Publishing; 2007. p. 101–240.
6. Guo L, Pribaz JR, Pribaz JJ. Nasal reconstruction with local flaps: a simple algorithm for management of small defects. Plast Reconstr Surg 2008;122(1): 130–9.
7. Zitelli JA. The bilobed flap for nasal reconstruction. Arch Dermatol 1989;125(7):957–9.
8. Burget GC, Menick FJ. Nasal support and lining: the marriage of beauty and blood supply. Plast Reconstr Surg 1989;84(2):189–202.
9. Menick FJ. Nasal reconstruction: forehead flap. Plast Reconstr Surg 2004;113(6):100E–11E.
10. Menick FJ. A 10-year experience in nasal reconstruction with the three-stage forehead flap. Plast Reconstr Surg 2002;109(6):1839–55.
11. Menick FJ. The use of skin grafts for nasal lining. Clin Plast Surg 2001;28(2):311–21.
12. DeQuervain F. About partial lateral rhinoplasty. Zentralbl Chir 1902;29:297–302.
13. Pribaz J, Stephens W, Crespo L, et al. A new intraoral flap: facial artery musculomucosal (FAMM) flap. Plast Reconstr Surg 1992;90(3):421–9.
14. Walton RL, Burget GC, Beahm EK. Microsurgical reconstruction of the nasal lining. Plast Reconstr Surg 2005;115(7):1813–29.
15. Taghinia AH, Pribaz JJ. Complex nasal reconstruction. Plast Reconstr Surg 2008;121(2):15e–27e.
16. Menick FJ. The nose. In: Achauer BM, Eriksson E, Guyuron B, editors. Plastic surgery: indications, operations, and outcomes. St. Louis (MO): Mosby; 2000. p. 1465–84.
17. Pribaz JJ, Falco N. Nasal reconstruction with auricular microvascular transplant. Ann Plast Surg 1993; 31(4):289–97.

18. Pribaz JJ, Weiss DD, Mulliken JB, et al. Prelaminated free flap reconstruction of complex central facial defects. Plast Reconstr Surg 1999;104(2): 357–65.

19. Pribaz JJ, Guo L. Flap prefabrication and prelamination in head and neck reconstruction. Semin Plast Surg 2003;17(4):351–62.

20. Lauer G, Schimming R, Gellrich NC, et al. Prelaminating the fascial radial forearm flap by using tissue-engineered mucosa: improvement of donor and recipient sites. Plast Reconstr Surg 2001; 108(6):1564–72.

21. Burget GC. Aesthetic reconstruction of the nose. In: Mathes SJ, editor. Plastic surgery. 2nd edition. Philadelphia: Elsevier; 2006. p. 573–648.

22. Burget GC, Walton RL. Optimal use of microvascular free flaps, cartilage grafts, and a paramedian forehead flap for aesthetic reconstruction of the nose and adjacent facial units. Plast Reconstr Surg 2007;120(5):1171–207.

The Evolution of Lining in Nasal Reconstruction

Frederick J. Menick, MD[a,b,c]

KEYWORDS

- Nasal lining • Folded forehead flap • Microvascular lining
- Skin graft lining • Hingeover flaps • Intranasal lining flaps

"In perusing the literature of this subject, one is struck chiefly with the lack of appreciation of the need for a lining for all mucous lined cavities... No nose, or portion of the nose, can be made without adequate skin for mucous lining, and the whole status of rhinoplasty, as practiced by the author and colleagues, has since that day undergone a change which is truly remarkable."
—H.G. Gillies, 1920.[1]

Historically, external skin has been the most obvious tissue deficiency after nasal trauma and skin cancer excision. The loss of underlying support or lining was less apparent and, practically speaking, an afterthought. A surgeon interested in nasal reconstruction might assume that nasal repair has always been about external skin replacement and its transfer, rather than the restoration of a nasal appearance.

Gillies,[1] after World War I, attributed the modern recognition of lining to the work of Keegan,[2] in India, before the turn of the twentieth century. Gillies found, independently, that the addition of lining to the repairs of the injured soldier prevented late retraction and loss of nasal shape.

Because of its ideal surface quality, forehead skin has long been acknowledged as the ideal donor to resurface major skin deficiencies. Five hundred years before the birth of Christ, the Indian median flap first transferred the midline forehead on paired supratrochlear arteries to resurface the nose.[3,4] Unfortunately, the underlying raw surface of the unlined flap contracted with late distortion, airway collapse, and stenosis. Slowly, surgeons addressed the problem.

Petralli (1842) folded the distal aspect of the flap to line itself. Volkman (1873) hinged over adjacent skin, bordering the defect, for lining. Both maneuvers increased the size of the defect and the size or length of the required forehead flap. The Indian flap, with a high pivot above the eyebrow, was too short to resurface the nose without carrying hairy scalp on its distal end.

To provide enough skin, the forehead flap was redesigned to increase its length and dimension. The oblique, horizontal, up and down, scalping, and sickle flaps are derivatives of this search for a bigger, longer flap. Each design increased the size or length of the flap. All also increased donor injury and scarring.[5,6]

Millard,[7,8] in the twentieth century, pivoted a "seagull" shaped flap, centered near the medial canthus, on a unilateral pedicle. This lowered the flap's base and brought the flap closer to the defect, effectively lengthening the flap and the skin available for transfer. Its narrow proximal stalk resurfaced the dorsum and its wings covered the alae. The residual donor defect was less visible high, under the hairline.

This paramedian forehead flap can be elevated on either the right or left supratrochlear pedicle.[9] The supratrochlear vessels exit the orbit over the periosteum and then pass through the corrugator muscles and into the overlying frontalis. About 2 cm above the superior orbital rim, the vessels pass through the frontalis muscle to run vertically, within the subcutaneous fat, almost adherent to skin at the hairline and into the scalp. The flap is perfused randomly, through the frontalis muscle and, most importantly, through its vertical axial vessels. Because of its axial blood supply, the width of its pedicle need only be 1 to 1.2 cm wide or less. This paramedian flap has vascularity, size, reach, reliability, efficiency, and relatively minimal morbidity. It can resurface the entire nose.

a Division of Plastic Surgery, St. Joseph's Hospital, Tucson, AZ, USA
b University of Arizona College of Medicine, Tucson, AZ, USA
c Private Practice, Tucson, AZ, USA
E-mail address: drmenick@drmenick.com

Clin Plastic Surg 36 (2009) 421–441
doi:10.1016/j.cps.2009.02.014

FLAPS IN USE TODAY

Today the nose can be lined with various flaps.[10,11]

Hingeover Flaps

Hingeover flaps of adjacent skin from the residual nose or within the medial cheek can be turned over to line a full-thickness defect. Healing of cover to lining, along the incised edges of the defect, must first occur to ensure survival through the scar along the margin of the defect.

Hingeover flaps are relatively poorly vascularized, although they usually survive if less than 1.5 cm in length. Unfortunately, contracture of the scar along the periphery of the defect narrows the airway. This stenosis persists after turning over the external skin for lining. Although the external nostril margin may seem satisfactory in size, the internal nose in the area of the hingeover flap base remains tight, limiting airflow. Later opening of the airway is difficult because of poor exposure deep within the nose, and unavailability of other tissues to fill the gap once the stricture is incised. A skin graft can be applied but recurrent contraction is frequent.

Such hingeover flaps are also stiff and thick. Their bulk occludes the airway and their rigidity prevents careful soft tissue contouring with support grafts. The unreliable vascularity of hingeover flaps contributed to the traditional hesitancy of surgeons to place primary support grafts. Lining necrosis often led to cartilage exposure and infection.

A Second Flap

Thiersch in 1879 used adjacent facial flaps. More recent choices are a second forehead flap, as suggested by Converse, or a nasolabial flap, championed by Millard. Both add additional scars to the face and are bulky.

Millard's nasolabial flaps were usually elevated as unpredictable random flaps, based on scar along the periphery of the defect. They are stiff and may die if more than 1 to 1.5 cm in length. He also elevated nasolabial tissue as axial subcutaneously based flaps. Bilateral flaps were swung medially to line the ala and then sewn together in the midline to line the back of the reconstructed columella. Unfortunately, they are also stiff and stuff the airway.

Skin Graft

A skin graft can be applied, at the time of transfer, to the deep raw surface of the forehead flap, as first used by Lossen in 1898. A full-thickness skin graft is thin and pliable. It has no intrinsic blood supply, however, and must be placed against a highly vascular bed for survival. A skin graft may not take and contracts unless braced by support. Primary support is excluded, however, because a skin graft does not survive on an avascular cartilage graft.

Early in the history of nasal repair, surgeons voiced concerns about skin graft "take" and late postoperative contraction. Kazanjian and Converse[12] noted "The septal composite (or a skin graft with separate buried cartilage graft), when placed under a scalping flap at the time of transfer, is associated with a disappointing distortion of the alar border."

Rather than place skin grafts primarily, others attempted to "build the nose on the forehead" with the prelamination technique (prefabrication). At least 6 weeks before transfer, a full-thickness skin graft, with separate cartilage pieces buried within the subcutaneous layer of the flap, or a composite skin graft were placed on the deep surface of a forehead flap. This prelaminated flap is transferred only after take is ensured. Graft shrinkage still occurred, however, in these poorly supported noses.

A prelamination delays the formal repair but does provide time to ensure graft survival. It also permits the placement of a support graft along the future nostril rim. The cartilage graft is buried in a subcutaneous pocket between the skin and frontalis of the flap and does not interfere with the vascularity of the deeper bed on which the lining skin graft is positioned.

The skin graft usually survives on raw frontalis muscle. If not, the repair is not irretrievably destroyed because the skin graft can be reapplied. The cartilage graft must be limited in size, however, and provides minimal rim support. Such support replacement does not replicate a complete, shaped, subsurface architecture or recreate a delicate three-dimensional contour.

Composite Skin Grafts

Composite skin grafts alone can be applied along the nostril margin.[13–15] They can restore limited cover and lining deficiencies along the nostril rim or within the columella.

Composite skin grafts, taken from the ear, are used to repair losses of the alar margin. Most often, a two-layered sandwich of skin containing cartilage or fat is taken from the helical root, helical rim, or lobule. They survive if placed on a well-vascularized recipient, sutured with care, and immobilized. They are most reliable if less that 1.5 cm in size.

Larger composite grafts have been recommended. Close examination reveals that they are, most often, large full-thickness skin grafts with a modest distal composite extension. The composite component is positioned as an "add on" to the full-thickness graft. Frequently, the edges of the wound are first allowed to heal secondarily. Later, adjacent normal tissue is hinged over to line the superior aspect of the full-thickness defect. This increases the surface dimension of the external defect and expands the size of the vascularized bed for the full-thickness graft. It is hoped that the revascularization of the composite component is increased by the enlarged surface area of contact of the adjoining full-thickness skin graft.

The advantages and disadvantages of both methods are now combined: stiff, questionably viable hingeover flaps and avascular skin grafts. Although the results can be good, graft "take," color and texture, and donor ear deformity are unpredictable.

Although championed by surgeons who have used them with great success, not all have been able to reduplicate these results. Nevertheless, small composite grafts can be useful if the defect is small and located along the alar rim. Their primary advantage is simplicity.

CHOOSING AMONG TRADITIONAL TECHNIQUES

Among these traditional choices, hingeover flaps remain useful to line small rim defects. Prefabricated flaps may be helpful in the elderly sick patient when a less aesthetic result is acceptable. They can be accomplished under very light monitored anesthesia.

Second flaps for lining are rarely used, although the facial artery musculomucosal flap, developed by Pribaz, which transfers intraoral mucosa based on the facial artery, is useful to line an isolated loss within the midvault in a nose injured by cocaine or Wegner's disease.

Traditional Folded Flap

The traditional folded flap folded the forehead onto itself. The cover flap was folded inward to line the nostril rim or the columellar and both alar margins, simultaneously. The flap supplies both cover and lining. Poor exposure and stiff soft tissue, however, make it impossible to position sophisticated support to shape the rim, tip, and other parts of the nose. Also, the folded flap contains two layers of folded skin, fat, and frontalis, and makes a very thick nostril margin.

Adding Support

Support, in all traditional methods of repair, has been a secondary concern. Most often, the cover and lining were left without support leading to soft tissue collapse, scar fixation, and distortion. Alternatively, cartilage grafts were designed as limited bulky cantilevers to lift the bridge, or crude, poorly shaped "cement blocks" to hold up the nostril margin and prevent the rim from falling into the airway. Excessive soft tissue bulk and fear of tissue necrosis precluded the primary placement of delicate support during initial flap transfer. Unfortunately, it was difficult or impossible to insert them secondarily once the soft tissues healed. Scarred cover and lining were stiff and not easily molded by cartilage grafts placed secondarily.

To decrease bulk and improve contour, others tried to excise excess soft tissue months later, after the soft tissues had matured. The flap edges were elevated along the peripheral margins of the flap in stages after the division of the forehead flap. Fat, frontalis, and scar were excised from one area of the nose. Some months later, while maintaining an alternate area of inset, another area was debulked. Poor exposure, piecemeal thinning, and contracted, scarred skin prevented significant improvements in contour.

Intranasal Lining Flaps

The modern revolution in nasal repair was the development of intranasal lining flaps, in the 1980s.[16,17] At first glance, there seems to be little excess residual lining within the remaining nose after a full-thickness loss. Burget realized, however, that residual intranasal lining could be elevated, based on named vessels. Equally importantly, because this lining was thin, supple, and highly vascular, primary cartilage grafts could be placed to support and shape these flimsy lining flaps at the time of their transfer. When combined with a regional unit approach to repair, the quality, border outline, and three-dimensional contour of a nose could be re-established.

A bipedicle flap of residual vestibular lining can be incised in the area of the intercartilaginous incision of cosmetic rhinoplasty. This flap is based on the septum, medially, and the alar base, laterally. Once released, it is swung inferiorly to replace the nostril margin. Its donor defect can be skin grafted or resurfaced with another lining flap (an ipsilateral or contralateral septal flap).

The ipsilateral septal mucosa can be elevated and pivoted from the septal surface to line the lower nose, based on the septal branch of the superior labial artery. Originating from the facial artery, a branch of the superior labial artery passes from the lip, just lateral to the nasal spine, near the philtral column to the base of the septum.

The contralateral septal mucosa can be elevated from the septum and swung laterally to line the opposite midvault. This flap is based dorsally on the superior ethmoidal vessels and passes through a slit in the ipsilateral septum or through a fistula created by the simultaneous elevation of an ipsilateral septal flap. The contralateral mucosal flap can line the lateral midvault but does not extend inferiorly to reach the nostril margin.

More dramatically, the entire septum can be incised deeply into the piriform aperture and swung out, based on both the right and left superior labial artery branches. This is a composite flap of bilateral septal mucosa and cartilage. It is maintained on a 1.5-cm pedicle, based at the nasal spine. Pulled out of the depths of the nasal cavity, it can be positioned anteriorly to supply central bridge support. More importantly, the septal mucosa along its free edge can be turned laterally, on each side, to fill a central lining defect for a subtotal or total nasal defect. This composite lining flap can line the upper nose within the narrower upper or middle vault. It is not long enough, however, to reach along the nostril margin to the alar base more distally. It must be sutured to a residual alar remnant or a nasolabial flap, at the nasal base, to augment lining for a defect of the inferior nasal vault.

Intranasal lining flaps are thin and supple. Equally importantly, they permit the placement of individual shaped cartilage pieces, which shape the covering skin. These support grafts, when seen through a conforming forehead flap, recreate the appearance of a nose. They also shape and support the restored lining and the airway.

Fortunately, the raw surface left in the wake of an ipsilateral flap heals spontaneously. The septal fistula, which follows the use of the combined ipsilateral and contralateral flap or a composite flap, is largely asymptomatic. Nasal bleeding is a risk and temporary nasal crusting is inconvenient.

Intranasal flaps are relatively morbid, however, especially in the elderly, and are destructive to the residual intranasal anatomy even though they work. Practically speaking, the primary limitation of intranasal flaps is their dimension. Although dramatically useful in smaller defects, as the size of the defect increases, the capability of the technique is easily overreached. An intranasal flap may be inadequate in dimension. Its distal margin may necrose. The reconstructed nostril can be too small, leading to stenosis and malposition of the nostril margin.

Intranasal lining flaps remain an important technique; however, I use them infrequently. The exception is the heminasal or subtotal loss when the combinations of ipsilateral and contralateral flaps or a composite septal flap are effective.

Three-Stage Full-Thickness Forehead Flap

More recently, forehead skin has been transferred as a three-stage full-thickness forehead flap.[10,18,19] The forehead is multilaminar, consisting of external skin, subcutaneous fat, frontalis muscle, and a thin underlying areolar layer. It is thick and stiff. Practically speaking, the surgeon needs its "skin," not the "forehead," to resurface the nose. The three-stage approach elevates a flap without initial thinning and adds an intermediate stage between transfer and pedicle division. During the intermediate operation, the flap is re-elevated with 2 mm of subcutaneous fat to create thin supple cover. Primary and delayed primary cartilage grafts are combined with extensive excision of the underlying soft tissue excess to shape a subsurface framework before pedicle division. The "thin" skin flap is returned to the recipient site. The pedicle is divided later at a third stage.

The technique maximizes the flap's vascularity and improves the final result. The need for late revisional surgery is minimized in major nasal defects, those with large skin losses, and those in which both skin and cartilage are missing. Just as importantly, it became apparent that the three-stage technique lent itself to a modification of the traditional folded method of nasal lining. This modified folded lining technique provides a simple, efficient, and widely applicable method for lining replacement that can be applied to most common nasal defects. The three-stage full-thickness flap with an intermediate operation permits the technique of the folded flap for lining to be reborn.

Modified Menick Folded Flap

The modified Menick folded flap method has unique characteristics. A full-thickness flap is highly vascular and can tolerate being turned in to line a defect. Once healed, the folded lining becomes integrated into the residual normal lining and is no longer dependent on the vascular supply of the proximal forehead flap for survival.

Importantly, the reconstructed lining remains soft and supple. Unless the subcutaneous fat is injured or the frontalis excised, wound healing is not initiated in a forehead flap. The soft tissues within a folded three-stage full-thickness flap remain soft and are easily manipulated during the intermediate operation, between initial transfer and division.

At the first stage, primary support grafts are placed only in areas in which adjacent vascularized lining is intact. They are not placed within the folded aspect of the flap, which replaces both cover and lining. Although primary support cannot be effectively placed to support and shape the folded flap initially, it can be placed in a delayed primary fashion, during the intermediate operation between transfer and flap division.

The flap, along the future nostril margin, is divided between its proximal cover and distal lining components 4 weeks after transfer. Proximal forehead skin is elevated completely off the nose with 2 to 3 mm of fat. This exposes excess soft tissue, composed of the doubled layers of frontalis, fat, and the underlying healed lining. The excess fat and frontalis are excised. The underlying soft and supple lining, healed to adjacent normal lining, is then shaped and supported with delayed primary support grafts in any area in which they were precluded at the time of initial transfer. Old primary cartilage grafts can be repositioned, carved, or augmented as needed during the intermediate stage, if they were imperfectly designed or had shifted.

Although forehead skin is used for cover and lining, the donor defect is minimally enlarged because the lining extension is harvested above distal edge of the traditional covering flap in an area normally discarded as a dogear on forehead closure. Even in a short forehead, if a few hairs are carried on the distal flap, they appear as inconsequential intranasal "vibrissae."

Although an additional intermediate stage is required to thin the flap and place delayed primary support, the interior of the nose is not injured, bleeding and crusting are avoided, and the initial transfer is less complicated and time consuming. During the intermediate operation, old primary grafts can be reshaped, augmented, or repositioned if necessary; soft tissue sculpted into a nasal shape; and delayed primary grafts placed to shape any unsupported areas. Practically speaking, thin vascular cover, shaped support, and missing lining are integrated, to the surgeon's advantage. The use of this modified technique of nasal lining has become the workhorse of my practice.

PRINCIPLES AND TECHNIQUE OF THE MENICK MODIFIED FOLDED FLAP FOR LINING
Stage 1: Flap Transfer

A full-thickness forehead flap is outlined to replace missing external skin (**Figs. 1–4**). The cover

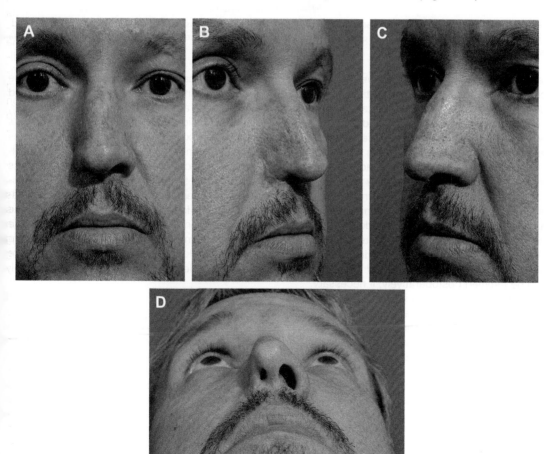

Fig. 1. (A–D) Nasal deformity after traumatic injury. The patient is missing the full-thickness of the right ala and adjacent nostril sill.

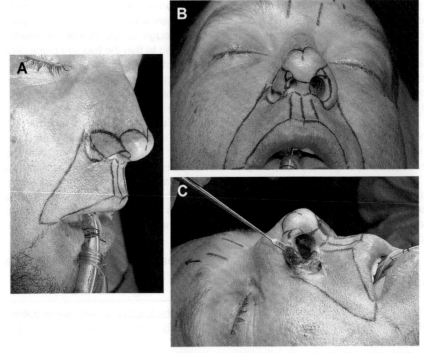

Fig. 2. (*A–C*) The nasal subunits are marked with ink. The scarred ala is released at its base. The defect is recreated. The defect includes cover and lining for the right ala and extends on to the nasal floor to the columella. The ala will be resurfaced as a subunit.

template is positioned vertically over its supratrochlear artery base. At the same time, the lining deficit is defined and a second exact template is positioned distally on the forehead, in continuity with the cover flap. The lining replacement is added as an extension of a full-thickness forehead flap. Two to 3 mm of extra length is added between these two templates to permit easy folding.

Forehead height is not a limiting factor. The lining extension lies in the area normally discarded, as a dogear, on closure of the donor site. The donor site suffers minimal extra injury. If the lining template must extend into the hairline, any transferred follicles simulate intranasal vibrissae and can be trimmed postoperatively, if necessary.

The forehead flap, as a single cover and lining unit, is elevated, with all its layers, from its distal end to its proximal base. The distal lining extension of the full-thickness forehead flap is folded inward and sutured to the residual mucosal lining about the margin of the defect with fine absorbable sutures. The more proximal aspect of the flap is folded back onto itself to supply nasal cover. It is sutured to the external skin of the recipient site in one layer. This creates, in the area of folding, an external layer of skin, subcutaneous fat, frontalis, and areolar tissue resting against an inner layer of areolar tissue, frontalis muscle, subcutaneous fat, and skin, which replaces the missing lining.

No primary cartilage support is placed within the folded flap. Primary cartilage grafts can be placed in neighboring areas of superficial injury, however, if normal residual vascularized lining remains intact. For example, if the defect combines a partial-thickness defect of the tip with a full-thickness defect of the ala, primary cartilage grafts are positioned to repair the tip loss, where vascularized lining remains. In the adjacent area of full-thickness alar loss, the lining is replaced with the distal extension of the forehead flap. No cartilage is placed within the folded flap. The proximal flap is turned back on itself to resurface the entire external skin deficiency.

Stage 2: The Intermediate Operation

Three to 4 weeks later, during an intermediate operation, the forehead flap is physiologically delayed (**Figs. 5–8**). Its blood supply is significantly augmented. The proximal aspect of the forehead flap, which was designed for cover, can be widely re-elevated and thinned with impunity. Even more importantly, its folded distal extension, which was designed to line the repair, is now integrated into the residual normal lining and is no longer dependent on the proximal forehead flap and its supratrochlear pedicle for blood supply.

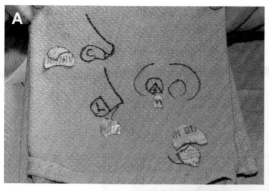

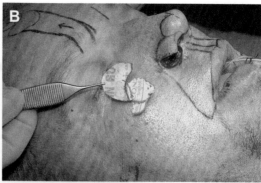

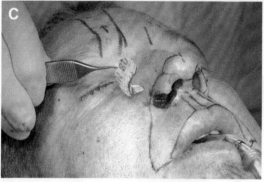

Fig. 3. (A–C) A template of the contralateral normal left ala is used to determine the correct dimension and outline of the required skin replacement for the right ala. Templates are also made of the missing alar lining and nasal floor. Subunit covering skin, nonsubunit lining, and adjacent nasal floor are replaced with the Menick modified folded flap technique. The three templates are combined. The lining template is positioned as a distal extension of the covering flap with a few millimeters of extra tissue between them as a hinge. The nasal floor template is designed as an extension of the lining template.

Because the frontalis muscle is not excised or the subcutaneous plane of the flap injured during transfer, its skin remains soft and supple. Wound contraction and scarring do not occur within the transposed flap. The forehead skin, which replaces both cover and lining, conforms to delayed primary cartilage grafts placed during the second stage. This shaped architectural framework shapes the soft tissues.

The proposed ideal nostril margin is marked with ink, based on templates of the contralateral normal alar rim or the ideal, a template of the opposite normal nostril, and by direct visualization.

Incising along the proposed alar rim, the flap is completely divided, separating the proximal covering aspect from its distal lining extension. The proximal flap is completely re-elevated with 2 to 3 mm of subcutaneous fat. The forehead flap becomes covering skin of nasal thinness. The proximal flap is temporarily placed to the side of the operative field.

The underlying double layer of soft tissue, residual subcutaneous fat, frontalis, areolar tissue and a second layer of areolar tissue, frontalis muscle, and subcutaneous fat are exposed. This

soft tissue overlies the underlying forehead skin, which was folded for lining. It is now integrated into the residual normal lining and dependent on adjacent intact lining, rather than the flap's pedicle, for blood supply. This excess soft tissue is excised. As the excess is trimmed, the newly transferred folded forehead skin is visualized. It is thin, supple, highly vascular, and approximately equal in thickness to the normal. It is difficult to distinguish from normal nasal lining and bleeds freely.

Unscarred, the reconstructed lining is now shaped, supported and braced against the future contraction of wound healing with delayed primary support grafts. Individual cartilage grafts are placed to recreate subunit support and shape.

The thin, supple, unscarred skin of the proximal flap is returned to resurface the recipient site. It covers the underlying fabrication of primary and delayed primary cartilage grafts and lining.

Stage 3: The Division

Three to 4 weeks later (6–8 weeks after beginning the nasal repair) the pedicle is divided (**Figs. 9** and **10**).

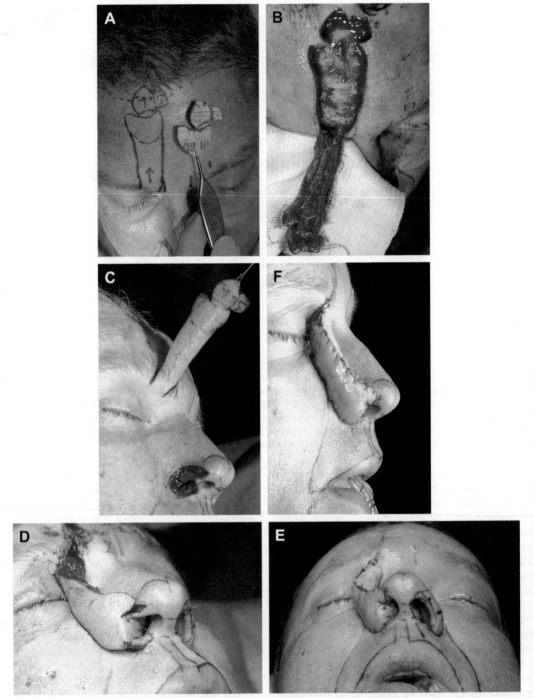

Fig. 4. (*A–F*) The combined pattern is positioned at the hairline and a forehead flap is marked with a 1.2-cm pedicle base. Any hairs carried on its distal extension simulate vibrissae. The forehead flap was elevated without thinning, as a full-thickness flap. Its distal extension is folded to supply nasal lining and floor. No primary cartilage grafts are placed. The raw pedicle is covered with a skin graft.

SKIN GRAFT INLAY METHOD

The use of skin grafts for lining[10] has also been revisited. Gillies developed the skin graft inlay

method. If lining and support were lost but the overlying skin remained intact, he released sca on the undersurface of the contracted and collapsed external skin envelope. He then applied

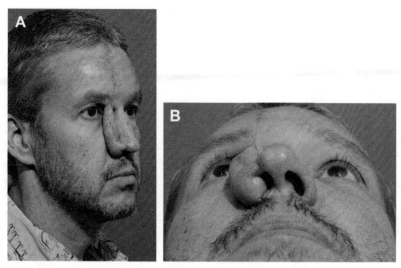

Fig. 5. (*A, B*) Four weeks later, the tissues are thick and unsupported.

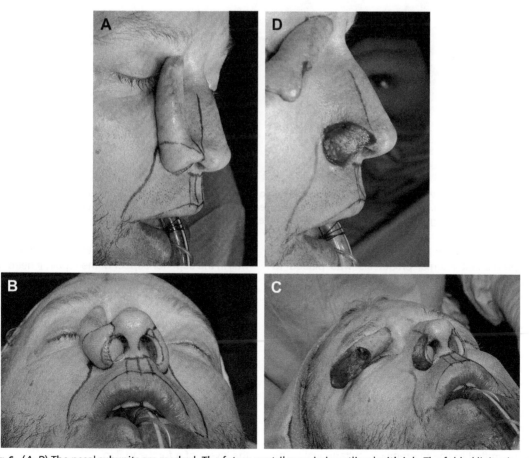

Fig. 6. (*A–D*) The nasal subunits are marked. The future nostril margin is outlined with ink. The folded lining is no longer dependent on the covering forehead flap pedicle or blood supply. The nostril margin is incised and the forehead covering skin is elevated with 2 mm of subcutaneous fat. The underlying excess double layer of subcutaneous fat, frontalis muscle, frontalis muscle, subcutaneous fat, and forehead skin lining are exposed.

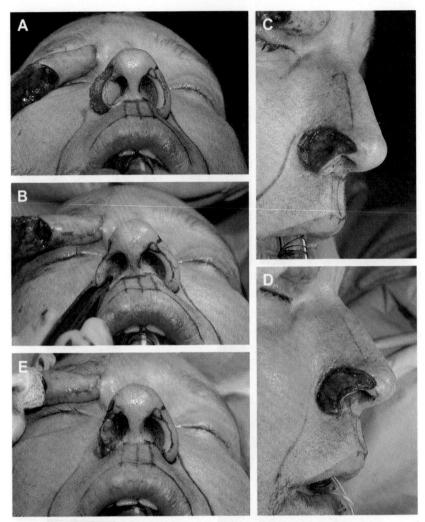

Fig. 7. (*A–E*) The excess soft tissue is excised leaving 1 to 2 mm of subcutaneous fat adherent to the underlying reconstructed lining. It is soft and supple and bleeds readily. Based on the contralateral normal alar template, a conchal cartilage graft is positioned to support, shape, and brace the right ala.

a skin graft to the raw underlying surface. When a permanent internal prosthesis was placed to splint the graft, the airway remained patent and the nasal shape was maintained. The technique was used to treat the saddlenose deformity of syphilis and leprosy.

Burget, realizing that a paramedian forehead flap is bilaminar, tunneled a cartilage graft within the subcutaneous fat between the frontalis and external skin. Completely surrounded by well-vascularized soft tissue, the cartilage graft survived. It supported and contoured the nostril margin. Because the raw undersurface of the frontalis muscle remained well vascularized, it could be skin grafted to line the repair simultaneously. The buried cartilage graft "stented" the skin grafted lining, much like Gillies' external splint. Four weeks later, the pedicle was divided. An additional

cartilage graft could be placed to support the sidewall in the superior aspect of the repair, if needed, at division.

Alternatively, a skin graft might be combined with an intranasal lining flap. In smaller unilateral defects, significant residual skin remains above the defect. A bipedicle flap of remnant vestibular skin, based on the septum medially and laterally at the alar base, is incised and transposed inferiorly to the level of the proposed alar margin. Because the marginal bipedicle flap has its own blood supply, a primary cartilage graft can be sutured to its vascularized external surface. The rim support graft does not need to be buried within the layers of a forehead flap.

After its transfer inferiorly, a secondary lining defect appears above the vascularized vestibular flap. It is repaired with a full-thickness skin graft

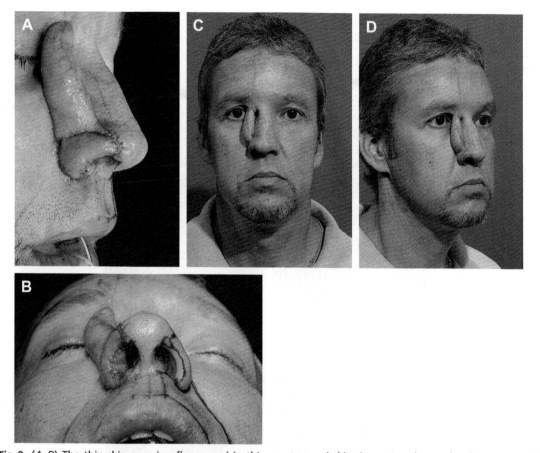

Fig. 8. (A–D) The thin skin covering flap, equal in thinness to nasal skin, is resutured over the thin supported lining. Four weeks later (8 weeks after flap transfer) the pedicle is ready for division.

The skin graft is vascularized by the undersurface of a full-thickness forehead flap. This precludes the placement of a primary cartilage graft, under the more superior aspect of the covering flap, to support the superior aspect of the defect. But 3 weeks later, the forehead flap can be partially re-elevated. The skin graft lining is now vascularized through the adjacent residual lining. A delayed primary cartilage graft can be placed over the previously unsupported area to shape the superior ala and sidewall at pedicle division or during an intermediate operation.

In both methods, rim support is supplied during the first stage (within a marginal pocket between the skin and frontalis of a full-thickness forehead flap or over a bipedicle vestibular flap). The superior aspect of the defect remains initially unsupported. At a second stage 3 weeks later, once the skin graft is vascularized, the flap's pedicle can be divided or an intermediate operation can be performed. Excess soft tissue and scar is excised in the superior aspect of the defect, and a shaped plate of cartilage or bone is inserted to support the nasal sidewall and middle vault. The delayed primary graft is placed above the previously tunneled rim support graft or above the primary graft positioned over the bipedicle flap. After two or three stages, a sheet of hard tissue lies within the defect to brace the entire repair against upward retraction or inward collapse.

These lining skin grafts retain most of their original dimensions, although the aesthetic result may be less precise. Some graft contracture does occur, causing minor distortion. Unfortunately, narrowing of the internal valve is not uncommon and difficult to fix.

Still, it is a simple technique and requires less intranasal dissection than intranasal septal lining flaps. It was recommended by Burget when the nasal mucosa has been injured or is unavailable (which precludes intranasal lining flaps); in the elderly or debilitated patient (when the risk of intranasal bleeding or crusting is best avoided); or for the less demanding patient who desires a simple, less elegant repair and accepts a lesser result.

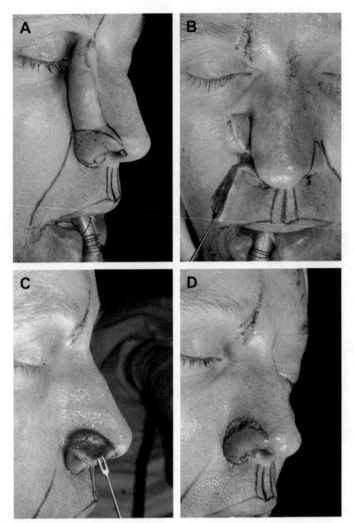

Fig. 9. (*A–D*) The pedicle is divided. The proximal aspect is reinserted as a small inverted "V" at the brow. Distally, the skin is elevated with 2 mm of subcutaneous fat. This exposes the underlying excess bulk within the superior ala. This is excised, recreating the convexity of the alar surface and the depth of the alar crease. Excess skin is trimmed and inset with quilting sutures and peripheral sutures.

THE MENICK MODIFIED METHOD OF SKIN GRAFT FOR LINING

The development of the three-stage forehead flap, with an intermediate operation, has broadened the application of skin grafts for nasal lining. The Menick modified method of skin graft for lining was developed to permit placement of a complete and ideally shaped cartilage framework, before the completion of wound healing. Its principles are similar to those of the folded flap lining technique.

Stage 1

A full-thickness forehead flap is highly vascular. A full-thickness skin graft routinely takes on the deep areolar surface of a full-thickness forehead flap. Unlike the raw bleeding surface of a two-stage

forehead flap in which the frontalis and subcutaneous fat have been excised, the areolar surface of a full-thickness forehead flap provides a reliable and dry bed onto which a skin graft can be applied with success.

An exact pattern of the lining defect is outlined and transferred from the postauricular area. The full-thickness skin graft is sutured with fine absorbable materials to the adjacent residual normal mucous membrane. The skin graft replaces missing lining in the area of full-thickness loss.

Because a primary cartilage graft placed between a skin graft and the undersurface of the flap interferes with revascularization, primary cartilage grafts are precluded in the area of skin graft lining replacement. Cartilage support can be placed over normal residual vascularized

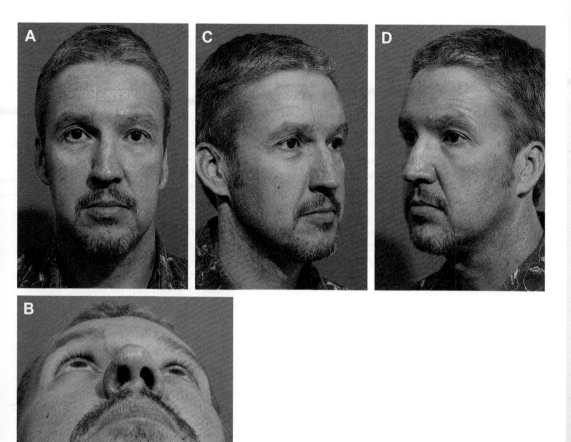

Fig. 10. (*A–D*) Postoperatively, overall quality, outline, and contour of the nose and nasal floor have been restored. The forehead scar is minimal. Subunit cover, non-subunit lining, and missing nasal floor had been restored with a folded forehead flap. No revision was performed.

lining, however, adjacent to the full-thickness defect.

Support grafts are not placed in soft tissue tunnels within the flap's subcutaneous tissue. This avoids a thick nostril rim and soft tissue injury and scar. It is also difficult to design a tunneled cartilage graft with the correct size and shape or to position it correctly within a tunnel. Although useful, pocketed cartilage grafts provide only limited control over nasal form. They are no longer used.

After placing the lining graft, a full-thickness forehead flap is transferred to resurface the nose, based on an exact template of the recipient cover requirement. It provides a vascular bed for the lining skin graft. The flap is sutured to the recipient site with a single layer of fine absorbable sutures. The skin graft is quilted to the overlying vascular bed of the forehead flap. It is also splinted with a sponge bolus, placed within the nostril for 3 to 4 days to immobilize the repair and apply stabilizing pressure.

Stage 2

At 4 weeks, the skin graft is integrated into the adjacent normal residual lining and is no longer dependent on the covering flap for its blood supply.

Occasionally, the skin graft fails. Practically speaking, it often takes 1 to 2 weeks to be sure. Once identified, the granulating bed on the undersurface of the forehead flap is sharply debrided and a second graft applied (the forehead flap does not need to be re-elevated from the recipient site). Because the frontalis muscle is not excised during the initial procedure, the subcutaneous plane of the full-thickness forehead flap remains uninjured. Wound healing and fibrosis are not initiated. The flap remains soft and noncontracted, even if the skin graft fails to take and must be reapplied. A full-thickness forehead flap is thicker and stiffer than forehead skin alone. The intrinsic thickness of the flap acts as a brace and limits early distortion caused by scarring on its undersurface. Significant early scar contraction does not occur. Although the final result is delayed and an additional stage required, the overall result is not impaired.

At the second stage (4 weeks after flap transfer), the covering skin with 2 to 3 mm of subcutaneous fat is incised along its periphery and completely re-elevated, creating thin supple cover of nasal thinness. It remains soft and supple. It is temporarily positioned to the side of the operative field.

Excess subcutaneous fat and frontalis, which lay over the skin graft, are exposed. This excess soft tissue is excised down to the newly reconstructed lining. The skin graft remains thin, relatively supple, and highly vascular. It is difficult to distinguish from normal lining and bleeds readily. Unscarred, it can now be shaped, supported, and braced against future wound contraction with delayed primary cartilage grafts. Individually designed subunit cartilage replacements are positioned to restore the aesthetics and function of the nose. An alar margin batten is fixed to support and shape the nostril margin and to support the airway against collapse. A sidewall brace is placed to support the middle vault and against upward retraction. A complex cartilage framework is restored in a single operation.

Once a complete cartilaginous framework has recreated a subsurface shape, the thin supple forehead skin flap is replaced over the delayed primary cartilage grafts, the sculpted soft tissue, and restored skin graft lining. It is sutured along its periphery and fixed with percutaneous quilting sutures to eliminate dead space and conform the flap to the recipient site bed.

Stage 3

Four weeks later (7–8 weeks after forehead flap transfer) the pedicle is divided. This modified skin graft technique for lining is reliable, efficient, and effective for the repair of small, full-thickness nasal defects. Most importantly, it permits the combination of skin graft lining and a complete, sculptured support framework.

Skin graft "take" is routine, although a second graft may be required in 20% to 30% of cases. All repeat grafts have taken. Even if the initial skin graft fails, the final result is not impaired, although an additional stage is required to replace the skin graft. An initial skin graft loss delays pedicle division for 12 weeks, however, rather than the routine 6 to 8 weeks normally required for an uncomplicated three-stage skin graft technique.

Scar contraction and secondary distortion are modest. A delicate alar rim can be created. The technique should be limited, however, to lining defects of 0.5 to 1.5 cm in size. The risk of poor skin graft take and subsequent contraction increases as the size of the lining defect increases. Moderation in the use of the method is recommended.

It is especially useful in the elderly or the debilitated patient when the risk of temporary nasal obstruction caused by crusting, edema, or intranasal bleeding should be minimized or when previous injury or rhinoplasty precludes the use of intranasal lining flaps. Overall morbidity, as in the folded flap technique for lining, is minimal. The occasional poor revascularization of skin graft lining and the requirement for another application, however, can make repair tedious. Equal or better results can be obtained with the folded forehead flap lining technique. The modified folded flap lining technique is the preferred option. The skin graft lining method is alluring, but not as attractive. I rarely use it anymore, but it should be in one's armamentarium and it can be helpful, especially in a salvage situation.

The modified folded forehead flap and modified skin graft lining techniques are recommended for moderate-sized defects of the nose. They are excellent choices for most common full-thickness nasal defects. Both methods are reliable, less complex, require little intranasal manipulation, shorten the operating time, and are associated with minimal morbidity. Because of their simplicity, they are applicable to almost all patients. They are especially attractive in the smoker, the elderly, those with unassociated medical illness, or when intranasal lining flaps are unavailable.

I rarely use skin grafts for lining today. I use the folded flap method for all defects less than 3 cm in size. The folded forehead flap lining technique is my everyday solution to complex nasal problems. The ease of its use and its good results make it my first choice. Because of its reliability, it is preferred over the skin graft technique for even small defects. All available lining options should be considered for any specific defect but, in my practice, the modified folded technique is my first choice for all small and moderate defects.

THE USE OF DISTANT MICROVASCULAR TISSUE

Distant tissue can provide large amounts of vascularized tissue to repair a large, complicated wound caused by trauma or massive cancer excision, to protect exposed vital deep structures, and to control infected or radiated beds. Distant skin, however, does not match facial skin in quality. Microvascular transfer of distant tissue is used for "invisible" requirements. Distant skin on an exposed visual surface always looks like a patch.

Microvascular distant flaps are used to line the nose and oral cavities and supply soft tissue bulk and vascularity. Then, conventional techniques, using local grafts and regional flaps, are applied to resurface facial units and the nose. Free flaps[20] can line the nose in complicated cases, but the external surface of the repair is restored with a forehead flap.

As long as the microvascular flap is thin enough to line the nose, without stuffing the airway, and has a long enough pedicle to pass from the defect to the available recipient vessels, the specific microvascular tissue or its exact design is of little importance. More critical is a careful preoperative analysis of the anatomic defect (the site, size, and position of missing tissues) and the aesthetic deficiencies that require replacement (the nose and lip-cheek platform).

A technique that permits modification of local and distant tissues to recreate conforming cover, shaped support, and thin lining is vital. Staged repairs are planned to recreate the defect; reposition the normal to its normal position; build a stable facial platform; and, sequentially, supply lining, support, and cover. The three stage full-thickness forehead method permits a timed integration of cover, lining, and support, which can restore the three-dimensional character of a normal nose. Success is determined by the surgeon's ability accurately to define the tissue and aesthetic requirements, his or her ability to coordinate available local and distant tissue, and the effectiveness of shaping these tissues into a nose. The specific microvascular donor or the number of paddles is secondary. Each defect is different. Only a thoughtful approach, which meets the needs of the specific problem, and careful modification of all transferred tissues work.

PRINCIPLES OF FREE FLAP LINING

The normal nose is projected and positioned on the lip and cheek. If missing, the facial platform must be restored, often at a preliminary operation.[10,21–23] Major defects are filled with the bulk of a truncal free flap (often a latissimus or scapular flap, which replaces soft tissue and bone) as needed. Then the nose is recreated on a stable facial base.

Identify the nasal needs (cover, support, and lining). Although visually enormous, the typical full-thickness defect is limited to a few centimeters of lining loss within the projecting aspect of the nose. Lining may be missing over the tip and dorsum, but the rest of the nose remains. The dorsal and caudal septum is largely intact. Such limited lining losses can be replaced with local tissue.

Massive, more complicated defects typically have lost lining for the nasal vault, columellar, and the nasal floor. The septum may be completely absent. The residual lining may be unavailable because of prior injury or irradiation. Such wounds require distant free-flap lining because simpler options are unavailable or less reliable.

The vault spans from alar base to alar base and projects anteriorly to the tip. Although easily underestimated, about 8 cm of skin is required to arc, transversely, from one alar base to the other, across the nasal tip. Vertically, 4 cm of skin is needed to span from nasal root to tip and an additional 3 cm is needed to line the back of the columella. Re-establishment of vault lining is straightforward. It must simply drape across a central support, which prevents its collapse into the pyriform aperture.

The columella, for practical purposes, requires only a soft tissue backing to envelope cartilage support and to line the posterior surface of a covering forehead flap. The columella must be long enough to project the nose and narrow enough to maintain patent nostrils and open airways without obstruction. If the internal septum is absent, the septal partition is not reconstructed. To avoid stuffing the airway with transferred tissue, a septal fistula is accepted.

The nostril floor (sill) is the skin platform onto which the nose is placed. In many cases, the floor remains intact. If it is absent, it is often restored before the nasal repair during a preliminary operation. It may also be reconstructed at the time of free-flap transfer with local tissue or part of the free flap.

A floor deficiency may be obvious after excision or trauma, especially if an open wound is present or, by history, if the lip has suffered extensive injury. The loss of the floor or sill is less apparent, however, when the injury is caused by cocaine or other intranasal processes. Clinically, the upper lip retrudes or retracts inward, creating a "monkey lip" deformity, because of the contraction, which follows intranasal lining injury. This is identified by displacement and posterior angulation of the upper lip. The lip is pulled inward and adheres to the pyriform aperture, across the lip and alar bases. This must be corrected by lip release and skin replacement under the future alar and columellar bases.

The reconstruction is planned in stages. The initial goal is to supply lining for the inner surface of the nose. A radial forearm flap is usually used as a skin-only flap. Its fasciocutaneous layer is excised, except for the fascia over the radial vessels. This soft tissue connection maintains its vascular connections to the overlying skin paddle.

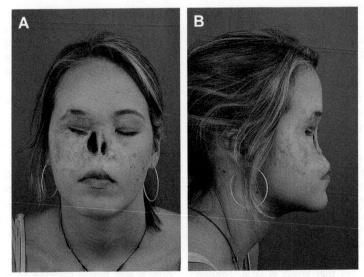

Fig. 11. (*A, B*) Shotgun injury with total nasal loss, skin grafted cheek, and exenteration.

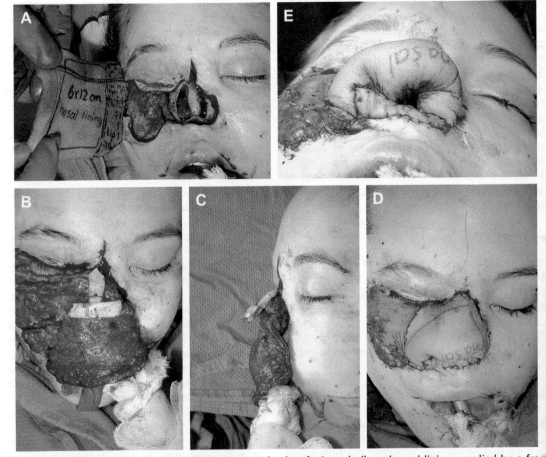

Fig. 12. (*A–E*) Skin excised from right cheek. Missing cheek soft tissue bulk and nasal lining supplied by a free radial forearm flap draped over a reconstruction plate and temporary cadaver rib grafts for dorsal support. The distal aspect of the radial flap is folded back on itself to provide its own covering skin. No columella lining is restored. A fasciocutaneous extension flap fills the nasal floor defect after the release of upper lip retraction. The raw cheek surface of the skin is grafted.

Survival of the free flap must be ensured. Swelling is allowed to resolve before going forward with cartilage grafts and cover. Later, during forehead flap transfer, the lining flap can be thinned more aggressively (and safely) and more extensive support placed.

Some months later, subcutaneous fat is excised under loupe magnification almost to forearm skin. The vascular leash is maintained. Then a complete, shaped support framework is placed. The lining and cartilage framework is resurfaced with forehead skin, which matches the face in color and texture.

The free flap is placed with its skin surface inward for lining. Its external surface is temporarily covered with a full-thickness skin graft or, more often, folded onto itself to provide vascularized skin for temporary external cover. Folding the flap on itself establishes a cleaner initial wound, initiates less scarring within the repair, and allows for greater flexibility at the time of forehead resurfacing.

If underlying support is completely absent, folding the lining flap onto itself also allows a cantilevered dorsal graft to be placed initially. This prevents the lining from collapsing into the pyriform aperture and establishes a preliminary projecting dorsal nasal line.

If the height of the residual native septum is adequate, the flap is simply draped over the remaining septum. The skin of the radial flap is sutured to the periphery of the defect, positioning the raw soft tissue externally.

If the septum remains but has been partially resected, it can be swung out of the nasal cavity as an inferiorly based composite septal flap. The septal flap is transferred during a preliminary operation. This helps restore the dorsal line and provides support for the free flap lining and additional dorsal unit grafts.

If residual central septal partition is missing (eg, cancer excision, cocaine injury, or immune disease), it is not reconstructed. Local or distant tissue is too thick to rebuild the septum without creating an airway obstruction. A large septal fistula is largely asymptomatic. The surgeon only provides lining for the vault and backing for the columella.

In smaller defects, the floor defect can be repaired with local tissue. If available, the cheek is advanced and the nasal floor defect repaired with a nasolabial skin.

Alternatively, external skin of the residual nose that will be discarded can be de-epithelialized on its deep surface and hinged on its lateral alar base. These bilateral local flaps are sutured in the midline of the lip to resurface the nasal floor.

A larger tissue loss within the floor is replaced with extensions of the nasal lining free flap. They can be designed in continuity, as an extension of the lining flap (a random or fasciocutaneous extension), or as a separate paddle with an axial pedicle of radial vessels.

Building a long thin columella and maintaining patent airways is the most difficult challenge. The goal is a lined soft tissue envelope that contains cartilage support, projects the tip, separates the airways, and provides a backing for the columellar extension of a forehead covering flap. The septal partition is not reconstructed.

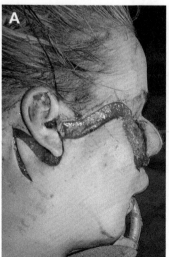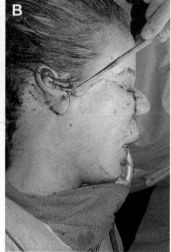

Fig. 13. (A, B) Subsequently, the skin graft is excised and the cheek resurfaced with an advancing Schrudde cheek flap.

SEVERAL OPTIONS EXIST TO RESTORE COLUMELLAR LINING

The lining flap can be designed with an incontinuity columella extension. Although slightly smaller in size, it has the same outline as the forehead flap used for external cover. Its skin surface is positioned inward to line the nose. Its external raw surface of the flap is skin grafted. This is considered if the septum is intact and strong central support remains to maintain projection and nasal length. Unfortunately, it is very easy to shortchange the defect and fail to re-establish a long columella and ample open nostril margins. Scar contraction and gravity are difficult to overcome,

if dorsal support is not in place initially. In general, this approach is avoided.

At the time of vault replacement, the free flap can be draped under a cantilevered dorsal graft, placed for initial support. The radial flap is folded back on itself distally, in the general area of the future nostril margin, to cover its own outer surface and protect the dorsal graft. Lining for the columella is not initially provided (**Figs. 11** and **12**).

Some months later, the folded external skin is hinged inferiorly and trimmed along the proposed nostril margins, except for a central extension of skin, which is unfolded, turned inward and "tubed" (opened outward) to create internal lining for the columella partition, which envelopes a columellar

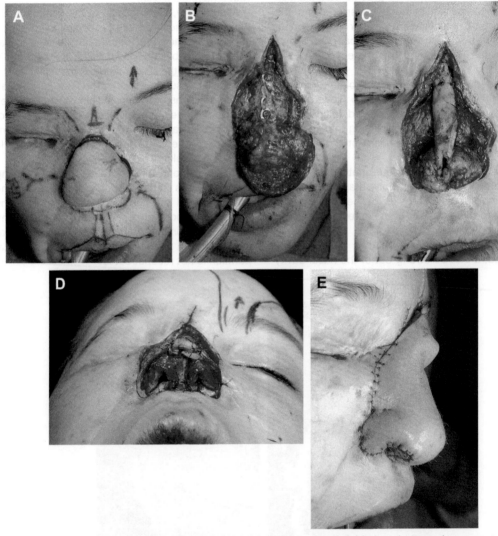

Fig. 14. (*A–E*) Subsequently, the external radial skin is hinged downward, folded, and trimmed to recreate nostril margins and a posterior backing for the future columella. Autogenous rib grafts are placed as a dorsal strut, columellar strut, tip graft, and bilateral alar margin battens. The nose is covered with a full-thickness three-stage paramedian forehead flap.

support graft. The distal tip of the columellar flap is sutured into a de-epithelialized columellar inset site in the midline of the lip (**Figs. 13–16**).

If care is taken to design a long columella and ample nostril apertures, this works. The results are better than in the previous method because edema has resolved, more aggressive thinning is possible after maturation of the free flap, and a strong complete support framework can be placed simultaneously with lining and a forehead flap. The rims and columella must be rigidly but trussed by cartilage grafts. Secondary revisions are likely, however, to revise the airways and open the nostril margins.

Lining is most successfully designed by infolding the free flap on itself to create columella, vault lining, and nostril margins. This is similar to the old traditional technique of folding a distal forehead flap on itself to provide its own cover and lining. This method can produce a long columella, arching vestibules, and elegant nostril rims.

The radial forearm flap is transferred to the defect and its blood supply re-established. The external skin side of the flap is pinched centrally, between the surgeon's fingers, along the planned distal nostril margin. This approximates the underlying raw flap surface to itself. The raw surfaces of the future columella are folded against each other

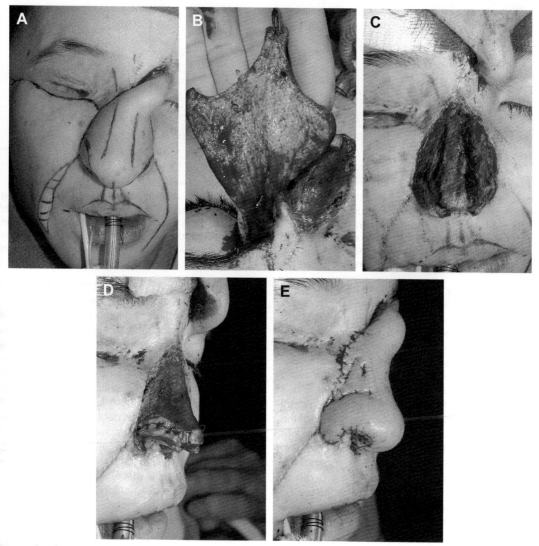

ig.15. (*A–E*) During the later intermediate operation, forehead skin was elevated with 2 mm of subcutaneous fat nd the underlying excess soft tissue and cartilage grafts sculpted into a nasal shape. The thin flap was returned o the donor site. The pedicle was later divided and a revision performed.

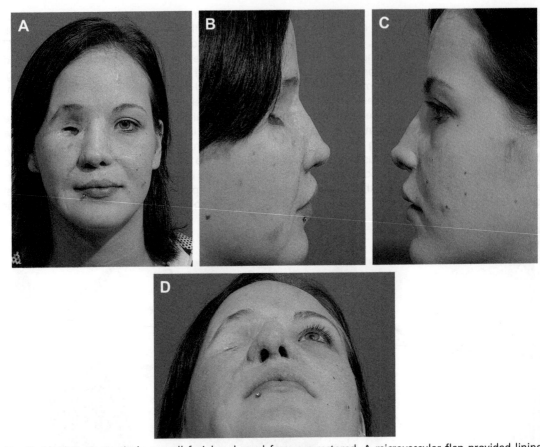

Fig. 16. (A–D) Postoperatively, overall facial and nasal form are restored. A microvascular flap provided lining Success, however, is dependent on the exact replacement of missing tissues and their modification from "unlike" to "like" tissue. Forehead flaps, rib grafts, and forearm skin have nothing in common with a "nose." The three-stage forehead flap technique with an intermediate operation permits the restoration of quality, two-dimensional border outline and three-dimensional contour. There is nothing magical about free flaps or their design. The surgeon only need identify and replace what is missing.

and sutured along their free margin to approximate the skin surfaces to one another. This creates a columella with an external skin surface and bilateral membranous septal epithelial surfaces. It length is adjusted by altering the height of the pinch and infolding, more or less. This soft tissue columella is advanced upward under the more proximal aspect of the flap. As the flap is folded under, it lines itself, creating vault lining and nostril margins. The deepest, most superior aspect of the fold is fixed centrally with an absorbable suture to the raw undersurface of the overlying free flap surface to maintain its position. The length of the columella, the nostril margins, and the depth of the membranous septum are easily adjusted by manipulation of the design.

Two months later, after resolution of edema and wound healing, the proposed nostril margins are marked. Excess external forearm skin is excised. Folded skin along the rim is hinged over, as needed, and trimmed to design the ideal nostril

rim. The external skin surface of the healed reconstructed columella is split to allow inset of the forehead flap. A complete cartilage support framework is placed to support, shape, and brace the repair.

This design is the first choice. It is simple, easily adjustable intraoperatively, and permits the creation of a long columella and capacious arching nostril margins. Smooth, arching, unscarred nostril margins and vestibular lining are established. The flap's infolding adds a degree of soft tissue support, which is invaluable in the early postoperative period. The continuity of the columella and nostril margin maintains an open airway until permanent support is placed. Temporary cadaver grafts can also be used, until definitive support is placed during a later stage. This method does not attempt to recreate a deep septum partition, which may occlude the inner airway.

In some cases, a remnant of the native columella and adjoining scarred dorsal skin can be cut from residual nasal skin, which is otherwise discarded.

It is shifted and made available to line the columella and back the external columellar repair. Such excess can also be used to resurface a retracted nostril floor or nasal base after its release.

If a stable platform is present or has been restored, a nose can be restored in four operations over 4 to 5 months. Lining is positioned with a free radial flap. Two months later, a complete support framework is established and the nose is resurfaced with a full-thickness three-stage forehead flap. One month later, the forehead flap is completely re-elevated and the soft tissues sculpted. One month later, the pedicle is divided. At this point, the overall result should be good. A revision, 4 to 6 months later, is needed to define the alar creases and nostril margins or debulk the airways. In general, if unexpected complications do not occur, the patient should be confident that his or her future is bright.

SUMMARY

The complexity of these reconstructions should not be minimized, but when carefully planned and executed, they progress with relatively few problems. Success is determined by the surgeon's ability to diagnose the anatomic and aesthetic deficiencies and to integrate soft and hard tissues, rather than by the ability to perform microvascular surgery.

My practice includes a great deal of nasal reconstruction. I use the folded forehead lining technique as my routine technique. It can repair most common defects. A free flap is used in more complex cases. Other techniques are used infrequently.

REFERENCES

1. Gillies H. Plastic surgery of the face. London: Oxford Medical; 1920.
2. Keegan D. Rhinoplastic operations with a description of recent improvements in the Indian method. London: Tindal and Cox; 1900.
3. Menick FJ. Aesthetic refinements in use of forehead for nasal reconstruction: the paramedian forehead flap. Clin Plast Surg 1990;17:607.
4. Kanzanjian V. The repair of nasal defects with the median forehead flap: primary closure of the forehead wound. Surg Gynecol Obstet 1946;83:307.
5. New G. Sickle flaps for nasal reconstruction. Surg Gynecol Obstet 1945;80:497.
6. Converse J. Reconstruction of the nose by the scalping flap technique. Surg Clin North Am 1959; 39:335.
7. Millard D. Aesthetic reconstructive rhinoplasty. Clin Plast Surg 1981;8:169.
8. Millard D. Reconstructive rhinoplasty for the lower two thirds of the nose. Plast Reconstr Surg 1976; 57:700 22.
9. MacCarthy J, Lorenc T, Cutting C, et al. The median forehead flap revisited: the blood supply. Plast Reconstr Surg 1985;76:866.
10. Menick F. Nasal reconstruction: art and practice. Elsevier Publishing; 2008.
11. Burget G, Menick F. Aesthetic reconstruction of the nose. Mosby; 1993.
12. Kazanjian V, Converse J. Surgical treatment of facial injury. Baltimore: Williams & Wilkins; 1949. p. 352.
13. Converse J. Composite graft from the septum in nasal reconstruction. Trans Lat Am Cong Plast Surg 1956;8:281.
14. Gillies HA. New free graft applied to the reconstruction of the nostril. Br J Surg 1943;30:305.
15. Gillies H, Millard DR. The principles and art of plastic surgery. Boston: Little Brown; 1957.
16. Burget G, Menick F Nasal support and lining: the marriage of beauty and blood supply. Plast Reconstr Surg 1989;84:189.
17. Kazanjian V. Reconstruction of the ala using a septal flap. Trans Am Acad Ophthalmol Otolaryngol 1937; 42:338.
18. Menick F. 10-Year experience in nasal reconstruction with the 3 stage forehead flap. Plast Reconstr Surg 2002;109:1839.
19. Menick FJ. A new modified method for nasal lining: the Menick technique for folded lining. J Surg Oncol 2006;94:509.
20. Menick F. Defects of the nose, lip and cheek: rebuilding the composite defect. Plast Reconstr Surg 2007;120:1228.
21. Menick F. Facial reconstruction with local and distant tissue: the interface of the aesthetic in reconstructive rhinoplasty. Plast Reconstr Surg 1999;102:1424.
22. Burget G, Walton R. Optimal use of microvascular free flaps, cartilage grafts, and a paramedian forehead flap for aesthetic reconstruction of the nose and adjacent facial units. Plast Reconstr Surg 2007;120:1228.
23. Burget G, Walton R. Microsurgical reconstruction of nasal lining. Plast Reconstr Surg 2005;115:1813.

Nasal Reconstruction with a Forehead Flap

Frederick J. Menick, MD[a,b,c]

KEYWORDS

- Forehead flap • Two-stage forehead flap
- Three-stage forehead flap • Nasal reconstruction
- Nasal defects

"The tint of forehead skin so exactly matches that of the face and nose that a forehead flap must be the first choice for reconstruction of a nasal defect."

—H.D. Gillies and D.R. Millard

The forehead makes by far the best nose. With some plastic surgery juggling, the forehead defect can be camouflaged effectively.

The use of a forehead flap, however, is not particularly indicated where only a new surface of the nose is required. Although its color is natural, the flap is liable to be a little too thick; if time and opportunity allow it to be thinned adequately, however, an acceptable contour can be achieved.[1]

PRINCIPLES

The forehead and scalp are richly perfused by the supraorbital, supratrochlear, superficial temporal, postauricular, and occipital vessels. These axial vessels permit its safe and effective transfer on multiple individual vascular pedicles.[2] The first "Indian" flap transferred forehead tissue on both the right and left supratrochlear vessels.[3] The midline forehead was pivoted on a high, wide base, positioned above the eyebrow. This technique, however, limited the length of available skin, if hair-bearing scalp was to be avoided on its distal end.

Employing a modern design, Millard[4–6] designed a "seagull"-shaped flap on a unilateral pedicle, centered on the medial canthus. A narrow, proximal, vertical stalk resurfaced the dorsum, and its distal wings covered the alae. Its low base brought the flap closer to the defect and effectively lengthened the flap's reach. It harvested forehead tissue in both vertical and horizontal directions. The majority of the donor site was closed as a T-shaped scar. The flap could resurface the entire nose. This paramedian flap has vascularity, size, reach, reliability, efficiency, and relatively minimal morbidity. It can be elevated on a right or left supratrochlear pedicle.

The supratrochlear vessels exit the orbit over the periosteum and then pass through the corrugator muscles. About 2 cm above the superior orbital rim, the vessels pass through the frontalis muscle to run vertically upward, within the subcutaneous fat, almost adherent to skin at the hairline and into the scalp. The flap is perfused from three sources: randomly, through the frontalis muscle, and, most importantly, through its vertical axial vessels. Because of its axial blood supply, the width of the pedicle can be narrowed to 1.0 to 1.2 cm or less at its base.[7]

The shortest distance between two points is a straight line. If skin harvest is not precluded by scar or pedicle injury, central nasal defects can be repaired, based on either the right or left brow. Lateral defects, however, are repaired with an ipsilateral rather than a contralateral pedicle. An ipsilateral pedicle places the base of the flap closer to a unilateral defect and shortens the distance from the donor site to the recipient site. The base of a contralateral pedicle is farther from the defect, making the recipient site harder to reach, so the flap must be longer.

Some suggest that a contralateral flap is easier to rotate, but the difference in "twist" is minimal,

[a] Division of Plastic Surgery, St. Joseph's Hospital, Tucson, AZ, USA
[b] University of Arizona College of Medicine, Tucson, AZ, USA
[c] Private Practice, Tucson, AZ, USA
E-mail address: drmenick@drmenick.com

Clin Plastic Surg 36 (2009) 443–459
doi:10.1016/j.cps.2009.02.015

perhaps 180° versus 160°. The most important maneuver in flap rotation is to incise the flap lower on its medial edge than on its lateral edge. It then is rotated, medially, toward the nose, regardless of flap's base. The problem with a contralateral flap is the extra length required, not the ease or difficulty of transfer.

To increase the length, some elevate a forehead flap obliquely, to slant across the forehead, or raise a vertical flap, which then passes transversely under the hairline. Unfortunately, both designs cross the midline and transect the vertical axial vessels. The "working" paddle becomes random. Although it may survive, the distal aspect is at greater risk. It is less vascularized, is more vulnerable to tension, and is more likely to necrose.

Patients often need a second nasal repair. A new cancer may develop in sun-injured skin, or an old cancer may recur. Occasionally, the initial reconstruction is inadequate, and the old forehead flap must be discarded and a second one harvested to improve the result. In most instances, a second flap can be taken easily from the contralateral

forehead after a prior vertical flap, but an initial oblique or angled design into the opposite forehead makes a second flap repair much more difficult. The pedicle is destroyed on one side, and the opposite hemi-forehead is scarred so that donor skin is unavailable. Pre-expansion or surgical delay may allow a second flap, but the repair will be delayed and more morbid. The potential need for a second flap may be the most important clinical reason to use a vertical flap.

The assumption, obvious in many discussions of nasal repair, is that most foreheads are short. Most foreheads, however, are 5 cm or more in height from eyebrow to hairline. A vertical paramedian flap can resurface the entire nasal unit easily without extending significantly into the hairline.

Most often, a template of the cover requirement is positioned just under the hairline, and the vascular pedicle is drawn downward and through the medial eyebrow. The distal flap is incised and elevated until it reaches the defect. The dissection is continued, little by little, incising skin, releasing fibrous restraints, and snipping corrugator muscles, while maintaining the visible vessels.

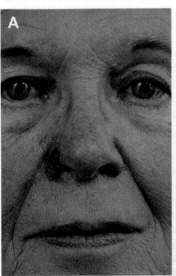
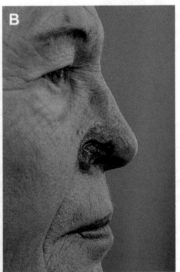
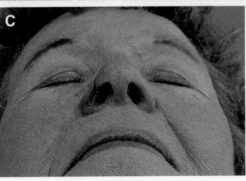

Fig. 1. (A–C) Skin over most of the right ala is missing after excision of a basal cell carcinoma by Mohs technique. This defect could be repaired with a nasolabial or forehead flap. Both will create linear scars, but a scar within the forehead will be less visible postoperatively than a distorted nasolabial fold. Because the defect is small, a forehead flap can be thinned at the time of transfer without risk to its vascularity and with the expectation that the final contour will be good.

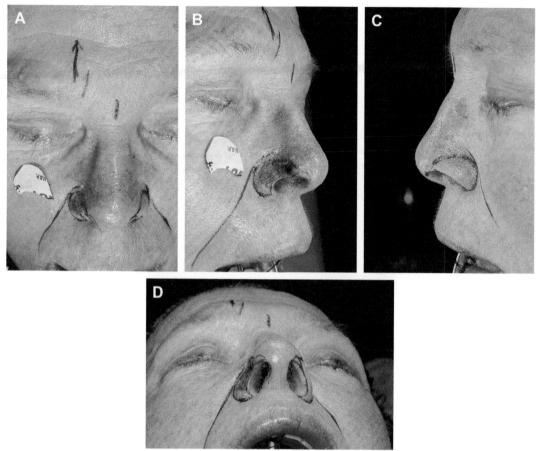

Fig. 2. (*A–D*) The alar subunits are marked with ink. A foil template based on the contralateral normal left ala will determine the dimension and outline of a forehead flap and of the alar margin support graft.

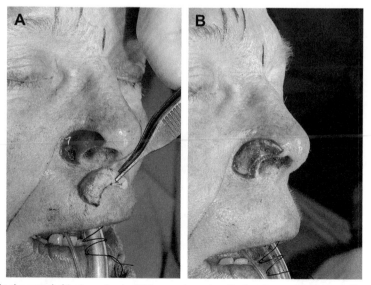

Fig. 3. (*A, B*) Residual normal skin is excised within an alar subunit. A primary conchal cartilage graft is fixed to support, shape, and brace the soft tissues.

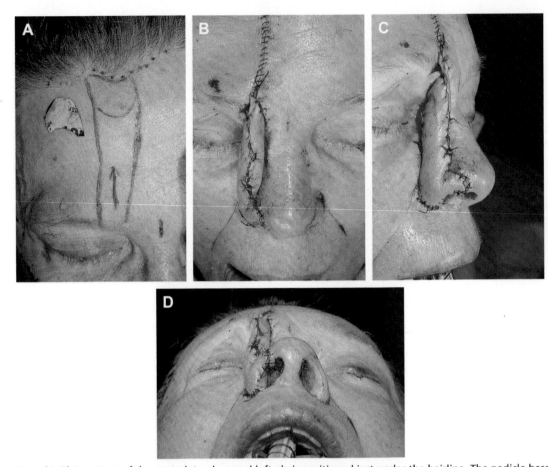

Fig. 4. (*A–D*) A pattern of the contralateral normal left ala is positioned just under the hairline. The pedicle base then is drawn over the ipsilateral supratrochlear vessels. The flap is elevated with 2 to 3 mm of subcutaneous tissue distally for 2 cm. The disection is carried through the frontalis muscle, over the periosteum, to the orbital rim. The flap is sutured to the recipient site with a single layer of fine suture. The raw surface of the pedicle is covered with a full-thickness skin graft. The forehead is closed in layers primarily.

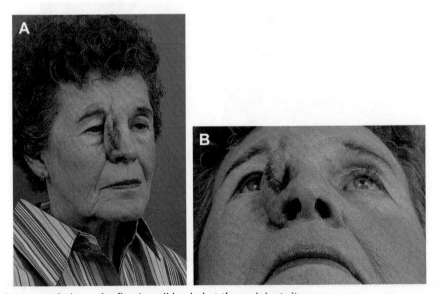

Fig. 5. (*A, B*) Four weeks later, the flap is well healed at the recipient site.

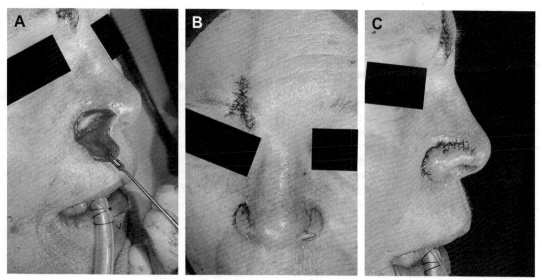

Fig. 6. (*A–C*) The pedicle is divided. The inferior forehead is reopened, and the proximal pedicle instead has a small inverted V replacing the medial brow. Distally, the skin is elevated superiorly with 2 mm of subcutaneous fat. The underlying soft tissue of fat, cartilage graft, and scar is sculpted to create a convex ala and the ala crease superiorly. It is trimmed and inset with quilting sutures and a single-layer skin closure.

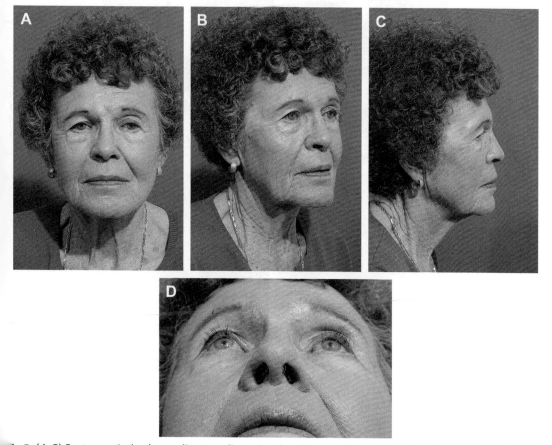

ig. 7. (*A–D*) Postoperatively, the quality, two-dimensional outline, and three-dimensional contour of the ala has •een restored. The forehead scar is almost invisible. No revision was performed.

The lower the pivot, the more hairless skin is available superiorly to cover the defect and the less hairless skin is wasted as a vascular "carrier."

If the forehead seems short preoperatively, the pivot of a paramedian flap can be lowered. The pedicle design is carried through the eyebrow to move the pivot point toward the medial canthus and nearer the defect. The closer the base of the flap is to the recipient site, the shorter is the flap required to reach it.

Alternatively, the flap design can be placed distally within the hairline, accepting a small amount of hair on the end of the flap. Hair can be plucked, depilated, or lasered. It is better to have a normal nose with a little hair than one with a poor shape.

All agree that the paramedian flap is axial. The supratrochlear vessels are the primary blood supply. Anastomoses to the dorsal nasal, supraorbital, and angular arteries create a rich surplus but are secondary. These less important vessels, however, add to the flap's superb blood supply and reassure the surgeon that prior injury to the supratrochlear vessels does not preclude its use.

Its axial nature also means that a vertical flap can be thinned distally without significantly diminishing its perfusion. The distal supratrochlear artery is bound tightly to the overlying skin and is not injured by the excision of frontalis and subcutaneous fat. Excessive tension—too short or too small a flap, too wide a pedicle or tight a twist, too complete an inset—or over-radical thinning

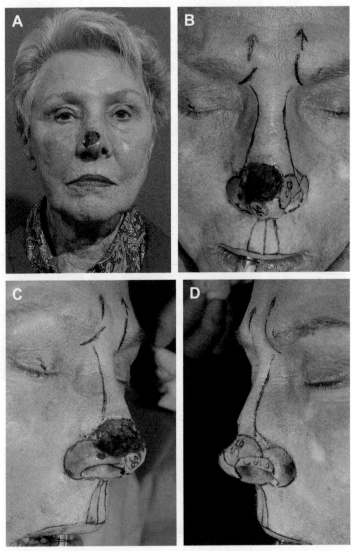

Fig. 8. (A–D) A Mohs defect lies within the distal nose, distorted by multiple previous skin grafts. The left nostril margin is retracted in an area of old composite graft.

can devascularize the flap and cause ischemia. If the repair is performed under general anesthesia without local epinephrine, worrisome blanching can be identified intraoperatively and can be avoided.

The resulting donor defect after a vertical flap is limited largely to the central/lateral forehead. The gap is closed by drawing the adjacent tissues together, vertically and horizontally. Any resultant defect is high in the forehead after closure and is left to heal secondarily. Although eyebrow distortion can occur, it usually can be avoided.

In contrast, oblique and transversely oriented flaps harvest skin within the opposite hemi-unit. The larger the nasal loss; the larger the flap, the bigger the resultant forehead defect, and the closer the defect lies to the brow. The risk of superior eyebrow malposition is significant when an oblique or horizontal oriented flap is used. As an alternative, any remaining forehead gap can be closed with a skin graft. Unfortunately, the skin graft always will look like a mismatched patch of shiny, irregularly pigmented skin within the remaining forehead and will not diminish with time.

FLAP TRANSFER IN TWO OR THREE STAGES

A forehead flap typically is transferred in two stages.[7] Because the forehead skin is thicker than nasal skin, the subcutaneous flap and frontalis muscle are excised distally to thin the flap during the first stage. Axial vessels in the superficial subcutaneous fat are preserved easily.

Although the frontalis muscle is excised, the supratrochlear vessels remain tightly adherent to the distal skin. The flap remains perfused by its axial supply. Its distal aspect is inset into the recipient defect, after restoring missing support or lining.

The pedicle is divided 3 or 4 weeks later during the second stage, once the inset has healed to the recipient bed. The skin over the superior aspect of the recipient site is elevated, and the underlying excess fat and frontalis is excised to debulk the more superior aspect of the repair. The proximal pedicle is trimmed and returned to the medial eyebrow, as a small, inverted V. Because the pedicle is narrow, it is returned easily to the donor site without drawing the eyebrows medially. Ideally, its scars blend into the normal frown lines.

Excellent results can be obtained with the two-stage transfer. Unfortunately, because the flap's blood supply is entirely dependent on its distal inset at the time of pedicle division, the distal and most aesthetic aspects of the repair—the tip and ala—cannot be altered after the flap is transferred. Revisions can be made only months later, in stages, by elevating the flap from the recipient site.

More recently, Menick[8,9] suggested that a forehead flap be transferred as a full-thickness flap in three stages, without initial thinning. This technique is especially useful when a large defect requires a large flap, complex contour restoration, or lining. It has become the primary approach used in major nasal repairs. The

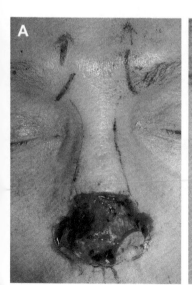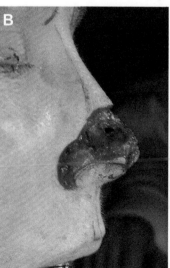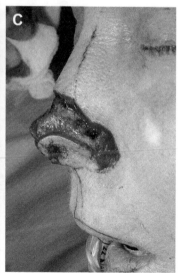

Fig. 9. (A–C) Rather than simply close the fresh defect, the distal nose will be resurfaced and the left nostril margin repositioned to restore the quality, outline, and contour of the nose. Skin within the dorsum tip and alae is discarded except for skin along the left nostril margin, which will be hinged over for lining.

two-stage method is used for smaller, and superficial defects that do not require thinning of the flap over a wide area or the re-establishment of complex three-dimensional (3D) contour with multiple cartilage support grafts or soft tissue shaping. A full-thickness flap, transferred in three stages, maintains maximal vascularity through the axial vessels, frontalis muscle, and a random skin blood supply. The flap is raised with all its layers, and thinning is avoided at the time of transfer. The technique is particularly useful if the patient is a smoker or has an old scar in the region of the flap.

After restoration of missing support and lining, a full-thickness flap is moved to resurface the defect. Four weeks later, the flap is physiologically delayed and has a robust blood supply. During the second intermediate stage, the skin of the flap is elevated with 2 to 3 mm of fat, creating an ideally thin and supple "skin only" flap to resurface the nose. Its elevation exposes the underlying excess fat and frontalis. This soft tissue is excised off the recipient site to sculpt a precise 3D contour. Previously placed cartilage support grafts are modified, if needed, and additional grafts are added, as appropriate. The flap then is replaced on the recipient site. Four weeks later (8 weeks after flap transfer), the pedicle is divided at a third stage.

In three stages, all anatomic components of a normal nose are integrated. During the intermediate operation, the repair is fine tuned, and the

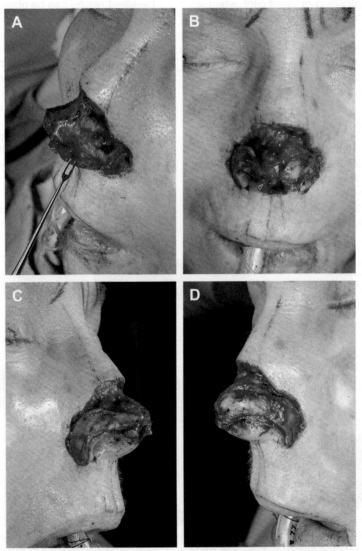

Fig. 10. (A–D) External residual skin along with a left nostril margin is turned over for lining. Conchal cartilage grafts are placed as alar margin battens and to shape, support, and brace the reconstruction.

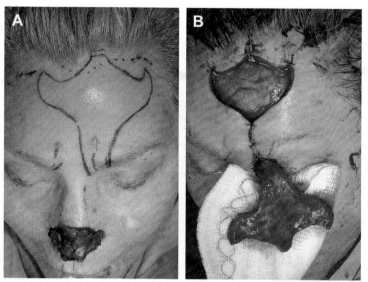

Fig. 11. (*A, B*) A full-thickness forehead flap without thinning is elevated.

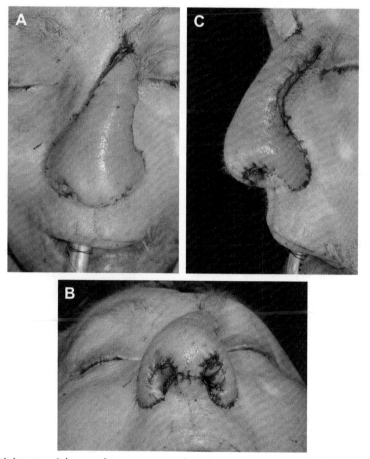

Fig. 12. (*A–C*) Containing an axial, musculocutaneous, and random blood supply, a forehead flap is sutured in one layer to the recipient site. Its raw surface is covered temporarily with a full-thickness skin graft.

hard and soft tissues of the nose are sculpted to create a 3D contour over the entire unit.

This three-stage technique has permitted the development of a new method of lining.[10] The traditional technique of folding a forehead flap for cover and lining is rarely effective because it precludes the placement of support and creates a thick nostril margin and collapsed airway. These limitations have been overcome with a three-stage modified technique.

To line a full-thickness defect, extra tissue is added distally as an extension of a full-thickness flap and is folded for lining. Within a few weeks, the distal folded lining incorporates into the adjacent residual lining and no longer depends on the forehead pedicle or its covering skin for blood supply.

In a three-stage full-thickness flap technique, regardless of how lining is reestablished, the skin of the full-thickness flap then is re-elevated completely off the recipient site with 2 to 3 mm of subcutaneous fat. The underlying exposed fat and frontalis now is adherent to the recipient site (and to any primary cartilage grafts that were placed initially over intact vascularized residual lining adjacent to the full-thickness lining defect during the initial flap transfer). The soft tissue excess and old cartilage grafts are sculpted to establish a contoured soft tissue and hard tissue recipient bed. Previously positioned support grafts are modified if insufficient, shifted, or poorly designed, and new delayed primary support grafts are placed to support the area of reconstructed lining. Delayed primary support is placed over the reconstructed folded lining to recreate a complete support framework. The thin cover flap then is returned to the donor site. Four weeks later (8 weeks after the initial operation), the flap's pedicle is divided.

The advantages of the three-stage flap technique are vascular safety, the capacity to modify the soft tissues and cartilage support of the distal, most aesthetically important tip and ala before pedicle division, and the ability to fold the flap effectively to supply thin, supple lining. This three-stage method has become the usual technique for all large, deep defects and is invaluable in the repair of moderate full-thickness losses.

TECHNIQUE

A major nasal repair is best performed under general anesthesia. Local anesthesia balloons recipient and donor tissues and makes precise contour evaluation almost impossible. Epinephrine blanches the tissue, making it difficult to evaluate

vascularity and tension, and this difficulty may cause tissue ischemia intraoperatively.

All important landmarks and reference points must be identified before the first incision. Once the operation is underway, intraoperative edema, gravity, and tension distort the soft tissues and make it impossible to identify facial landmarks. The hairline, frown lines, location of the supratrochlear vessels by Doppler, the outline of the defect, and nasal and lip subunits are marked with ink.

Exact templates then are made. The normal contralateral side of the missing nasal subunit is used to determine the dimension and outline of the required forehead flap and support grafts. A pattern of the contralateral upper lip is designed also, if the alar base is malpositioned and must be identified.

Quarter-inch adhesive strips are placed over the contralateral subunit, which has been outlined with ink. The strips are consolidated with an outer layer of collodion. Marking ink adheres to the deep surface of the pattern. The paper "mold" is removed and trimmed along the inked border. The paper pattern is used to create a foil pattern from a suture pack. It is flattened on the forehead to outline the exact tissue dimension required to resurface the nose. Later, the template can be used to design a cartilage graft with the correct size and outline of nostril margin needed to support and shape the alar margin.

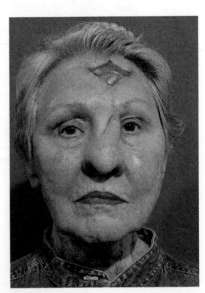

Fig.13. At 4 weeks, the flap has healed to the recipient site, and the donor defect is healing secondarily. The reconstruction is bulky and shapeless. The flap has been effectively physiologically delayed by its elevation and transfer.

Debris, granulation tissue, and irregular margins of the defect are trimmed. If the remaining tissues have been displaced by scar within a healed or previously repaired wound, normal landmarks are returned to their normal position. Extra residual tissue within the subunits is excised, if a subunit excision is planned to alter the size and outline of the defect that requires repair.

The lining must be intact or, if missing, restored before or simultaneously with the restoration of nasal cover with a forehead flap. Then, septal, ear, or rib cartilage is used to replace missing bone and cartilage support. Although the ala normally contains no cartilage, a cartilage graft must be placed to support and shape the nostril margin when significant skin is missing. The alar grafts also brace against wound contraction to avoid alar rim retraction postoperatively.

Usually, the cover template is positioned just under the hairline, and the vascular pedicle is drawn downward and through the medial eyebrow.

The pedicle is then drawn inferiorly, centered over the supratrochlear vessels. Because the flap is an axial flap, its base can be tapered to a pedicle 1.2 cm wide.

A vertical flap design maintains the vascularity of the axial vessels and permits the harvest of

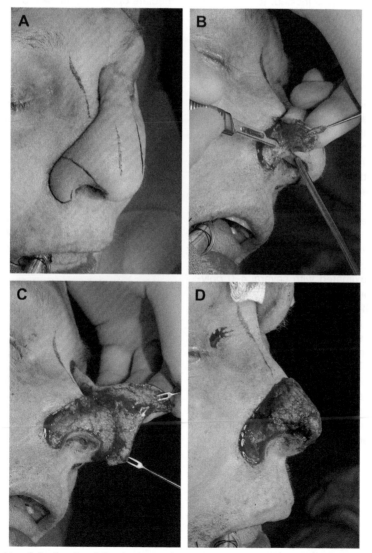

ig. 14. (*A–D*) The skin of the forehead flap is elevated completely off the recipient site with 2 to 3 mm of subcuaneous fat. This elevation exposes the underlying excess subcutaneous fat and frontalis muscle, which now is dherent to the underlying cartilage grafts.

a second flap from the opposite forehead in the future, should another forehead flap be needed.

Unless the donor site has been injured by prior trauma, scars, or flap harvest, prior expansion is not needed. Pre-expansion adds an additional stage, morbidity, and the risk of extrusion or infection. If the forehead is excessively short (4 cm), tight (usually because of a prior flap harvest), or scarred, pre-expansion is a useful tool.

THE TWO-STAGE FLAP

Traditionally, a forehead flap is transferred in two stages.[7] A forehead flap is thicker than nasal skin. Frontalis muscle and some subcutaneous fat must be excised to thin the flap (**Figs. 1–7**).

The border of the flap is incised. It is elevated from distal to proximal. Distally, the flap is lifted off the frontalis for 1.5 to 2 cm. The dissection then passes through the muscle and over the periosteum to the superior orbital rim. Inelastic periosteum is not elevated because it will restrict flap rotation and reach.

As the dissection reaches the brow, the skin borders of the flap are incised, snipping fibrous bands and corrugator muscle while preserving visible vessels. The flap is released, little by little, until the flap reaches the defect without tension.

If support is absent and vascularized lining is intact or has been restored, primary cartilage support grafts with a subunit outline are placed.

The pedicle of a two-stage flap is divided 3 to 4 weeks later.

The donor site is closed after wide undermining under the frontalis muscle into the temples. The forehead is approximated with several 4–0 polypropylene tension sutures, placed just at the wound edges. Then the frontalis is repaired with 4–0 clear slowly absorbing sutures, followed by 5–0 subcuticular sutures and 6–0 sutures for the skin. Any gap under the hairline is allowed to heal secondarily. The wound fills with granulation, epithelializes, and contracts over several weeks. It heals well. Months later, any residual scar can be excised secondarily after the residual forehead has relaxed. A skin graft is not applied to avoid a visible permanently discolored patch.

THE THREE-STAGE FULL-THICKNESS FOREHEAD FLAP

A large defect requires a large flap. A large flap must be widely thinned. A large defect encompasses multiple subunits, each requiring individual complex contour restoration. Multiple cartilage grafts and extensive soft tissue shaping will be needed. The greater the size of the defect, the

more likely it is to extend through the underlying lining. In such cases, the author prefers to transfer a full-thickness forehead flap in three stages,[8,9] with an intermediate operation to provide thin cover and a shaped middle support layer and lining, if needed (**Figs. 8–21**).

The flap is elevated over the periosteum, containing skin, fat, and frontalis muscle with the thin deep areolar layer. It maintains its axial, musculocutaneous, and random blood supply. The flap is not thinned. Missing support is replaced with cartilage and bone grafts over intact vascularized lining. Then the flap, with all its layers, is sutured to resurface the nasal defect.

Three to 4 weeks later, the flap is physiologically delayed. Its vascularity is maximized. At an intermediate operation, the skin of the flap is elevated off the entire recipient site with 2 to 3 mm of subcutaneous fat. The underlying excess of soft tissue then is excised to sculpt the healed fat and frontalis from the surface of the recipient site. Additional cartilage grafts can be applied, or old grafts can be sculpted or repositioned, if necessary. The flap, now of ideal nasal thickness, is resutured to the recipient site. This three-stage approach ensures maximal blood supply, ideal contouring of the soft and hard tissue, and better results.

Its pedicle is divided at a later third stage.

During the first stage of either a two- or three-stage transfer, the flap is inset with one layer of fine suture. It is sutured at the columella and rim. It is not necessary to inset the flap completely. If blanching occurs, placement of the inset should stop, and any tight sutures should be removed.

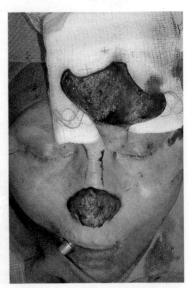

Fig. 15. The thick and stiff forehead flap has been converted to thin, supple forehead skin that matches the normal nasal skin in quality and thickness.

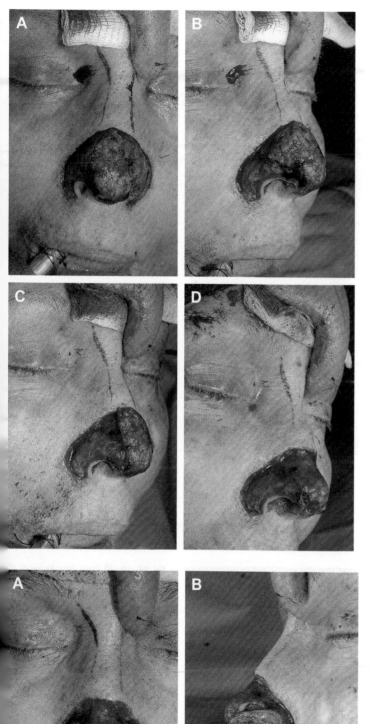

Fig. 16. (*A–D*) The excess soft tissue, cartilage support, and lining now are rigidly healed together. The excess can be sculpted by excision to remove bulk and improve contour.

Fig. 17. (*A, B*) A rigid subsurface architecture with a correct contour and outline is created.

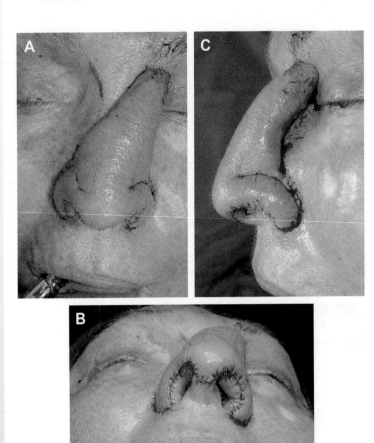

Fig. 18. (*A–C*) The thin forehead skin is returned to the contoured recipient site and fixed with quilting sutures and peripheral sutures.

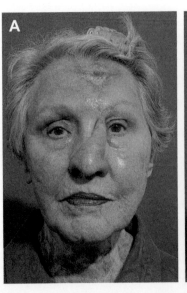
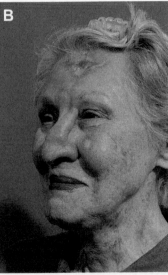

Fig. 19. (*A, B*) Four weeks later (8 weeks after flap transfer), the contour of the distal, most aesthetic aspect of the nose has been established by the intermediate operation.

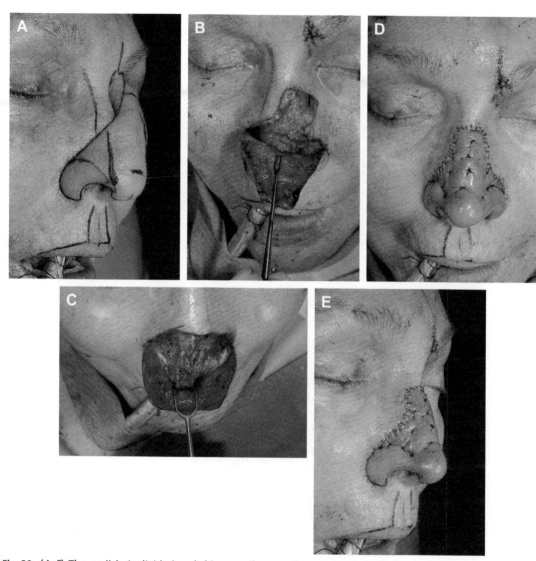

Fig. 20. (*A–E*) The pedicle is divided and skin over the superior aspect of the defect is elevated. Distinct dorsal lines, a flat sidewall, and alar creases are created by soft tissue excision. The inset is completed with quilting sutures and peripheral sutures.

The flap is sutured to the columella and along the nostril margins. Any lateral gaps along the lateral aspects of the defect are allowed to heal spontaneously. A forehead flap is very vascular, but a too small, too short, too tightly inset, or a too aggressively thinned flap will die.

Although not vital, the raw undersurface of the exposed pedicle is skin grafted. This procedure maintains a cleaner wound between each surgical stage.

The next day, the patient can wash and shampoo. Skin sutures are removed in 5 days.

An extension of a full-thickness flap also can be used to replace nasal lining, if lining also is missing. A template of the external skin loss is

created. Then another template of the lining defect is added as a distal extension to the covering flap. At transfer, the distal skin is folded inward to line the wound, and the proximal covering skin is turned back on itself to resurface the nose. Four weeks later, the lining component has healed and revascularized to residual normal lining. It no longer depends on the proximal forehead flap for blood supply. At the intermediate operation, the flap is divided along the ideal nostril margin. The proximal covering skin is elevated completely from the nasal surface with 2 to 3 mm of subcutaneous flap. The folded frontalis and subcutaneous fat, which overlie the skin lining, are excised. Delayed primary support grafts are

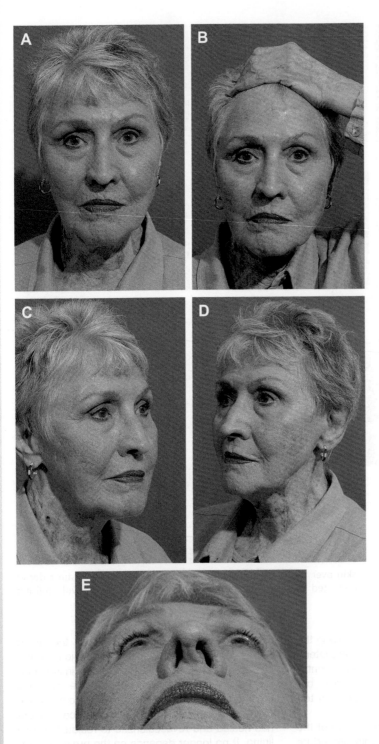

Fig. 21. (*A–E*) Postoperatively, the expected uniform quality of nasal skin and the two-dimensional outline and three-dimensional contour of the nose had been reestablished. The forehead healed uneventfully. No revision was performed.

placed to shape and brace the reconstruction. Lining and a 3D cartilage support skeleton are restored.

This modified folded lining technique now is the author's preferred method of repairing small and moderate full-thickness defects.

Pedicle division is similar for a two-stage or three-stage flap. Three to 4 weeks later (6–8 weeks after the initial transfer of a three-stage flap), old scars and units are marked with ink under general anesthesia. No local anesthesia is used. The site of pedicle division is marked to ensure adequate tissue to resurface the recipient site and to replace the medial eyebrow in its correct position.

The proximal pedicle is untubed. The inferior forehead is reopened. Excess soft tissue at the base of the flap and under the medial brow is excised. The forehead is re-closed, in layers, to create a small, inverted V-shaped recipient site, inferiorly. The excess proximal flap skin is trimmed to fit the defect in the medial brow and returned to the donor site. This procedure replaces the eyebrow.

The distal flap is partially re-elevated over the superior inset with 2 to 3 mm of subcutaneous fat. The underlying soft tissue is sculpted to restore the expected contour of the recipient site. The flap is reapplied to the defect with quilting sutures and peripherally with a single layer of fine sutures. The quilting sutures are removed in 2 days, and the skin sutures are removed in 5 days.

Complex repairs of large or deep defects may require a later revision at 4 months to define the alar crease, thin a thick nostril margin, or revise the forehead, if a gap has been allowed to heal secondarily. Such revisions are not considered a failure but are a necessary part of the repair of difficult defects.

REFERENCES

1. Gillies H, Millard DR. The principles and art of plastic surgery. Boston: Little Brown; 1957.
2. McCarthy J, Lorenc T, Cutting C, et al. The median forehead flap revisited: the blood supply. Plast Reconstr Surg 1985;76:866–9.
3. Menick F. Aesthetic refinements in use of forehead for nasal reconstruction: the paramedian forehead flap. Clin Plast Surg 1990;17(4):607–22.
4. Millard D. Principlization of plastic surgery. Boston: Little Brown; 1986.
5. Millard D. Aesthetic reconstructive rhinoplasty. Clin Plast Surg 1981;8(2):169–75.
6. Millard D. Reconstructive rhinoplasty for the lower two-thirds of the nose. Plast Reconstr Surg 1976; 58(3):283–91.
7. Burget G, Menick F. Aesthetic reconstruction of the nose. Mosby; 1993.
8. Menick F. Nasal reconstruction: art and practice. Elsevier Publishing; 2008.
9. Menick F. A 10-year experience in nasal reconstruction with the three-stage forehead flap. Plast Reconstr Surg 2002;109:1839–55.
10. Menick F. A new modified method for nasal lining: the Menick technique for folded lining. J Surg Oncol 2006;94:509–14.

Maximizing Results in Reconstruction of Cheek Defects

Marc A.M. Mureau, MD, PhD[a],*,
Stefan O.P. Hofer, MD, PhD, FRCS(C)[b,c]

KEYWORDS
- Cheek • Reconstruction • Flap • Aesthetic • Unit
- Outcome

The face is exceedingly important, as it is the medium through which individuals interact with the rest of society. The unique character of the facial skin and the close anatomic and functional association with the underlying muscles allow the face to express emotions critical to social interaction. Sustaining a major deforming injury to the face is one of the most devastating injuries suffered in terms of social interaction and quality of life.[1]

Reconstruction of major facial soft tissue deformities or deficits after trauma or surgery is a continuing challenge for surgeons who wish to reliably restore facial function and appearance. Important in aesthetic facial reconstruction are the aesthetic unit principles,[2] by which the face can be divided into central facial units (nose, lips, and eyelids) and into peripheral facial units (cheeks, forehead, and chin). It is essential to make this difference in central and peripheral facial units, since these aesthetic facial unit principles are less appropriate in the reconstruction of a peripheral cheek unit than in the reconstruction of a central facial unit.[3]

This article summarizes established options for reconstruction of cheek defects and provides an overview of several modifications and tips and tricks to avoid complications and maximize aesthetic results.

CONTOUR AND OUTLINE OF THE CHEEK

The aesthetic surface anatomy characteristics of the cheek have been described eloquently by Menick:

*The face can be divided into adjacent topographic areas of characteristic skin quality (color, texture, hear bearing), outline, and contour that define its regional units. The skin quality of the cheek matches the face in color and texture. The peripheral outline of the cheek unit is formed by the contours of the bordering units (forehead, eyelids, nose, lips, neck, and ear). Its outline follows the preauricular contours of the tragus and helix; goes around the sideburn, across the zygomatic arch, and into the lower eyelid-cheek junction; and then passes inferiorly along the nasal sidewall into the nasolabial fold and marionette line, around the chin and toward the submental crease. It then extends laterally along the jawline, passing superiorly up the angle of the jaw and back to the ear (**Fig. 1**). In contour, the cheek is a relatively flat, expansive surface, except for the soft roundness of the nasolabial folds and cheek prominences.[3]*

[a] Department of Plastic and Reconstructive Surgery, Erasmus University Medical Center Rotterdam, PO Box 2040, 3000 CA Rotterdam, The Netherlands
[b] Division of Plastic Surgery, Department of Surgery, University of Toronto, University Health Network, 200 Elizabeth Street, 8N-865, Toronto, ON, Canada M5G 2C4
[c] Department of Surgical Oncology, University of Toronto, University Health Network, 200 Elizabeth Street, 8N-865, Toronto, ON, Canada M5G 2C4
* Corresponding author.
E-mail address: m.mureau@erasmusmc.nl (M.A.M. Mureau).

Clin Plastic Surg 36 (2009) 461–476
doi:10.1016/j.cps.2009.02.003
0094-1298/09/$ – see front matter © 2009 Elsevier Inc. All rights reserved.

AESTHETIC FACIAL UNIT PRINCIPLES IN CHEEK RECONSTRUCTION

To achieve an aesthetically pleasing result, the aesthetic facial units should be taken into account.[4] The reconstructed requirements of central facial units (nose, lips, and eyelids), which have complex and subtle contours and which are seen in primary gaze with their contralateral normal (sub)unit available for visual comparison, should have the highest priority in reconstruction.[3,5] In contrast, the units of the facial periphery (cheek, forehead, and chin) are a lesser focus of attention. The cheek is a flat expansive area with a variable outline; therefore, it is of secondary visual interest, like a picture frame.[5] Because the outline of the contralateral cheek cannot be fully compared with the other cheek, exact symmetry is not vital. Therefore, the preoperative plan should distinguish between central and peripheral features with regard to guidelines for unit reconstruction (**Fig. 1**).[3,4]

In cheek reconstruction, the most important element in restoring normal facial surface appearance is uniformity of skin color and texture, not contour and outline. Therefore, cheek defects preferably are reconstructed with tissue from adjacent units, such as neck, submental area, or chest, using local or regional flaps.[3] These flaps may be anterior-based rotation advancement flaps vascularized by the facial and submental vessels (**Fig. 2**)[6,7] or posterior-based rotation advancement flaps supplied by the superficial temporal and preauricular vessels (**Fig. 3**).[8] Although the presence and position of facial scarring are less important in a peripheral unit,[3] vertical incisions anterior to a line drawn from the lateral canthus should be avoided.[9] Furthermore, an attempt should be made to plan the position of future dog-ear excisions in inconspicuous contour lines.[3]

Large, deep, complex, or compromised wounds often have to be reconstructed with distant or free flaps, but they usually lead to poor color and texture match for facial skin.[10]

DEFECT ANALYSIS

Location and amount of locoregional skin laxity should be assessed first as they dictate design and position of the flap. Defect site, size, shape, and depth should be assessed carefully for the same reasons. Preoperative management should consist of identifying patients who have risk factors for flap failure, especially smoking, a history of irradiation, and previous surgery.

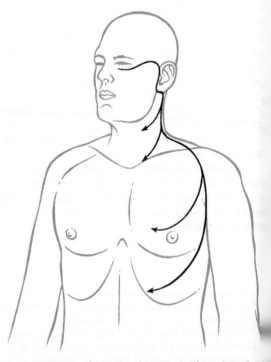

Fig. 1. Diagram of the aesthetic facial units, which are outlined with dashed lines. The solid lines depict the cheek unit borders.

Fig. 2. Diagram of incisions for anterior-based cervicofacial and cervicopectoral flaps, with back-cut oriented in a cervical crease, in the supraclavicular region, above the areola, and along the costal margin.

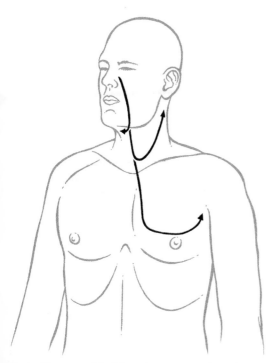

Fig. 3. Diagram of incisions for posterior-based cervicofacial and cervicopectoral flaps, with back-cuts oriented in the submental crease, in the supraclavicular region, and above the areola.

Primary closure or local flaps may repair small cheek defects, but most defects greater than 30% of the cheek unit require transposition or rotation of residual cheek and neck skin. In areas of burn scarring or past excisions, defect size may appear smaller than it actually is after scar excision and replacement of neighboring structures to their anatomic position.

The site of the cheek defect influences the direction of skin flap transposition, pedicle base location, and risks to underlying structures. Small to moderate anterior cheek defects are reconstructed with posterior-based rotation-advancement flaps. Posterior or large anterior cheek defects are covered with anterior-based rotation-advancement flaps.[3]

Deeper wounds have an increased risk for facial nerve involvement. In addition, there may be a need for soft tissue bulk or intraoral lining. Most lining defects are closed primarily or with small local flaps[3]; however, sometimes a second regional or a microvascular free flap is required.[11,12]

A highly contaminated or infected wound may require delayed primary reconstruction after serial débridements or temporary split-thickness skin grafting (**Figs. 4** and **5**). After cancer excision, clear margins must be ensured before definite repair.[3]

LOCAL FLAPS
Anterior-Based Cervicofacial Flaps

Since the first description of a local cheek rotation flap by Esser in 1918,[13] several modifications have been described by, among others, Mustardé[14] and Converse[15] to overcome the problem of noticeable scars and donor sites. Juri and Juri[6,7] combined the concept of cervical advancement as described by Stark and Kaplan[16] with a cheek rotation flap, converting their flap into an advancement rotation flap. This anterior-based flap is nourished by the facial and submental arteries and advances upward from the cervical area and rotates forward. There is no need to skin graft the donor site and scars are placed

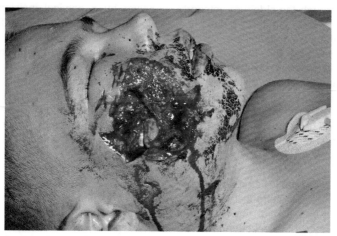

Fig. 4. Contaminated dog bite injury of the right cheek of a 12-year-old boy who had damage of facial muscles and facial nerve branches.

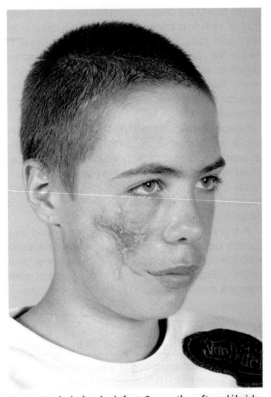

Fig. 5. Healed cheek defect 8 months after débridement and temporary split-thickness skin grafting. Note the decrease in original defect size because of secondary wound contracture.

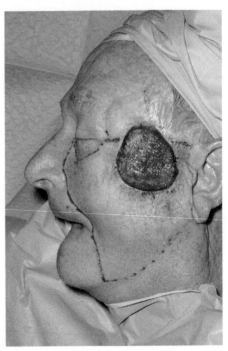

Fig. 6. Posterior cheek defect measuring 6 cm after Mohs' excision of a recurrent basal cell carcinoma in a 76-year-old man. The borders of the cheek unit are marked.

inconspicuously. Now, most local cervicofacial flaps are a combination of rotation and advancement flaps.

Anterior-based rotation-advancement cervicofacial flaps are useful for posterior and moderate-sized anterior cheek defects. The incision passes transversely from the superior aspect of the defect, around or through the sideburn, inferiorly in the preauricular crease and then around the earlobe to follow the occipital hairline, with or without a back-cut inferiorly (**Fig. 6**).[3] Classically, these flaps are widely undermined in the subcutaneous plane, including the cheek, chin, neck, and retroauricular regions down to the clavicular line.[6] A deep-plane dissection to enhance the blood supply was introduced because of the unfortunate tendency for the distal edge to develop necrosis (especially in smokers, in large wounds under tense closure, and after previous radiation).[17,18] After standard flap design and incision, 2 cm anterior to the tragus, the plane shifts just below the parotid fascia, which is a part of the superficial musculoaponeurotic system. Dissection over the parotid gland is relatively safe for the facial nerve, but once the anterior margin of the gland is

reached, care must be taken to avoid injuring the nerve, which no longer is protected by parotid tissue.[17] Careful dissection with blunt-tipped scissors in a plane perpendicular to that of the skin is a safe and effective way to perform the anterior portion of the dissection. Bipolar electrocautery is recommended to minimize the risk for facial nerve injury. Dissection passes beneath the platysmal plane in the portion of the flap lying below the border of the mandible. This step is made easier by a cervical incision, which allows for good exposure.[18] Inclusion of the platysma transforms the flap into a composite musculocutaneous flap vascularized by branches of the facial artery. The platysma may be sectioned transversely in the lower part of the flap to allow adequate flap transposition.[18] Disadvantages are the increased difficulty of dissection, risk for facial nerve injury, and increased operating time. In addition, this thicker flap must be thinned if applied to the lower eyelid or nasal sidewall.[3]

A modification of the deep-plane cervicofacial flap is the so-called hike flap, described by Longaker and colleagues,[19] which was specifically designed to cover defects over the lateral aspect of the zygoma, the lower eyelid, and the temporal region without making an incision along the nasolabial fold (**Fig. 7**). The deep-plane hike flap i

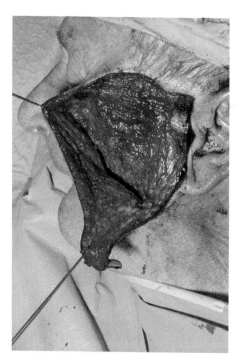

Fig. 7. Intraoperative situation after elevation of cervicofacial hike flap. Note that only the borders of the aesthetic cheek unit were incised.

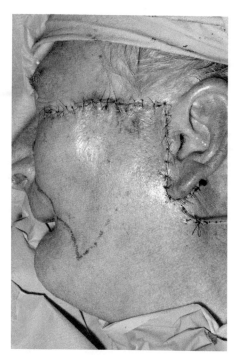

Fig. 8. Result immediately after closure of the anterior-based cervicofacial hike flap. All suture lines follow the borders of the aesthetic cheek unit.

designed similar to conventional anterior-based cervicofacial flaps and its dissection technique is similar to the previously described deep-plane flap. After identifying the lateral border of the orbicularis oculi muscle, the soft tissue is cleared off the zygomatic major muscle, by transecting the firm fibers of the zygomatic restraining ligaments, which come through the muscles and the superficial musculoaponeurotic system and continue into the dermis. This maneuver releases and mobilizes the entire cheek flap, allowing for considerable vertical advancement.[19] Next, the dissection progresses downward, but the modiolus is left undisturbed. The mobilized flap then is hiked into an overcorrected position, which prevents late downward vector forces thereby avoiding ectropion of the lower eyelid (**Figs. 8** and **9**). The resulting dog-ear is oriented in a horizontal instead of vertical direction. The flap must be anchored in its overcorrected position to the zygoma and periorbital area while avoiding damage to the frontal branch of the facial nerve.[19] No fixation should be performed along the zygomatic arch for 3.5 cm anterior to the external auditory canal because the temporal branches of the facial nerve pass through that zone.[19] The horizontal dog-ear can be excised incorporating it into upper or lower blepharoplasty incisions.

Recently, the yin-yang principle was described; it combines a classical Mustardé cheek rotation flap with a second temporoparietal scalp flap, which is rotated in an opposite direction to close the preauricular donor-site defect of the Mustardé cheek flap (**Fig. 10**).[20] Anterior cheek defects up to 7 cm in diameter can be closed using this technique. Advantages are limited subcutaneous undermining of the cheek until the lower border of the mandible without undermining of the neck and a natural suspension of the cheek flap by the opposing temporoparietal scalp flap preventing secondary sagging of the cheek flap. Classical complications of wide undermining, such as hematoma and distal edge necrosis, are greatly reduced using this yin-yang technique.[20]

Another modification to optimize outcome is the angle rotation cheek flap, originally described by Schrudde and Beinhoff in 1987[21] and recently recommended by Boutrous and Zide as the first-choice flap for combined cheek–lower eyelid reconstructions.[22] The angle rotation cheek flap elevates and rotates simultaneously using a postauricular "angle" flap (as a Burrow's triangle) leaving an inconspicuous donor site while placing the angled flap ideally in the preauricular zone. Its design can be used in combination with tissue expansion (especially in children) and its value is

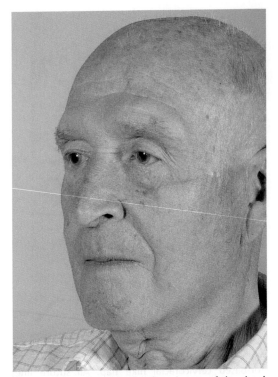

Fig. 9. Final result 9 months after closure of the cheek defect. Because incisions were planned along the borders of the cheek unit, they healed inconspicuously. Note the absence of downward pull of the flap and ectropion of the lower eyelid.

best seen in leaving no scars on the neck or chest and its ability to be redeployed for future advancement (**Figs. 11–15**).[22]

To prevent lower eyelid ectropion, cheek flaps should be overcorrected, tension should be minimized, and the lateral superior border of an anterior-based rotation advancement flap should be planned above the lateral canthal-helical root plane, suspending the flap higher than the eyelid margin.[3,22] The flap should be sutured to fixed deep underlying structures, using Mitek mini anchors if necessary.

Posterior-Based Cervicofacial Flaps

Posterior-based cervicofacial cheek flaps typically are used for small and moderate-sized anterior cheek defects (**Figs. 16–18**). In particular, these flaps are useful for reconstruction of small medial cheek defects next to the nose or lips.[3] Excess skin of the inferior face, jowl, and submental areas is transferred along an incision that follows the nasolabial fold to the commissure. If necessary, the incision can be continued to or across the jawline and anteriorly into the submental crease ending with a back-cut.[3,8] The exact design must conform

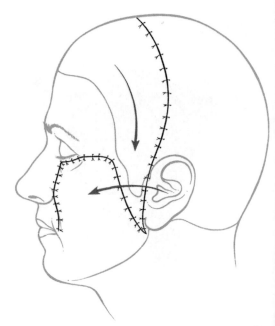

Fig. 10. Diagram of a classical Mustardé rotation flap in combination with a temporoparietal flap, which is undermined under the galea and rotated toward the preauricular region in an opposite direction to close the donor defect of the Mustardé flap. The temporoparietal flap naturally suspends the Mustardé flap avoiding the risk for lower eyelid ectropion.

to what the flap has to cover and where it has to be rotated. It is not strictly necessary to include the platysma in the cervical region for blood supply. The superficial temporal artery and vessels in the preauricular region supply the flap. Therefore, in all posterior-based flaps, undermining should stop at least several centimeters anterior to the ear.[3] This flap can be raised safely after

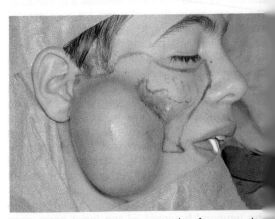

Fig. 11. Same patient as in **Figs. 4** and **5** after expansion of a previously subcutaneously inserted preauricular tissue expander. The proposed incision lines follow the cheek unit borders.

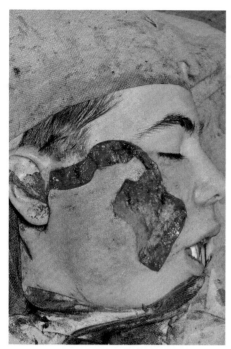

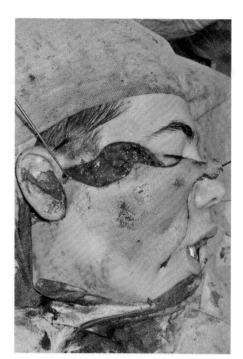

Fig. 12. Intraoperative situation after excision of the split-thickness skin graft, removal of the tissue expander, and wide undermining of a Schrudde cheek advancement rotation flap. Note the postauricular angle flap, which will be transposed to the preauricular region enhancing cranial advancement of the cheek flap.

Fig. 13. Intraoperative situation after upward advancing and forward rotating the Schrudde flap, using the postauricular angle flap to cover the preauricular region.

simultaneous parotidectomy or neck dissection.[8] The donor site is closed primarily in a V-Y manner or occasionally with a skin graft.

LOCOREGIONAL FLAPS
Anterior-Based Cervicopectoral Flaps

Larger posterior or lower cheek defects up to 10 cm can be closed if the incision of an anterior-based cervicofacial flap is extended, converting it into a cervicopectoral flap, which moves neck and chest skin to the face.[3,23–26] The lower border of the cheek defect is taken as the upper border of the cervicopectoral flap. From the back of the defect, marks are made around the earlobe and back to the hairline behind the ear, then down along the cervical hairline parallel to and 2 cm behind the anterior border of the trapezius muscle to avoid late scar webbing (**Figs. 2 and 19**). This broad curvilinear incision then is extended down lateral to the acromioclavicular joint and deltopectoral groove and along the lateral edge of the pectoralis major muscle. The inferior border of the flap is made parallel to the clavicle, approximately 3 cm above the male nipple or the third to fourth intercostals space where a back-cut can

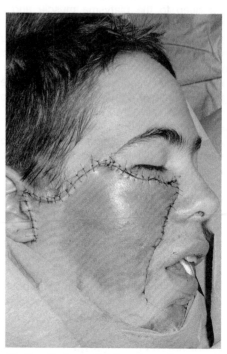

Fig. 14. Result immediately after closure of the Schrudde flap. All suture lines follow the borders of the aesthetic cheek unit.

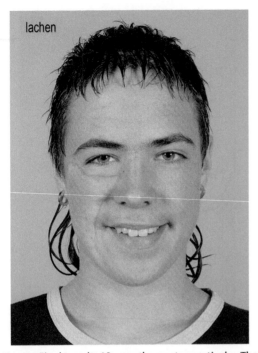

Fig. 15. Final result 10 months postoperatively. The scars that follow the aesthetic cheek unit border are beginning to fade. Note the spontaneously fully recovered facial nerve function and the absence of lower eyelid ectropion.

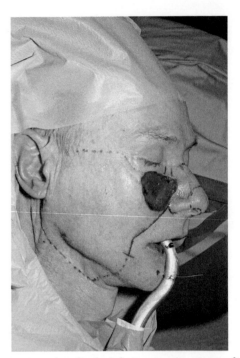

Fig. 16. Anterior cheek defect measuring 5 cm after Mohs' excision of a fifth recurrence of a basal cell carcinoma. The proposed incision is marked with a solid line. The cheek unit borders are marked with dashed lines. Note an old transverse neck scar and post irradiation skin damage resulting from treatment for a previous intraoral malignancy.

be made in the parasternal area.[3,24,25] The flap is raised deep to the platysma muscle and with deltoid and pectoral fasciae. The flap is vascularized by the internal mammary perforators. Simultaneous parotidectomy and radical neck dissection can be performed. After rotating and suturing the flap into position without any tension, the anterior dog-ear is trimmed as necessary and the donor site is closed primarily in a V-Y fashion at the lateral pectoral area (**Figs. 20 and 21**).[3,24,25]

Advantages of this anterior-based cervicopectoral flap are its reliability; good skin color, texture, and hair-bearing match; the favorable location of the scars; the one-stage nature of the reconstruction; wide exposure facilitating simultaneous tumor excision, parotidectomy, and radical neck dissection; and the ability to close the donor site without a skin graft.[3,24,25] These favorable characteristics make this somewhat underused flap an excellent technique, which should be strongly considered when confronted with large posterior or lower cheek defects below a line connecting the tragus and oral commissure.[25]

Posterior-Based Cervicopectoral Flaps

For larger anterior cheek defects, the vertical midline incision of the posterior-based

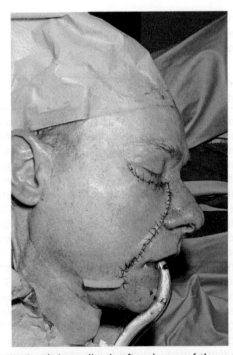

Fig. 17. Result immediately after closure of the posterior-based cervicofacial flap. All suture lines follow the borders of the aesthetic cheek unit.

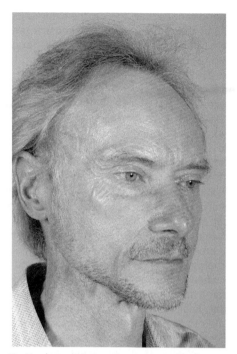

Fig. 18. Final result 9 months postoperatively. Because incisions were planned along the borders of the cheek unit, they healed inconspicuously.

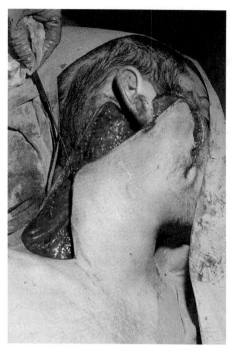

Fig. 20. Intraoperative situation after transposition of the cervicopectoral flap.

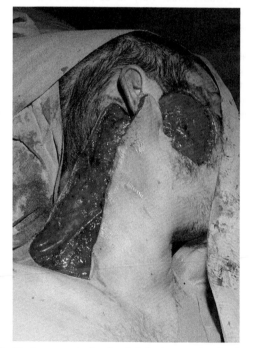

Fig. 19. Large posterior cheek defect measuring 6 × 9 cm after wide local excision of a dermatofibrosarcoma pro-tuberans in a 26-year-old man. An anterior-based cervi-copectoral flap is elevated, including the platysma muscle to enhance its blood supply.

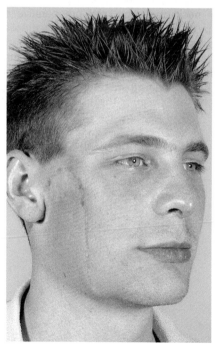

Fig. 21. Final result 7 months postoperatively and after radiotherapy. Note the postirradiation skin hypopig-mentation and alopecia. The neck scar is well hidden behind the anterior border of the trapezius muscle.

cervicofacial flap can be continued inferiorly along the sternum, then laterally down across the chest, above the nipple areola-complex and toward the axilla (see **Fig. 3**). This flap is vascularized by the superficial temporal artery and vessels, the vertebral and occipital arteries, and the perforators of the trapezius muscle and thoracoacromial vessels.[3,27] A Z-plasty may be needed secondarily where the scar crosses the mandibular border. The donor site is closed primarily in a V-Y manner or occasionally with a skin graft.

REGIONAL FLAPS
Platysma Musculocutaneous Flap

The platysma musculocutaneous flap (PMF) was first described for intraoral reconstruction.[28] Since then it has been used for various head and neck defects. As the flap can be superior or posterior based, it can provide an adequate amount of islanded skin that is sufficient for small to medium-sized skin or mucosal defects in the face, oral cavity, and pharynx.[29] The PMF is easily harvested and has low donor-site morbidity but has not gained widespread acceptance because of problems with vascularity.[29,30] Flap necrosis rates (partial and total) ranging from 0% to 29% have been reported in literature.[29,30] The arterial and venous blood supply may be compromised by the harvesting technique and pre-existing incisions, neck dissection, and preoperative radiotherapy.[31] The superior-based flap is supplied by branches from the facial and submental arteries but has less efficient venous drainage through small anterior communicating veins that drain into the superior thyroid vein, anterior jugular vein, or facial vein.[32] The posterior-based PMF

has good venous drainage into the external jugular vein, but the arterial supply is almost a random pattern through branches from the superior thyroid, occipital, and posterior auricular arteries (**Figs. 22–24**).[29,30]

An ipsilateral superior-based PMF can be used for reconstruction of defects of the cheek, parotid and mastoid, or ear regions. The skin incision during harvesting corresponds to the incisions made for neck dissection if needed. Skin flaps are developed superficial to the platysma muscle. Adequate exposure of the platysma muscle is necessary to establish the proper arc of rotation. Dissection should stop 1 to 2 cm below the lower border of the mandible, to protect the facial and submental arteries emerging from and anterior to the submandibular gland, respectively. The external jugular vein also should be preserved inferiorly whenever possible. The width of the pedicled platysma muscle should at least be 4 cm. The skin paddle itself is designed depending on the distance to the skin defect, bearing in mind that the fulcrum of the flap at the most anterior margin of the platysma is at the lower border of the mandible. When necessary, the inferior aspect of the skin island can be placed as far inferiorly as the level of the clavicle.[29]

The main complication of the PMF is venous congestion, which may cause partial or total skin necrosis. The main venous drainage is through the external jugular and submental veins; therefore, care should be taken to preserve both vessels, which usually is feasible.[29] Venous congestion may be treated through removal of stitches, with leeches, or by widening the subcutaneous tunnel over the pedicle. Advantages of this flap are its easy harvesting, its minimal

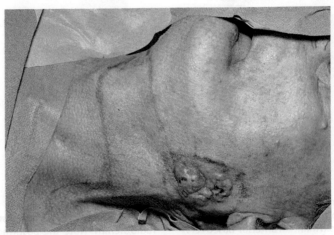

Fig. 22. Proposed excision margins of a squamous cell carcinoma and design of a posterior-based PMF in a 76-year-old man.

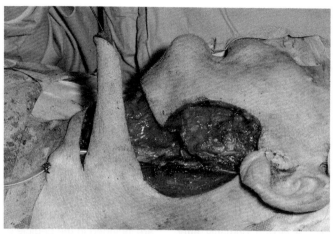

Fig. 23. Intraoperative situation after wide local excision of the squamous cell carcinoma, an ipsilateral neck dissection, and elevation of the posterior-based PMF.

donor-site morbidity, and its thin and pliable skin with good color and texture match.

DISTANT FLAPS
Supraclavicular Flap

In situations where healthy regional tissue to reconstruct a cheek defect is not available (eg, after burns or radiation), other donor sites should be looked for. The shoulder area is a potentially suitable distant donor site from which a thin fasciocutaneous flap with an acceptable skin color and texture match can be elevated. Flap skin color and texture match especially match the lower face, neck, and the upper chest wall region. In 1842, Mutter was the first to describe a random patterned flap of the supraclavicular region extending toward the shoulder.[33] After closer

examination of the vascularization, the flap was described as a supraclavicular axial pattern flap.[34] Anatomically, this neck/shoulder flap was based on the supraclavicular artery. Recently, Pallua and Noah[35] renewed attention to the supraclavicular flap with their study on its surgical anatomy, surgical technique, and clinical experience with this island flap.

Preoperatively, the supraclavicular vessels are marked using a handheld Doppler probe. The supraclavicular artery, originating from the transverse cervical artery, can be found in the triangle between the dorsal edge of the sternocleidomastoid muscle, the external jugular vein, and the medial part of the clavicle.[35] Next, the pedicle and flap are outlined. During flap elevation the patient lies on his side at an angle of approximately 45°. The incision is taken down to the deltoid muscle in a subfascial plane and

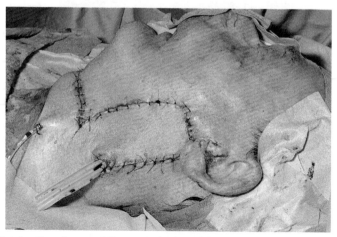

Fig. 24. Result immediately after closure of the posterior-based PMF.

the flap is raised from lateral to medial. In the medial third of the flap the pedicle can easily be identified by transillumination. Reaching the previously outlined medial edge of the required skin island, the skin is incised superficially, taking care not to damage the pedicle at the supraclavicular level.[35] Further preparation of the pedicle is at the subcutaneous level on the upper side, forming a tunnel, and on the lower side of the pedicle at the subfascial level. Dissection can be continued to the pivot point at the origin of the supraclavicular artery.[35] The aim of preparing a tunnel is to avoid visible scars on the medial part of the neck; however, if there is too much compression of the pedicle the flap may be inset without making a tunnel.[36] After insetting of the flap, the donor site usually can be closed primarily after extensive subcutaneous undermining of the wound edges, even in extreme wide flaps of 16 cm.[35]

To increase size (especially in children in whom the cheek area is large and the supraclavicular area is relatively small) the supraclavicular flap may be pre-expanded first.[1] After 3 months, when the flap has the right size and the capsule has matured, it may be transferred as an island flap or as a peninsular flap, which needs to be divided and inset 2 weeks later.[1]

Deltopectoral Flap

In cases where no other options are available, the medially based deltopectoral flap, described for the first time by Bakamjian in 1965,[37] may be used for defects of the lower cheek. The flap derives its primary blood supply from the perforating branches of the internal mammary artery through the second, third, and fourth interspaces. The medial part of the flap has an axial blood supply but the skin overlying the deltoid region derives its blood supply from the anterior perforating branch of the acromiothoracic artery, which is transected during elevation of the flap, making the distal third randomly vascularized through the subdermal plexus. Therefore, it is safer to delay the distal part overlying the deltoid muscle lateral to the deltopectoral groove approximately 1 week before elevation of the flap (**Fig. 25**). The superior flap incision starts at the sternoclavicular joint and continues laterally over the clavicle up to the acromial end where it turns caudally over he deltoid region. The width and length of the flap depend on the size and location of the defect; however, the second and third intercostal perforators usually are included in the pedicle of the flap. Raising this flap on a single perforator has developed a further refinement of this flap. This flap is known as the internal mammary artery perforator flap.[38] After insetting of the flap, the donor site is closed with skin grafts. Approximately 3 weeks later the pedicle is divided and may be transferred back to the chest, improving the donor site appearance by decreasing the skin grafted area. At the recipient site the flap is trimmed and inset further, completing the reconstruction of the cheek.

Disadvantages of the deltopectoral flap are the random vascularization of the distal third, usually making a delay procedure necessary; the multiple staged nature of the reconstruction; and a conspicuous skin grafted donor site.

FREE FLAPS

Although technologically complex, free flaps have become a first choice for large, composite through-and-through cheek defects[11,12] and

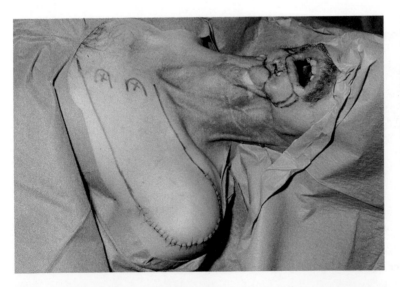

Fig. 25. Preoperative markings for a left-sided deltopectoral flap 1 week after a delay procedure of the randomly vascularized distal part of the flap overlying the deltoid muscle lateral to the deltopectoral groove. The second and third intercostal perforators from the internal mammary vessels were included in the flap design.

extensive composite facial skin defects with exposed bone, dura, sinuses, or orbit.[10] The reliable blood supply of free flaps ensures survival without marginal necrosis. In addition, revascularization of the recipient-site improves wound healing, closing wounds in one stage with minimal risk for wound breakdown and fistulization.[4] Free flaps have no restraint of a fixed, distant vascular pedicle; problems with pedicle bulk and limitations of an arc of rotation are eliminated by careful planning.[4] The choices in design, size, and composite materials for cover, lining, and bony support have been expanded to the limits of imagination, with a wide range of potential donor sites, especially with the advent of perforator flaps.[4] Free flaps have become indispensable to reconstructive surgery. Unfortunately, distant tissue usually does not match facial skin in color, texture, or thickness or have a facial shape.[4,10]

AESTHETIC USE OF FREE FLAPS IN CHEEK RECONSTRUCTION

Carefully tailored and thinned free flaps, using a template, sometimes may lead to acceptable aesthetic results,[39] especially in Asian patients, in

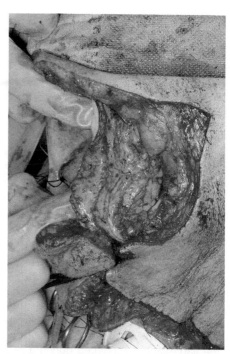

Fig. 27. Intraoperative situation after inset of a radial forearm free flap for intraoral lining reconstruction.

whom flap color mismatch and flap bulkiness often is less apparent.[10,39] For obtaining an optimal aesthetic cheek reconstruction result, however, free flaps ideally should be used only to protect vital structures, fill a cavity, reconstruct inner lining and bony structures, or rebuild a stable platform.[4] Skin cover of the defect ideally should be reconstructed using aforementioned local or locoregional flaps, whenever possible. This can be achieved primarily by covering the free flap immediately during the same procedure. For example, a radial forearm free flap may be used to reconstruct the

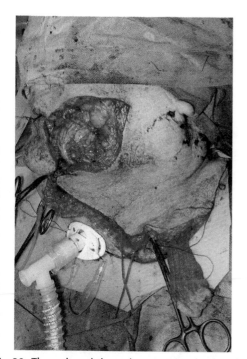

Fig. 26. Through-and-through composite cheek defect after wide local excision of a large intraoral squamous cell carcinoma in a 67-year-old woman. Note that the incisions for the ipsilateral neck dissection were planned according to a posterior-based cervicopectoral flap design.

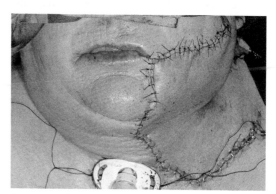

Fig. 28. Result immediately after closure of a through-and-through cheek defect with a radial forearm free flap for intraoral lining and a posterior-based cervicopectoral flap for external skin defect closure.

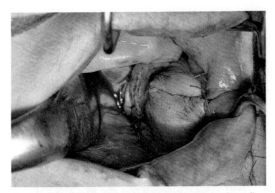

Fig. 29. Intraoral view of the radial forearm free flap for intraoral lining reconstruction.

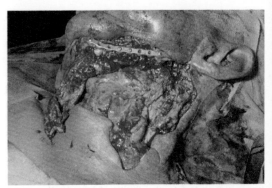

Fig. 30. Intraoperative situation after a left-sided segmental mandibulectomy for osteoradionecrosis in a 63-year-old man. The mandibular defect and intraoral lining were reconstructed with a free osteocutaneous fibula flap. The external skin of the lower cheek and neck had to be excised because of severe radiodermatitis and poor vascularization after re-elevation of the neck dissection skin flaps. The resulting skin defect was reconstructed with a second free anterolateral thigh flap.

inner lining of a through-and-through cheek defect in combination with a posterior-based cervicofacial flap to reconstruct the facial skin defect (**Figs. 26–29**). An ipsilateral neck dissection can be performed through the same incisions, if needed. Alternatively, the external (skin) part of the free flap may be resurfaced during a second stage using a (pre-expanded) locoregional transposition flap.[4] At the first stage the composite through-and-through cheek defect is reconstructed using a bipaddle, double island, or chimeric free flap for inner lining and external skin cover.[11,40,41] At the second stage, some time later, the external skin part of the free flap is excised and the defect is reconstructed with a locoregional transposition flap with or without the use of pre-expansion. A disadvantage of this approach may be that most patients receive radiotherapy after the first operation, because these extensive defects usually are a result of wide resection of large malignant tumors, making the use of tissue expanders troublesome.

Reconstruction of extensive composite mandibular defects, including external skin, usually after tumor or osteoradionecrosis resection, may even require double free flap reconstruction.[42,43] Usually, an osteocutaneous fibula free flap for reconstruction of oral mucosa and the segmental mandibular defect in combination with a fasciocutaneous free flap (radial forearm or anterolateral thigh flap) for external skin coverage is used.[42,43] Reconstruction of these major composite through-and-through defects often results, however, in modest functional and aesthetic outcome (**Figs. 30 and 31**).[43]

PREFABRICATED FLAPS

Flap prefabrication means the implantation of a vascular pedicle into a new territory, followed

by a period of maturation and neovascularization and the subsequent (microsurgical) transfer of that tissue based on its implanted pedicle.[44] Flap prefabrication occurs in two stages.

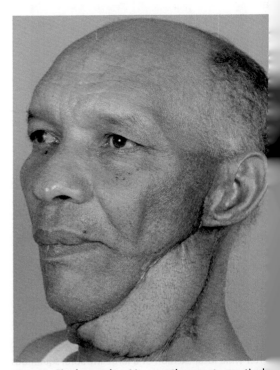

Fig. 31. Final result 11 months postoperatively showing a moderate aesthetic result due to flap bulkiness, flap pin cushioning, skin color, and texture mismatch.

In stage 1, a vascular pedicle is transferred to a new area of tissue and is simply implanted with the distal end ligated and with no vascular anastomoses. Vascular connections occur spontaneously between the implanted pedicle and surrounding tissue creating a new vascular territory. At the first stage an expander may be additionally introduced beneath the vascular pedicle to obtain a thinner, larger, and delayed flap with improved perfusion and to facilitate later donor-site closure.[44–46] Usually, Silastic or Gore-Tex sheets are wrapped around the base of the vascular pedicle to facilitate the transfer of the flap at the second stage.[44,45] Although using the prefabrication technique any donor site area in the body may be chosen, flaps preferably are prefabricated as near the recipient site (ie, cheek) as possible to obtain a flap with good color and texture match.[44,46] Another benefit of prefabrication near the recipient site is the possibility of using multiple sequential prefabricated flaps for complex reconstructions of multiple facial subunits, transferred sequentially by the same pedicle, using the vascular crane principle.[47] Usually, a local vascular pedicle of the superficial temporal vessels (together with the temporoparietal fascia) is used for implantation in the upper cervical or supraclavicular area. If local vessels are not available, however, a vascular pedicle from a remote site (eg, descending branch of lateral femoral circumflex vascular pedicle) is transferred as a mini–free flap to the upper cervical area.[44]

In stage 2, after flap maturation and neovascularization (at least 6 weeks later), the flap is (microsurgically) transferred based on the implanted pedicle.[44] These prefabricated flaps usually suffer from some venous congestion, which resolves in 36 hours to 8 days.[44,46] During this time period most of these flaps require (chemical) leeching to ensure complete survival.[44] If during the first stage a tissue expander is introduced beneath the vascular pedicle, venous congestion is less of a problem during transferal of the flap at the second stage,[46] especially if larger expanders are used.[44] Because tissue expansion and flap prefabrication are two-stage procedures, it makes sense to combine these techniques not only to enhance the vascular response but also to help thin out the flaps and assist with donor site closure.[44–46]

In conclusion, cheek reconstruction using flap prefabrication should be used only if more conventional reconstructive solutions (described previously) are not available (eg, after extensive burns or trauma), because it is a complex, multistaged procedure, often requiring more than one microsurgical tissue transfer with increased risk for complications.

REFERENCES

1. Spence RJ. An algorithm for total and subtotal facial reconstruction using an expanded transposition flap: a 20-year experience. Plast Reconstr Surg 2008;121(3):795–805.
2. Menick FJ. Artistry in aesthetic surgery. Aesthetic perception and the subunit principle. Clin Plast Surg 1987;14(4):723–35.
3. Menick FJ. Reconstruction of the cheek. Plast Reconstr Surg 2001;108(2):496–505.
4. Menick FJ. Facial reconstruction with local and distant tissue: the interface of aesthetic and reconstructive surgery. Plast Reconstr Surg 1998;102(5):1424–33.
5. Menick FJ. Defects of the nose, lip, and cheek: rebuilding the composite defect. Plast Reconstr Surg 2007;120(4):887–98.
6. Juri J, Juri C. Advancement and rotation of a large cervicofacial flap for cheek repairs. Plast Reconstr Surg 1979;64(5):692–6.
7. Juri J, Juri C. Cheek reconstruction with advancement-rotation flaps. Clin Plast Surg 1981;8(2):223–6.
8. Kaplan I, Goldwyn RM. The versatility of the laterally based cervicofascial flap for cheek repairs. Plast Reconstr Surg 1978;61(3):390–3.
9. Zide BM. Deformities of the lips and cheeks. In: McCarthy JG, editor, Plastic surgery, vol. 3. Philadelphia: WB Saunders; 1990. p. 2009–56.
10. Mureau MAM, Posch NAS, Meeuwis CA, et al. Anterolateral thigh flap reconstruction of large external facial skin defects: a follow-up study on functional and aesthetic recipient- and donor-site outcome. Plast Reconstr Surg 2005;115(4):1077–86.
11. Huang WC, Chen HC, Jain V, et al. Reconstruction of through-and-through cheek defects involving the oral commissure, using chimeric flaps from the thigh lateral femoral circumflex system. Plast Reconstr Surg 2002;109(2):433–41.
12. Jeng SF, Kuo YR, Wei FC, et al. Reconstruction of concomitant lip and cheek through-and-through defects with combined free flap and an advancement flap from the remaining lip. Plast Reconstr Surg 2004;113(2):491–8.
13. Esser JFS. Rotation der Wange. Leipzig: Vogel; 1918.
14. Mustardé JC. Repair and reconstruction in the orbital region. A practical guide. Edinburgh (UK): E & S Livingstone; 1966. p. 117.
15. Converse JM. Reconstructive plastic surgery. Philadelphia: WB Saunders; 1977. p. 1586.
16. Stark RB, Kaplan JM. Rotation flaps, neck to cheek. Plast Reconstr Surg 1972;50(3):230–3.

17. Kroll SS, Reece GP, Robb G, et al. Deep-plane cervicofacial rotation-advancement flap for reconstruction of large cheek defects. Plast Reconstr Surg 1994;94(1):88–93.

18. Delay E, Lucas R, Jorquera F, et al. Composite cervicofacial flap for reconstruction of complex cheek defects. Ann Plast Surg 1999;43(4):347–53.

19. Longaker MT, Glat PM, Zide BM. Deep-plane cervicofacial "hike": anatomic basis with dog-ear blepharoplasty. Plast Reconstr Surg 1997;99(1): 16–21.

20. Belmahi A, Oufkir A, Bron T, et al. Reconstruction of cheek skin defects by the 'Yin-Yang' rotation of the Mustardé flap and the temporoparietal scalp. J Plast Reconstr Aesthet Surg 2007; doi:10.1016/j.bjps.2007.11.012.

21. Schrudde J, Beinhoff U. Reconstruction of the face by means of the angle-rotation flap. Aesthetic Plast Surg 1987;11(1):15–22.

22. Boutros S, Zide BM. Cheek and eyelid reconstruction: the resurrection of the angle rotation flap. Plast Reconstr Surg 2005;116(5):1425–30.

23. Crow ML, Crow FJ. Resurfacing large cheek defects with rotation flaps from the neck. Plast Reconstr Surg 1976;58(2):196–200.

24. Becker DW Jr. A cervicopectoral rotation flap for cheek coverage. Plast Reconstr Surg 1978;61(6): 868–70.

25. Shestak KC, Roth AG, Jones NF, et al. The cervicopectoral rotation fla—a valuable technique for facial reconstruction. Br J Plast Surg 1993;46(5): 375–7.

26. Moore BA, Wine T, Netterville JL. Cervicofacial and cervicothoracic rotation flaps in head and neck reconstruction. Head Neck 2005;27(12):1092–101.

27. Garrett WS Jr, Giblin TR, Hoffman GW. Closure of skin defects of the face and neck by rotation and advancement of cervicopectoral flaps. Plast Reconstr Surg 1966;38(4):342–6.

28. Futrell JW, Johns ME, Edgerton MT, et al. Platysma myocutaneous flap for intraoral reconstruction. Am J Surg 1978;136(4):504–7.

29. Puxeddu R, Dennis S, Ferreli C, et al. Platysma myocutaneous flap for reconstruction of skin defects in the head and neck. Br J Oral Maxillofac Surg 2008; 46(5):383–6.

30. Peng LW, Zhang WF, Zhao JH, et al. Two designs of platysma myocutaneous flap for reconstruction of oral and facial defects following cancer surgery. Int J Oral Maxillofac Surg 2005;34(5):507–13.

31. Coleman JJ 3rd, Nahai F, Mathes SJ. Platysma musculocutaneous flap: clinical and anatomical considerations in head and neck reconstruction. Am J Surg 1982;144(4):477–81.

32. Agarwal A, Schneck CD, Kelley DJ. Venous drainage of the platysma myocutaneous flap. Otolaryngol Head Neck Surg 2004;130(3):357–9.

33. Mutter TD. Cases of deformities from burns, relieved by operation. Am J Med Sci 1842;4: 66–80.

34. Lamberty BG. The supra-clavicular axial patterned flap. Br J Plast Surg 1979;32(3):207–12.

35. Pallua N, Noah EM. The tunneled supraclavicular island flap: an optimized technique for head and neck reconstruction. Plast Reconstr Surg 2000; 105(3):842–51.

36. Hartman EHM, Van Damme PA, Sauter H, et al. The use of the pedicled supraclavicular flap in noma reconstructive surgery. J Plast Reconstr Aesthet Surg 2006;59(4):337–42.

37. Bakamjian VY. A two-stage method for pharyngoesophabeal reconstruction with a primary pectoral skin flap. Plast Reconstr Surg 1965;36:173–84.

38. Vesely MJ, Murray DJ, Novak CB, et al. The internal mammary perforator flap: an anatomical study and a case report. Ann Plast Surg 2007; 58(2):706–7.

39. Lee JT, Hsiao HT, Tung KY, et al. Successful one-stage resurfacing and contouring of an extensively burned cheek by using a scar template free anterolateral thigh flap: a case report and literature review. J Trauma 2008;65(1):E1–3.

40. Disa JJ, Liew S, Cordeiro PG. Soft-tissue reconstruction of the face using the folded/multiple skin island radial forearm free flap. Ann Plast Surg 2001;47(6): 621–9.

41. Yokoo S, Tahara S, Tsuji Y, et al. Functional and aesthetic reconstruction of full-thickness cheek, oral commissure and vermillion. J Craniomaxillofac Surg 2001;29(6):344–50.

42. Wei FC, Demirkan F, Chen HC, et al. Double free flaps in reconstruction of extensive composite mandibular defects in head and neck cancer. Plast Reconstr Surg 1999;103(1):39–47.

43. Posch NAS, Mureau MAM, Dumans AG, et al. Functional and aesthetic outcome and survival after double free flap reconstruction in advanced head and neck cancer patients. Plast Reconstr Surg 2007;120(1):124–9.

44. Pribaz JJ, Fine N, Orgill DP. Flap prefabrication in the head and neck: a 10-year experience. Plast Reconstr Surg 1999;103(3):808–20.

45. Khouri RK, Ozbek MR, Hruza GJ, et al. Facial reconstruction with prefabricated induced expanded (PIE) supraclavicular skin flaps. Plast Reconstr Surg 1995;95(6):1007–15.

46. Teot L, Cherenfant E, Otman S. Prefabricated vascularised supraclavicular flaps for face resurfacing after postburn scarring. Lancet 2000;355(9216): 1695–6.

47. Pribaz JJ, Maitz PKM, Fine MA. Flap prefabrication using the "vascular crane" principle: an experimental study and clinical application. Br J Plast Surg 1994;47(4):250–6.

Strategies in Lip Reconstruction

Peter C. Neligan, MB, FRCS(I), FRCSC, FACS

KEYWORDS

• Lip • Reconstruction • Defect • Function • Aesthetics

Injury or surgical trauma can result in significant alterations of normal lip appearance and function that can profoundly impact the patient's self-image and quality of life. Subtle changes in the appearance of the vermilion border, oral commissures, or Cupid's bow are easily detected by the casual observer. Neuromuscular injury can lead to asymmetry at rest and, even more particularly, during facial animation, and distressing functional disabilities are common. Loss of labial competence may interfere with the ability to articulate, whistle, suck, kiss, and contain salivary secretions. Lip reconstruction is not new. Surgeons have been trying to reconstruct lips functionally and cosmetically for centuries. For smaller defects, reconstruction can be very effective. The larger the defect, however, the more difficult it is to create an aesthetically pleasing and functional lip.

ANATOMIC AND FUNCTIONAL CONSIDERATIONS IN LIP CONSTRUCTION

The lips are trilaminar in nature and consist of mucosa, muscle, and skin. The external construct combines skin with a transition to mucosa at the mucocutaneous ridge or vermilion border. At the midline of the upper lip, there is a U-shaped indentation of the mucocutaneous ridge called "Cupid's bow." Above Cupid's bow, the philtrum is a vertical groove-shaped depression that is bordered on either side by elevations known as "philtral ridges" or "columns." The mucosa of the vermilion is unique in that it lacks minor salivary glands. The characteristic hue of the vermilion stems from a rich vascular supply that underlies an especially thin epithelial architecture. Sensation to the upper and lower lips is provided by branches of the maxillary and mandibular divisions of the

trigeminal nerve. The boundaries of the upper lip are defined by the base of the nose centrally and by the nasolabial fold laterally. The mental crease defines the inferior margin of the lower lip, although one thinks of the lip and chin as being a single aesthetic unit.[1] The lower lip is composed of only one aesthetic unit. The upper lip, however, consists of multiple subunits. According to Burget and Menick,[2] each side of the upper lip has two aesthetic subunits: the medial topographic subunit is one half the philtrum; the lateral subunit is bordered by the philtrum medially, the nostril sill and alar base superiorly, and the nasolabial crease laterally. Other authors maintain that the upper lip is composed of three subunits, with the entire philtrum constituting a single subunit.[3]

The orbicularis oris muscle is responsible for most of the bulk of the lip. This muscle forms a sphincteric ring around the mouth. It consists of superficial and deep fibers that function to hold the lips away from the facial plane and to approximate the lips to the alveolar arch, respectively.[4] The buccinators decussates as it approaches to oral commissure and merges with orbicularis fibers of both upper and lower lips.[4] The two most important elevator muscles of the lip are the zygomaticus major and the levator anguli oris. The zygomaticus minor and the levator labii superioris also contribute. The depressor muscles include the depressor anguli oris and the platysma, with minor contributions from the depressor labii inferioris. Contractions of these muscles result in modification of the shape of the lips associated with facial expression and function. The modiolus is situated just lateral to the oral commissure and is approximately a 1-cm thick fibrovascular region of muscle fiber intersection of the levator muscles and the depressor

University of Washington Medical Center, 1959 NE Pacific Street, Seattle, WA 98195, USA
E-mail address: pneligan@u.washington.edu

Clin Plastic Surg 36 (2009) 477–485
doi:10.1016/j.cps.2009.02.013
0094-1298/09/$ – see front matter © 2009 Published by Elsevier Inc

plasticsurgery.theclinics.com

muscles that attach firmly to the dermis. The modiolus can actually be felt in this location when pinched between thumb and index finger.[5] Movement of the modiolus results from the contractile forces of the levator muscles (zygomaticus major and levator anguli oris) and the depressor muscles (depressor anguli oris and platysma).[6,7] Sometimes there is a dimple in this location. The elevators and depressors of the lips are innervated by the buccal and mandibular branches of the facial nerve, respectively. Disruption of the musculature that attaches to the modiolar region (or their neural supply) can alter the appearance of the labial commissure at rest and during function secondary to imbalanced muscular contraction. Modiolar motion has also been analyzed to measure the success of facial reanimation in patients with facial paralysis.[8]

The superior and inferior labial arteries, branches of the facial artery, supply the lips. The superior labial arteries from each side tend to anastomose in the midportion of the upper lip, coursing between the mucosa and orbicularis muscle in half of the patients and through the muscle in the other half. The inferior labial artery, however, routinely courses between the mucosa of the inner aspect of the lip and the muscle.[9]

LIP FUNCTION

The lips are an important aesthetic feature of the lower face and any deformity of the lips is instantly recognizable. Even minor deformities are easily noticed. More important are the functional characteristics of the lips. The lips play a very important part in speech articulation, as anyone who has tried to speak after extensive local anesthesia at the dentist can attest. Also, the lips are vital for the maintenance of oral competence.[10] Sensation allows the lips to monitor the texture and temperature of substances before oral intake.

GOALS OF LIP RECONSTRUCTION

The goals of lip reconstruction are multiple. The primary goal of reconstruction is functional. No matter how good a lip reconstruction looks, if the lips do not function well and if oral competence is lost, the reconstruction is not successful. In addition, it is important that an adequate aperture be maintained to allow for a normal diet and to allow for adequate oral hygiene. This may also include the necessity to remove and replace dentures. A sensate lip functions better than a nonsensate one, so preservation of sensation is an important feature of an adequate reconstruction. Usually, if all of these requirements have been

met the lip is also aesthetically pleasing but cosmesis is a very important part of lip reconstruction even though it does take second place to function.

If the orbicularis has been disrupted it is imperative carefully to reapproximate the muscle in the repair. Otherwise, the sphincteric function of the orbicularis may be lost or disrupted. The best results are achieved if the sphincter is reconstructed and sensation preserved.[2,10,11] In cases where reconstruction of the sphincter is not feasible, an adynamic reconstruction must be pursued that provides some degree of oral competence. Decreases in the shape or depth of the labial vestibule can exacerbate oral incompetence and drooling, and may preclude patients from wearing a removable prosthesis. It is important to preserve or restore the labial vestibule; after all, it is there for a purpose.

Because of the unique anatomy of the upper lip, reconstruction presents some unique challenges. Loss of the philtral ridges and Cupid's bow creates a noticeable cosmetic deformity that presents a significant reconstructive challenge. The relationship of the upper and lower lip is also important to appreciate. Normally, the upper lip protrudes anterior to the lower lip. If this relationship is lost, as it may be with a tight closure of an upper lip defect, the aesthetic outcome of the reconstruction is compromised. This is not as big an issue with the lower lip and one can usually get away with a bigger resection of lower lip without compromising aesthetics in the repair.

Burget and Menick[2] brought attention to reconstruction of aesthetic subunits. Failing to appreciate these subtleties can result in an inferior reconstruction that is instantly recognizable by even the casual observer. Whenever possible, the height, projection, and relationship between the white and red portions of the lip should be duplicated. This is most easily achieved by using tissue from the adjacent or opposing lip.[1,12] Because the face is so visible and cosmesis is so important, the best possible aesthetic result is desirable. For this reason, one should use local tissue where at all possible. Local tissue provides the best color and texture match and provides tissue of similar thickness and with similar skin characteristics as the tissue being reconstructed.

DEFECT-SPECIFIC RECONSTRUCTION OF THE LIP
Defects of the Vermilion

Vermilionectomy involves resection of the vermilion. It is only used for very superficial lesions. Occasionally, if the vermillion is very dysplastic as in actinic cheilitis, vermilionectomy can be a very effective treatment. Reconstruction i achieved by an advancement flap of mucosa from labial or buccal surface. The undermined mucosa is advanced forward to re-establish the mucocutaneous junction. The procedure is called a "lip-shave." It is a very effective way to resurface the vermillion and the esthetic results are excellent (**Fig. 1**). Occasionally, patients complain of dryness and must be prepared regularly to use some sort of moisturizer or lip salve to prevent desiccation and discomfort. The patient must be warned of a tendency for thinning of the vermillion and some reduction in the sensitivity of the vermillion.[1] It is important to undermine and advance the labial mucosa adequately to minimize the risk of thinning and to prevent entropion of the lip. Other approaches to reconstruction of the vermillion include the mucosal V-Y advancement flap,[13,14] the cross-lip mucosal flap, and transposition flaps harvested from the buccal mucosa or the ventral surface of the tongue.[15] A facial artery musculomucosal flap can also be used to provide a vermillion in situations where the vermillion has been excised.[16] Buccal mucosal flaps tend to be more erythematous than natural vermilion, resulting in a color mismatch with the remaining vermilion. Mucosal tongue flaps require a second procedure 14 to 21 days later to release and inset the flap.

Small Full-Thickness Defects

Direct closure of defects that involve as much as a quarter of the upper lip or one third of the lower lip can be achieved.[10] A V-shaped wedge usually permits closure of smaller defects. In the lower lip, to avoid impinging on the chin and transgressing the mental crease, changing the V wedge to a W wedge keeps the scar high while allowing for a wider excision (**Fig. 2**). Wedge-shaped defects of the lateral lip should be more obliquely oriented so that the line of closure parallels the relaxed skin tension lines. Closure of all of these defects is achieved in three layers: mucosa, muscle, and skin. The aesthetic result following repair of a wedge excision is often less satisfactory in the upper lip, because the upper lip is able to withstand much less tissue loss before tightness becomes clinically apparent and the normal

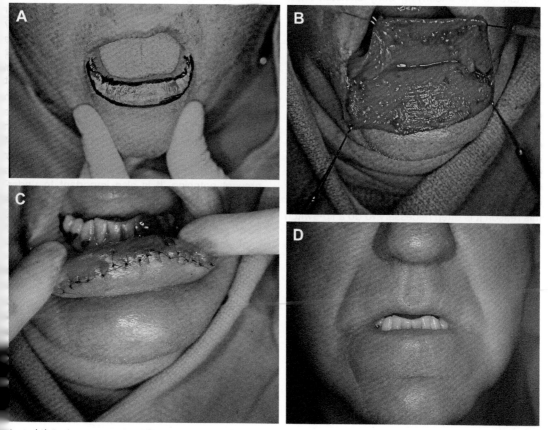

ig. 1. (A) Patient presents with severe actinic cheilitis. Extent of vermilionectomy is outlined. (B) Vermillion has ·een excised and mucosal flap undermined and advanced. (C) Immediate closure. (D) Final result. Note some thin-·ing of the lip but otherwise excellent aesthetic result.

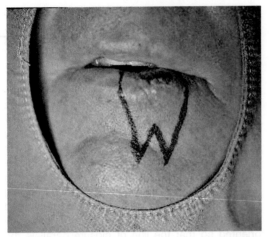

Fig. 2. W-shaped wedge excision planned for squamous cell carcinoma. Note how the W prevents the scar from impinging on the mental crease and keeps the scar on the lip.

overhang of upper and lower lip is lost as a consequence of closure-induced tension. In addition, the anchorage of soft tissues around the pyriform aperture to the underlying bony skeleton limits compensatory movement of the remaining lip. A "T"-shaped excision minimizes this effect by allowing the lateral lip elements to be advanced. Further advancement can be achieved by incorporating crescentic perialar excisions as described by Webster.[17] This technique not only allows advancement of the lip elements, but also some recruitment of cheek tissue, which allows further advancement of the lip elements (**Fig. 3**). There is a lot less leeway when dealing with upper lip defects. This is because of the specific aesthetic subunits within the upper lip. A wedge resection that is perfectly acceptable in the lower lip may cause significant deformity of the upper lip. For this reason it is often necessary to do a lip-switch operation for the upper lip to produce the optimal functional and cosmetic outcome (see later). This is particularly true of mid-upper lip defects in which a standard wedge and repair produces a very noticeable deformity because of tightness and loss of the philtrum with consequent disruption of the Cupid's bow.

Intermediate Full-Thickness Defects

For larger defects involving as much as two thirds of either lip, local flaps are the best reconstructive option. Three different technical approaches are used to achieve these reconstructions: (1) switching tissue from one lip to the other, (2) rotating tissue from one lip to the other, and (3) advancing cheek or neck tissue into the defect. The cross-lip (lip-switch) flaps are axial pattern local flaps that transfer labial tissue from the opposing lip based on an arterial pedicle from one of the labial arteries. Cross-lip flaps permit reconstruction with similar tissue from the opposite lip. The Abbe flap can be used to reconstruct lip defects with a full-thickness composite flap that reconstructs the mucocutaneous border and the orbicularis oris.[18] Although the Abbe flap is traditionally described as triangular in shape, the flap can also be designed to accommodate wedge- or rectangular-shaped defects. It is most usual for Abbe flaps to be transferred from lower to upper lip. Although it is technically feasible to do it the other way around (ie, from upper to lower lip), this is rarely done because of the constraints on resection of the upper lip and the potentially inferior cosmetic results that such a maneuver can produce. Because of the elasticity of tissue there are certain mathematical guidelines to lip-switch operations: the width of the flap should be half the width of the defect, and the height of the flap should be the same as the height of the defect to prevent notching. It is also important to understand where the pedicle will be placed. For the pedicle to be placed correctly the Abbe flap should be centered toward the edge of the excision on the contralateral lip on the desired pedicle side

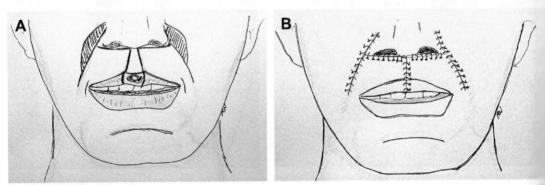

Fig. 3. (A) Schematic of carcinoma of upper lip with planned T excision with Webster's modification. (B) Schematic excision and closure.

(Fig. 4). Division of the pedicle and revision of the flap is performed 14 to 21 days later. The Estlander flap is in essence an Abbe flap that is brought around the commissure. Once again, the width of the flap is usually one half the width of the defect and is the same height as the defect (Fig. 5). Defects that involve the commissure and as much as 50% of the lower or upper lip can be adequately reconstructed with an acceptable functional and cosmetic result.

There are, however, several limitations to the cross-lip flaps. Blunting of the commissure regularly occurs with the Estlander flap, but this blunting frequently diminishes over time. Commissuroplasty is rarely necessary and should not be considered until at least 6 months following reconstruction. Even though the orbicularis muscle is reconstructed, disruption of the motor supply leads to varying degrees of oral competence. Pin cushioning frequently develops at the recipient site, and the cross-lip flap tends to appear thicker than the adjacent lip, at least initially. The fan flap, initially described by Gillies and Millard in 1957, is based on a technique described by von Bruns that used quadrilateral inferiorly based nasolabial flaps.[19] This flap rotates tissue around the commissure in the same fashion as an Estlander flap, but more tissue from the nasolabial region is included.[20] A vertical releasing incision is made in the donor lip and this results in at least some denervation.[21] A unilateral flap can be

performed to reconstruct a lip defect, but bilateral fan flaps are more frequently used to reconstruct total or near-total defects. Although defects involving up to 80% of the lip can be reconstructed with the Gillies fan flap, significant microstomia and vermilion deficiency are frequent sequelae. Denervation can worsen oral incompetence, although partial reinnervation seems to occur within 12 to 18 months.[21] The older von Brun's circumoral advancement-rotation flap, initially described in 1857, resulted in extensive denervation of the orbicularis muscle with a consequent loss of oral competence and cosmesis.[19] In 1974, Karapandzic[22] published a modification of von Bruns's technique. The incisional design of the Karapandzic flap is similar to that advocated by von Bruns, but full-thickness flaps are not created, and the neurovascular supply to the lip is preserved (see Fig. 5). The Karapandzic flap can successfully replace 80% of the total lip length.[22] The larger the defect, however, the greater the risk of inducing significant microstomia. Careful dissection of the peripheral muscle fibers and concentric undermining allows advancement without any dissection of the mucosa. A unilateral flap is adequate for smaller defects, whereas defects that constitute more than 50% of the lip require bilateral flaps. Function is restored because only the peripheral rim of orbicularis oris muscle is incised and the buccinator muscle is preserved. The Karapandzic flap results

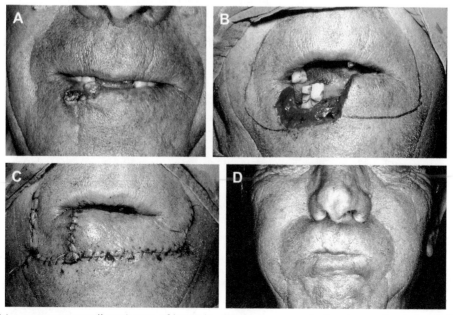

Fig. 4. (A) Large squamous cell carcinoma of lower lip. (B) Carcinoma excised and reconstructed with Abbe flap from lower lip. (C) Appearance before pedicle division. (D) Postoperative appearance showing good oral continence on pursing. Note blunted commissures not noticeable.

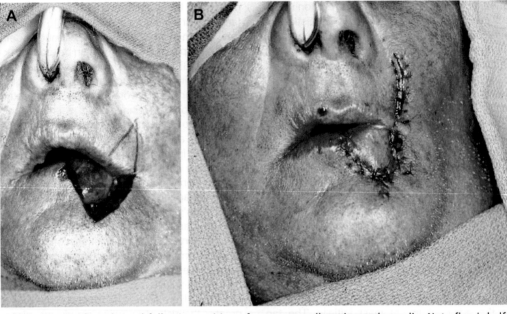

Fig. 5. (*A*) Estlander flap planned following excision of squamous cell carcinoma lower lip. Note flap is half the width of the defect but the same height. (*B*) Appearance on rotation of the flap and closure. Note blunting of commissure.

in blunting or rounding of both commissures, which is usually less noticeable than alteration of only one commissure (see **Fig. 4**). Some degree of microstomia is also inevitable. In extreme cases this may preclude the use of dentures. Based on the superior functional and cosmetic results that can be achieved, the Karapandzic flap is arguably the flap of choice for most defects. Frequently, a defect is too wide to close primarily but is not wide enough to require a flap, such as the Estlander flap, which interferes with the commissure. The stair-step advancement flap, described by Johanson and colleagues,[23] can be used for such defects and is capable of reconstructing defects that constitute as much as two thirds of the lower lip (**Fig. 6**). This technique involves the excision of two to four small rectangles arranged in a stair-step fashion that descends from medial to lateral at a 45-degree angle from either side of the base of the defect. The lateral-most excision

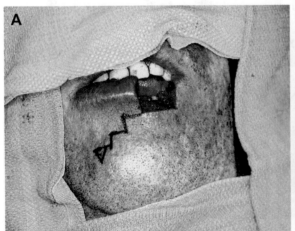
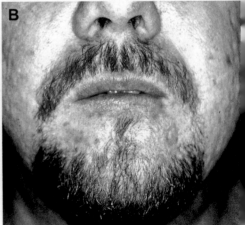

Fig. 6. (*A*) Planned step reconstruction following excision of squamous cell carcinoma, unilateral flap only planned. (*B*) Postoperative appearance.

in the stair-step is a triangle with its apex inferior (see **Fig. 6**). For lateral defects, the step incision is outlined exclusively on the remaining long side of the lip and advancement from that single side may be all that is required to close the defect.[24] If the defect is located near the midline the staircase pattern is marked on both sides of the lower lip. Although the original description described full-thickness excision of the rectangles, it is often possible to excise skin only and preserve the orbicularis and its motor supply. By placing the step incisions outside of the mental crease, the aesthetic unit of the chin can be preserved.

Large Full-Thickness Defects

Defects that involve up to 80% of the total lip length may be reconstructed with bilateral Gillies fan flaps or the Karapandzic flap.[20,22]

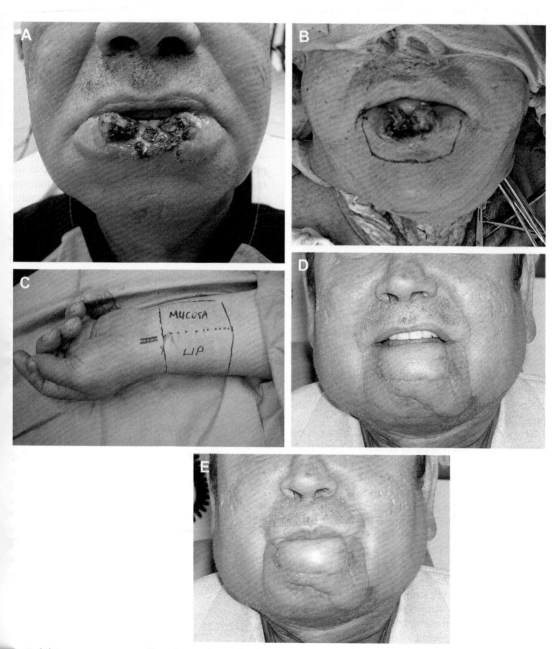

Fig. 7. (A) Large squamous cell carcinoma lower lip. (B) Planned excision combined with bilateral neck dissection. (C) Planning of the flap. Note mucosal element smaller than skin element. (D) Postoperative appearance showing good cosmesis and (E) continence on pursing.

Reconstruction of total or near-total defects constituting more than 80% of the lip typically leads to an inferior aesthetic outcome, significant microstomia, and compromised labial competence that is largely adynamic. Before free-tissue transfer, nasolabial flaps played a prominent role in total lip reconstruction. In 1845, Dieffenbach initially described the use of nasolabial flaps for upper lip reconstruction.[1] The rectangular-shaped nasolabial flaps that von Bruns described in 1857 for lower lip defects were inferiorly based. The "gate flap" design, originally published by Fujimori in 1980,[25] rotates two nasolabial island flaps that are based on the angular artery. Although Fujimori's technique was fashioned for the lower lip, modifications of the gate flap have also been proposed for total upper lip reconstruction.[26] Reconstruction with any of these nasolabial flap designs is associated with suboptimal oral competence and aesthetics, and denervation of the flaps routinely occurs. More recently, free-tissue transfer has been used to reconstruct total or subtotal lip defects. The radial forearm flap is most frequently used for the reconstruction of total lower lip defects. Sakai and colleagues[27] in 1989 reported the reconstruction of a lower lip defect with a composite radial forearm-palmaris longus tendon free flap. The forearm flap is folded over the tendon sling to resurface the internal and external surfaces of the lip and cheek.[1,28] A microneural anastomosis between the lateral antebrachial cutaneous nerve and the cut end of the mental nerve can be performed to achieve sensory reinnervation.[28] A ventral tongue flap may be used to recreate the vermilion border, although a second procedure is necessary.[29,30] Following flap reconstruction, medical tattooing can also be used to create the vermilion with acceptable cosmetic results.[31]

There are certain mathematical guidelines in the use of radial forearm flaps for lip reconstruction. As with lip-switch flaps, the width of the flap should be one half the width of the defect. It is important, however, that the height be the same or even slightly greater. This is because of the postoperative scarring that tends to reduce the height of the reconstruction. One other technical fact is important to appreciate. The height of the skin defect is often different from the height of the mucosal defect and this has to be taken into account when the flap is being planned.[28] Oral competence and aesthetics are optimized by placing the palmaris longus tendon under the appropriate degree of tension. Lip entropion can develop if the palmaris longus tendon is inset too tightly (bow-strung), and ectropion may develop if inadequate tension is placed on the tendon. The author weaves the

palmaris sling through the remaining orbicularis muscle, suturing the tendon to itself (**Fig. 7**). If adequate tension is placed on the tendon by the facial musculature at the modioli, the muscle action from the remaining facial muscles is transferred to the new lip, resulting in a more dynamic suspension. Optimal suspensory support for the tendon is achieved by slightly overcorrecting the tension. The ultimate free flap reconstructive technique of the lip, which also incorporates muscle between the inner and outer layers and restores the vermilion component, has not been described. Nevertheless, the composite radial forearm-palmaris longus tendon free flap has several advantages over pedicled flaps. This reconstruction allows for a single-stage procedure that results in complete skin coverage and intraoral lining. The large amount of skin that can be used with the radial forearm flap usually results in an adequate stomal size. This technique can also be used where a segmental mandibulectomy has been performed by incorporating radial bone into the flap, resulting in a very acceptable functional and cosmetic result. Although the color match between the radial forearm flap and surrounding facial tissue is frequently suboptimal, acceptable cosmetic results are attainable by respecting the borders of the aesthetic subunits during surgical resection and reconstructive planning.

SUMMARY

The importance of restoring normal lip appearance and function following cancer resection is undeniable, and surgeons must be able to appreciate the nuances of surgical reconstruction that make the greatest impact on the ultimate reconstructive outcome. Lip reconstruction should be guided by a defect-specific approach that strives to optimize oral competence and recreate the aesthetic appearance of the lips. A sensate dynamic flap that restores normal lip height, volume, and sphincteric function is optimal, and the aesthetic subunits of the lip should be respected. Limited defects are best reconstructed with local flaps from the remaining labial tissue or the adjacent cheek. Larger defects may require free-tissue transfer or multiple local reconstructive techniques. The goal remains normal or near-normal oral function and optimal cosmesis.

REFERENCES

1. Neligan P, Gullane P, Werning J. Lip reconstruction. In: Werning J, editor. Oral cancer. New York: Thieme Medical Publishing Inc.; 2006. p. 180–93.

2. Burget GC, Menick FJ. Aesthetic restoration of one-half the upper lip. Plast Reconstr Surg 1986;78(5): 583–93.

3. Iwahira Y, Maruyama Y, Yoshitake M. A miniunit approach to lip reconstruction. Plast Reconstr Surg 1994;93(6):1282–5.

4. Wijayaweera CJ, Amaratunga NA, Angunawela P. Arrangement of the orbicularis oris muscle in different types of cleft lips. J Craniofac Surg 2000; 11(3):232–5.

5. Zufferey J. Anatomic variations of the nasolabial fold. Plast Reconstr Surg 1992;88:225–31.

6. Ewart C, Jaworski NB, Rekito AJ, et al. Levator anguli oris: a cadaver study implicating its role in perioral rejuvenation. Ann Plast Surg 2005;260–3.

7. Marinetti C. The lower muscular balance of the face used to lift labial commissures. Plast Reconstr Surg 1999;104:1153–62.

8. Johnson P, Bajaj-Luthra A, Llull R, et al. Quantitative facial motion analysis after functional free muscle reanimation procedures. Plast Reconstr Surg 1997;100:1710–9.

9. Pinar Y, Bilge O, Govsa F. Anatomic study of the blood supply of the perioral region. Clin Anat 2005; 18:330–9.

10. Langstein H, Robb G. Lip and perioral reconstruction. Clin Plast Surg 2005;32:431–45.

11. Cordeiro PG, Santamaria E. Primary reconstruction of complex midfacial defects with combined lip-switch procedures and free flaps. Plast Reconstr Surg 1999;103(7):1850–6.

12. Williams E, Setzen G, Mulvaney M. Modified Bernard-Burow cheek advancement and cross-lip flap for total lip reconstruction. Arch Otolaryngol Head Neck Surg 1996;122:1253–8.

13. Kolhe PS, Leonard AG. Reconstruction of the vermilion after lip-shave. Br J Plast Surg 1988; 41(1):68–73.

14. Carvalho LM, et al. V-Y advancement flap for the reconstruction of partial and full thickness defects of the upper lip. Scand J Plast Reconstr Surg Hand Surg 2002;36(1):28–33.

15. McGregor I. The tongue flap in lip surgery. Br J Plast Surg 1966;19:253–63.

16. Pribaz J, Stephens W, Crespo L, et al. A new intra-oral flap: the facial artery musculo-mucosal (FAMM) flap. Plast Reconstr Surg 1992;90:421–9.

17. Webster J. Crescentic peri-alar cheek excision for upper lip flap advancement with a short history of upper lip repair. Plast Reconstr Surg 1955;16:434–64.

18. Abbe R. A new plastic operation for the relief of deformity due to double harelip. Plast Reconstr Surg 1968;42(5):481–3.

19. Hauben D. Victor von Bruns (1812–1883) and his contributions to plastic and reconstructive surgery. Plast Reconstr Surg 1985;75:120–7.

20. McGregor IA. Reconstruction of the lower lip. Br J Plast Surg 1983;36(1):40–7.

21. Rea JL, Davis WE, Rittenhouse LK. Reinnervation of an Abbe-Estlander and a Gillies fan flap of the lower lip: electromyographic comparison. Arch Otolaryngol 1978;104(5):294–5.

22. Karapandzic M. Reconstruction of lip defects by local arterial flaps. Br J Plast Surg 1974;27(1):93–7.

23. Johanson B, Aspelund E, Breine U, et al. Surgical treatment of non-traumatic lower lip lesions with special reference to the step technique: a follow-up on 149 patients. Scand J Plast Reconstr Surg 1974;8:232–40.

24. Sullivan D. Staircase closure of lower lip defects. Ann Plast Surg 1978;1:392–7.

25. Fujimori R. Gate flap for the total reconstruction of the lower lip. Br J Plast Surg 1980;33(3):340–5.

26. Aytekin A, Ay A, Aytekin O. Total upper lip reconstruction with bilateral Fujimori gate flaps. Plast Reconstr Surg 2003;111:797–800.

27. Sakai S, Soeda S, Endo T, et al. A compound radial artery forearm flap for the reconstruction of lip and chin defect. Br J Plast Surg 1989;42:337–8.

28. Carroll CM, Pathak I, Irish J, et al. Reconstruction of total lower lip and chin defects using the composite radial forearm–palmaris longus tendon free flap. Arch Facial Plast Surg 2000;2(1):53–6.

29. Serletti JM, Tavin E, Moran SL, et al. Total lower lip reconstruction with a sensate composite radial forearm-palmaris longus free flap and a tongue flap. Plast Reconstr Surg 1997;99:559–61.

30. Sadove R, Luce E, McGrath P. Reconstruction of the lower lip and chin with the composite radial forearm–palmaris longus free flap. Plast Reconstr Surg 1991; 88:209–14.

31. Furuta S, Hataya Y, Watanabe T, et al. Vermilion-plasty using medical tattooing after radial forearm flap reconstruction of the lower lip. Br J Plast Surg 1994;47:422–4.

Maximizing Results for Lipofilling in Facial Reconstruction

Juan P. Barret, MD, PhD[a,b,]*, Neus Sarobe, MD[b],
Nelida Grande, MD[b], Delia Vila, MD[b], Jose M. Palacin, MD[b]

KEYWORDS

- Reconstruction • Fat • Graft • Lipostructure
- Transplantation • Face

Fat grafting has been used by plastic surgeons for more than 100 years. Fat is autologous and biocompatible; as such, it has been used extensively with different results all of which are technique-dependent. Fat tissue transplantation has been performed in many different ways but, in general, the use of a blunt cannula to perform the harvest and transfer has remained the instrument of choice. New advances in techniques and instrumentation have produced renewed interest in fat transplantation. Through the design of new small blunt cannulas and the use of centrifugation, the technique published and popularized by Dr. Sydney Coleman[1] has become the gold standard of fat tissue autotransplantation.

Fat grafting by means of small cannulas with or without centrifugation (ie, lipostructure) is a natural, long-lasting method of filling and supporting tissues that require contouring and augmentation for complete restoration of the natural aspect of the deformed anatomic area. Lipostructure has become an excellent tool in the armamentarium of the reconstructive surgeon. It can be used alone, as the definitive treatment for certain deformities (contour deficits, Parry-Romberg syndrome, involutive angiomas, etc.) or as an adjunct or finishing touch for complex reconstructions. Fat tissue, however, is extremely fragile, and successful transplantation demands careful attention to every step of the technique, such as the

method of harvesting and the transfer and placement of the small tissue parcels. Some of the permanent results of fat grafting have been attributed to several different mechanisms of action. Adult adipose tissue stem cells, stromal cells, growth factors, hormones, angiogenesis, among others have been pointed out to benefit this technique.

HISTORY OF FAT TRANSPLANTATION

The origin of fat transplantation is difficult to establish. It may be as old as the development of the new era of surgical practice in the mid and late nineteenth century. However, in contrast to the current surge of interest in lipostructure—mainly in the application of augmentation in cosmetic surgery—the development of fat transplantation has played a less important part in the development of reconstructive surgery.

At the turn of the nineteenth century, Neuber[2] recognized that fat could be transplanted in small tissue parcels; however, he warned that fat tissue was very fragile, and that careful manipulation of the tissue was necessary. A few years later, Lexer[3] reported survival of large fat tissue transplantations, with similar comments regarding the fragility of fat tissue. Peer[4] was the first surgeon who demonstrated that fat transplantation had a survival rate of 50%, mainly by diffusion and

[a] Department of Plastic Surgery and Burns, University Hospital Vall d'Hebron, Universidad Autonoma de Barcelona, Passeig de la d'Hebron, 119-129, 08035 Barcelona, Spain
[b] Centro Medico Teknon, Consultorios Marquesa Desp 39-40, Marquesa de Vilallonga 12, 08017 Barcelona, Spain
* Corresponding author. Department of Plastic Surgery and Burns, University Hospital Vall d'Hebron, Universidad Autonoma de Barcelona, Passeig de la Vall d'Hebron, 119-129, 08035 Barcelona, Spain.
E-mail address: jpbarret@hotmail.com (J.P. Barret).

Clin Plastic Surg 36 (2009) 487–492
doi:10.1016/j.cps.2009.02.005
0094-1298/09/$ – see front matter © 2009 Elsevier Inc. All rights reserved.

neovascularization. Plastic surgeons have used fat grafting with varying success over many decades, but the general, nonevidence-based consensus was that fat graft survival was very poor.

Over the last two decades of the twentieth century, Coleman[5] developed a new method of fat graft transplantation. This new technique transplanted fat as tissue and not as individual cells. The manipulation of fat tissue was kept at a minimum because of its fragility. For this reason, fat was harvested with a small cannula yielding small tissue parcels that could be easily injected by way of a small needle. In Coleman's method, oil, lidocaine, infiltrate solution, blood, and detritus were removed with sedimentation or centrifugation. The excellent fat graft survival rates and longevity of fat transplanted with Coleman's lipostructure has been demonstrated in a high number of cases with long-term follow-up of more than 8 to 10 years.[5,6]

FAT TISSUE AND ADULT STEM CELLS

Many surgeons have observed that transplanted fat not only adjusts facial volume and proportion but also improves the surrounding tissues where the fat has been infiltrated. Surgeons have observed the improvement of aging skin, scars, radiation damage, chronic ulcers, breast capsular contracture, and so forth. The role of adipose-derived stem cells and preadipocytes in fat survival and in the improvement of the quality of tissues is still unclear. Initial research implies these cells may be used in tissue remodeling and even in the development of other tissues such as bone, cartilage, and skin in the laboratory.[7] Human adipose tissue has emerged as an important source for adult stem cells, with the highest percentage of these cells of any tissue in the body. There are as many as 5000 adipose-derived stem cells per gram of fat compared with 100 to 1000 stem cells per milliliter of bone marrow.[8–10] These adipose cells differentiate into adult fat tissue. However, under certain circumstances, they have the ability to undergo multilineage differentiation, both in vitro and in animal models.[11–13] Little is known about what happens with these cells when they are transplanted into tissues and their real role and ability to change or repair tissue. Future studies will need to investigate the possible role of these cells for adult tissue engineering and cell and gene therapy.

INDICATIONS

Although lipostructure in reconstructive surgery follows similar rules as those mentioned for cosmetic surgery, indications for this technique in reconstruction are more patient dependent. Some patients will benefit from this option as an isolated treatment, whereas in the majority of cases it serves as an adjunct to other treatments or as a finishing touch to maximize the cosmetic enhancement of the reconstruction. More than ever, with this technique the line between reconstructive surgery and cosmetic surgery is crossed in both directions.

In general, lipostructure is indicated in the following situations:

Correction of scars (either depressed or hypertrophic)
Replacement of missing volume
Asymmetry (either as a whole or in individual anatomic areas)
Enhancement of facial elements or camouflage

A myriad of diseases and pathologic conditions can be treated with lipostructure. It would be impossible to list all potential facial deformities that can be treated with this technique. However, certain conditions merit special attention:

Parry-Romberg syndrome[14]
Post-radiotherapy scars or depressions[15]
Involutive angiomas
Enhancement of fat atrophy following:[16]
    Motor vehicle accidents
    Complex facial fractures
    Correction of gunshot wounds
Asymmetry after flap reconstruction
Asymmetry after tumor ablation
The skeletonized orbit
Donor sites for local flaps
The severely scarred face
Burn sequelae
Retroviral treatment related (HIV lipodistrophy.[17]

Over the past 11 years, we have treated these conditions in reconstructive surgery following strict cosmetic guidelines achieving excellent and permanent results that compare with those published previously by Coleman.[5]

THE TECHNIQUE OF FACIAL LIPOSTRUCTURE FOR RECONSTRUCTIVE PATIENTS

Over the past decade, there have been many reports of different techniques for fat procurement and manipulation. Even though many surgeons claim similar results to those achieved by the original Coleman technique, we follow the same guidelines published and popularized by Coleman.[1,5–7]

The technique for harvesting fat grafts should observe a strict sterile technique. Current studies do not indicate increased viability of adipocytes depending on the donor site chosen for a given patient.[18,19] Therefore, donor sites should be used to enhance and improve body contour as for any cosmetic indication and avoid postoperative deformity. In our practice, the most commonly used donor sites are the abdomen, flanks, and trochanteric areas. In most complex reconstructive cases lipostructure is performed at the end of the major reconstructive procedure; hence it is performed under general anesthetic and local infiltration. In smaller cases, intravenous sedation and local anesthetic are the anesthetic technique of choice. Ringer's lactate with 1:400,000 of epinephrine and 0.5% lidocaine are infiltrated bluntly through a stab incision before harvesting. Through 3 mm stab incisions, a two-hole Coleman harvesting cannula with a blunt tip, attached to a 10 mL syringe, is inserted. Gentle negative pressure is exercised to harvest the fat grafts while the surgeon pushes the cannula back and forth. When the 10 mL syringe is filled, a new one replaces it until the total amount of fat tissue required is obtained. More rapid harvest of fat grafts has been proposed with liposuction cannulas. The Coleman technique, however, has shown superior results in structural fat grafting.[20]

All syringes are capped and placed into the sterile central rotor of a centrifuge and spun at about 3000 rpm for 3 minutes. The centrifugation separates the aspirate in layers. The upper layer is less dense and consists merely of oil. The middle layer is the fat tissue that should be transplanted, and the bottom layer (the most dense) is blood, infiltrate, and water. The top layer is decanted, the syringe plug is removed, and the bottom layer is discarded by way of the opening at the end of the syringe. Absorbent material is used to wick off any remaining oil (**Fig. 1**).

The refined fat is then transferred into syringes that are used for transplantation. In our practice, 1 mL and 5 mL syringes are commonly used.

The instruments used for injection of fat tissue are very thin cannulas with only one hole at the distal end. The most useful cannula size for injection to the face is the 17 gauge, with different tip shapes, lengths, and curves. Blunt cannulas are used in deep tissues and in areas with normal fatty tissue. However, less blunt or sharp cannulas may be necessary for placement under the dermal plane, fibrous tissue, and scars. Sharp cannulas can also be used to free up adhesions. Through mm incisions, cannulas are inserted and

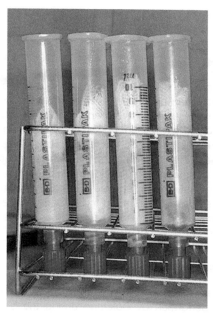

Fig. 1. Common appearance of fat grafts ready for transfer after centrifugation. Note the absorbent gauze to remove any remaining oil.

advanced in the recipient tissues. Small fat tissue parcels are injected only on withdrawing the cannula. Crosshatch patterns are often necessary to create a natural shape and appearance. The injection of fat parcels has to be very accurate, since it is not possible to change their shape with instrumentation or manual manipulation once they have been injected.

SAFETY AND COMPLICATIONS

Lipostructure is relatively safe with few complications, especially in experienced hands,[19] compared with other open surgical techniques. Infections are very rare in fat grafting procedures and when present usually relate to the major reconstructive case rather than to the lipostructure. In general, the infection rate is similar to that reported for cosmetic facial fat grafting procedures. Blunt cannulas have the potential to damage underlying structures such as nerves, muscles, glands, and blood vessels with potential intravascular injection. In our series, no cases of infection or permanent damage to deep structures in more than 400 cases of fat grafting have occurred.

Other common features of structural fat grafting are similar to those observed in liposuction: swelling, bruising, edema, and cosmetic irregularities. If present, they are self-limiting and less than when seen in liposuction.[19] Major bruising or swelling in the facial recipient site is rare. In our experience, bruising is seen in the donor area, especially in flanks and abdomen, and in male patients.

Cosmetic issues are the most common problems observed in lipostructure. The most frequent complications are injection of too much or too little fat, followed by cosmetic irregularities, which are more difficult to prevent and to correct. Not all outcomes can be controlled as they depend on the recipient site and the reaction of the injected tissues. The few patients that we encountered with cosmetic complications exhibited too little augmentation and required a second fat grafting procedure. Patients need to be made aware that a second procedure may be necessary as the final touch of the reconstruction.

PERSONAL EXPERIENCE

The first lipostructure at Centro Medico Teknon was performed by Coleman during the biennial Aesthetic Plastic Surgery Course organized by Palacin in 1997. Since then, 404 cases (of which 248 were facial lipostructures) following a strict Coleman technique, have been performed.

We have performed an objective analysis of all cases. We have seen minimal resorption of fat grafts and results were permanent. It is our impression that the stability of results over time is related to the technique used in this long series. We followed the exact Coleman technique for lipostructure and believe that the deposition of small fat parcels with careful manipulation is the gold standard to obtain these results (**Figs. 2** and **3**). Histologic studies have described a greater than 90% survival of fat grafts using the Coleman

technique with a blunt cannula and centrifugation.[10,21] In vivo studies are still required to produce further evidence to this viability. Our clinical impression after 11 years of experience with lipostructure is that the volume provided and the improvement of quality of tissues is permanent.

The method of placement is also a very important consideration in fat grafting.[7] Relatively pure fat should be transplanted and very small aliquots distributed in each pass of the small cannula when it is withdrawn. The surgeon needs experience to understand the small aliquots that are needed for each case, which are also related to the plane of infiltration (subdermal, muscular, supraperiosteal). Combining a cosmetic and reconstructive practice will yield good results. The surgeon can gain sufficient experience with the harvesting, manipulation and application of fat grafts before the application of this technique for complex reconstructions.

In 11% of patients (n = 44), a two-step procedure was necessary (two sessions were planned as part of their treatment). In 30 patients, a secondary minor procedure was performed to correct small deficiencies (two of them required a small liposuction to correct fat excess). The procedure was well tolerated by all patients with minimal pain.

We have treated facial atrophy, posttraumatic deformities, postoncologic defects, radiotherapy deformities, scarred and fibrotic tissues, and lipodystrophy with this technique. Even though the quality of recipient tissue plays an important role in the final outcome in cosmetic patients, reconstructive cases exhibit an excellent outcome in tissues with bad quality. Stem cells, angiogenesis, and growth factors may play a role in this effect.[22,23] Literature regarding the effect and the

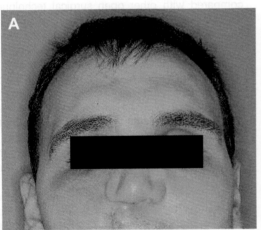
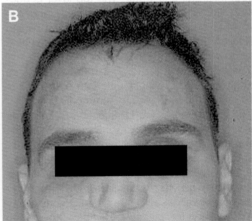

Fig. 2. (A) Appearance of upper-third of facial contour following gunshot wound to the face. Note the atrophy of soft tissues in the frontal and fronto-temporal areas, which is common to complex traumatic deformities. (B) Result following lipostructure to the fronto-temporal areas and endoscopic forehead lift.

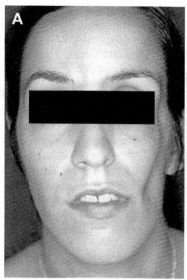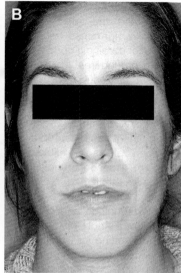

Fig. 3. (*A*) Parry-Romberg syndrome defect on the left side of the face and coup de sabre effect on the right frontal area. (*B*) Results following one session of facial lipostructure. Note that only lipostructure was performed to correct the defect (mandibular angle 8 ml, left cheek 27 ml, left upper eyelid 5 ml, right frontal area 4 ml, left temporal area 8 ml).

positive application of fat grafts in reconstructive cases is still scarce. The effect of fat grafts on damaged skin and soft tissues is remarkable. End-stage radiation dermatitis in breast reconstruction has been improved with fat grafts,[24] which is also our experience with this condition and other radiation therapy changes in the head and neck area. Chronic ulcers of Crohn's disease and perianal fistulas have been also treated with expanded stem cells from fat grafts with success,[25] although the real effect of lipostructure in this situation is still to be studied. Other conditions that have been clinically studied are correction of cicatricial ectropion,[26] and anophthalmic and enophthalmic sockets[27] by fat grafting. The Coleman technique was used in 14 orbits with excellent results, avoidance of alloplastic material, and good tolerance by the patients without complications.[27] Two patients required a second procedure to repeat some grafting, which is comparable to our series. Similarly, we have obtained good permanent results and good volume rehabilitation with improvement of the quality of the tissues in complex posttraumatic deformities. Fat grafts tend to be well accepted by the recipient tissues and patients return to a more natural look.[16]

Facial lipoatrophy in patients with HIV has been treated successfully in our center. It is important to realize that even though good results are usually obtained immediately following fat grafting, and stable results are commonly observed at 1 year after lipostructure, patients may exhibit new signs of lipoatrophy in the long run. We have no data to confirm our observations; however, it is our clinical impression that this condition is not stopped by the structural fat grafting, and that lipoatrophy continues after the procedure. Whether or not it occurs in the transplanted fat is a topic for future research. Others have shown the efficacy of this technique by a patient satisfaction of 93% in a series of 33 patients and good results at 1-year follow-up.[17]

Parry-Romberg syndrome or hemifacial atrophy is a local syndrome that presents with a severe change in facial features and atrophy of soft tissues in the face. It has also been treated successfully with lipostructure.[28] We also managed to improve the facial contour and volume with repeated fat grafting procedures in these patients. This experience is similar to others in the literature. It is possible to perform fat grafting procedures in the affected tissues and it is not necessary to perform any surgery or procedure to create space for the fat grafts.

SUMMARY

Fat grafting, structural fat grafting, lipofilling, or lipostructure has obtained an excellent reputation among plastic surgeons. Fat grafting is as old as the development of our specialty. However, refinements in the harvesting, manipulation and placement of small fat grafts developed in the last two decades have produced a reproducible and safe technique. Prospective research will have to produce evidence-based data regarding the longevity of fat grafts and the implication of adult-derived fat stem cells, hormones, angiogenesis, and growth factors for obtaining good results in structural fat grafting procedures. There is an extensive experience in cosmetic procedures, but the literature regarding the application of fat grafts in reconstructive patients is scarce. We have performed more than 240 facial fat-grafting procedures with permanent and reproducible effects. The complication rate is negligible, and the necessity to perform a second, unplanned, fat grafting procedure is less than 10%.

We believe that the production of excellent results depends on the technique and on good surgical planning. We follow a strict Coleman technique for structural fat grafting or lipofilling in reconstructive surgery cases and have produced good cosmetic results with long-lasting effects on facial contouring, changes in volume, and improvement of tissue quality.

REFERENCES

1. Coleman SR. Facial augmentation with structural fat grafting. Clin Plast Surg 2006;33:567–77.
2. Neuber FF. Bericht uber die Verhandlungen der Deutschen Gesellschaft fuer Chirurgie [German]. Zentralbl Chir 1893;22:66.
3. Lexer E. Free transplantation. Ann Surg 1914;60: 166–94.
4. Peer LA. The neglected free fat graft, its behavior and clinical use. Am J Surg 1956;92:40–7.
5. Coleman SR. Facial recontouring with lipostructure. Clin Plast Surg 1997;24:347–67.
6. Coleman SR. Long-term survival of fat transplants: controlled demonstrations. Aesthetic Plast Surg 1995;19:421–5.
7. Coleman SR. Structural fat grafting: more than a permanent filler. Plast Reconstr Surg 2006;118: 108S–20S.
8. Aust L, Devlin B, Foster SJ, et al. Yield of human adipose-derived adult stem cells from liposuction aspirates. Cytotherapy 2004;6:7–14.
9. Strem BM, Hicok KC, Zhu M, et al. Multipotential differentiation of adipose tissue-derived stem cells. Keio J Med 2005;54:132–41.
10. Von Heimburg D, Hemmrich K, Haydarlioglu S, et al. Comparison of viable cell yield from excised versus aspirated adipose tissue. Cells Tissues Organs 2004;178:87–92.
11. Gimble J, Guilak F. Adipose-derived adult stem cells: isolation, characterization, and differentiation potential. Cytotherapy 2003;5:362–9.
12. Zuk PA, Zhu M, Mizumo H, et al. Multilineage cells from human adipose tissue: implications for cell-based therapies. Tisue Eng 2001;7:211–28.
13. Lee JA, Parrett BM, Conejero JA, et al. Biological alchemy: engineering bone and fat from fat-derived stem cells. Ann Plast Surg 2003;50:610–7.
14. Grimaldi M, Gentile P, Labardi L, et al. Lipostructure technique in Romberg syndrome. J Craniofac Surg 2008;19:1089–91.
15. Coleman SR. Structural fat grafts: the ideal filler? Clin Plast Surg 2001;28:111–9.
16. Clauser L, Polito J, Mandrioli S, et al. Structural fat grafting in complex reconstructive surgery. J Craniofac Surg 2008;19:187–91.
17. Burnouf M, Buffet M, Schwarzinger M, et al. Evaluation of Coleman lipostructure for treatment of facial lipoatrophy in patients with human immunodeficiency virus and parameters associated with the efficiency of this technique. Arch Dermatol 2005;141: 1220–4.
18. Ullmann Y, Shoshani O, Fodor A, et al. Searching for the favorable donor site for fat injection: in vivo study using the nude mice model. Dermatol Surg 2005;31: 1304–7.
19. Coleman SR. Structural fact grafting. Quality Medical Publishing, Inc. St Louis (MO); 2004.
20. Pu LL, Coleman SR, Cui X, et al. Autologous fat grafts harvested and refined by the Coleman technique: a comparative study. Plast Reconstr Surg 2008;122:932–7.
21. Wolter TP, Von heimburg D, Stoffels I, et al. Cryopreservation of mature human adipocytes: in vitro measurement of viability. Ann Plast Surg 2005;55: 408–13.
22. Neels JG, Thinnes T, Loskutoff DJ. Angiogenesis in an in vivo model of adipose tissue development. FASEB J 2004;18:983–5.
23. Nakagami H, Maeda K, Morishita R, et al. Novel autologous cell therapy in ischemic limb disease through growth factor secretion by cultured adipose tissue-derived stromal cells. Arterioscler Thromb Vasc Biol 2005;25:2542–7.
24. Rigotti G, Marchi A, Galie M, et al. Clinical treatment of radiotherapy tissue damages by lipoaspirates transplants: a healing process mediated by adipose derived adult stem cells. Plast Reconstr Surg 2007; 119:1409–22.
25. Garcia-Olmo D, Garcia-Arranz M, Herreros D. Expanded adipose-derived ítem cells for the treatment of complex perianal fistula including Crohn' disease. Expert Opin Biol Ther 2008;8:1417–23.
26. Caviggioli F, Klinger F, Villani F, et al. Correction of cicatricial ectropion by autologous fat graft. Aesthetic Plast Surg 2008;32:555–7.
27. Hardy TG, Joshi N, Kelli MH. Orbital volume augmentation with autologous micro-fat grafts. Opthal Plast Reconstr Surg 2007;23:445–9.
28. Xie Y, Li Q, Zheng D, et al. Correction of hemifacial atrophy with autologous fat transplantation. Ann Plast Surg 2007;59:645–53.

Prefabrication and Prelamination Applications in Current Aesthetic Facial Reconstruction

Jon A. Mathy, MD, Julian J. Pribaz, MD*

KEYWORDS

- Prefabrication • Prelamination • Tissue flap
- Aesthetic facial reconstruction
- Composite tissue allotransplantation

Prefabrication and prelamination techniques can offer significant advantage in aesthetic facial reconstruction. Specifically, they can be applied to expand the recruitment and assembly of optimal tissues for better approximation of aesthetic ideals. This article begins by defining prefabrication and prelamination in the context of facial reconstruction. Perspective into their historical influences is provided. Clinical cases then exemplify some of their unique capabilities, highlighting their relevant advantages and limitations. Important technical features are pointed out. Lastly, the place for prelamination and prefabrication in the burgeoning era of composite tissue transplantation (CTA) is addressed. Interdependencies among these procedures as they relate to aesthetic facial reconstruction are discussed.

DEFINING "PREFABRICATION" AND "PRELAMINATION"

The terms "prefabrication" and "prelamination" are both used to describe surgical techniques that are performed on tissues before the transfer of those tissues for reconstructive purposes. They are performed with the intention of optimizing certain reconstructive goals. This article focuses on their applications for aesthetic facial reconstructive goals.

Both techniques are limited in their capacity to render useful changes in donor tissue by the natural pace of wound healing. Consequently, they must always be performed before a separate surgical procedure in which they are transferred.

Specifically, prefabrication refers to the pretransfer implantation of a nonnative vascular pedicle into tissue desired for reconstruction.[1] It is used when the tissue desired for reconstruction cannot be practically transferred by alternate means. For optimizing aesthetics in facial reconstruction, prefabrication is typically used to hand-pick thin tissues with cutaneous qualities most similar to the predisfigured part. A representative example is provided in **Fig. 1**.

Whereas prefabrication refers to pretransfer implantation of a vascular pedicle, prelamination is used to describe the pretransfer implantation of anything else.[2] Implantation typically creates a distinct layer or tissue plane. It is performed when wound healing between layers is desired before transfer. In aesthetic facial reconstruction, prelamination is often used to assemble composite flaps that can be transferred as a unit that more closely approximates the predisfigured part. A representative example is provided in **Fig. 2**.

It is worth mentioning that the term "prefabrication" has occasionally strayed from its original definition in its usage within the reconstructive

Division of Plastic Surgery, Department of Surgery, Brigham and Women's Hospital, Harvard Medical School, 75 Francis Street, Boston, MA 02115, USA
* Corresponding author.
E-mail address: jpribaz@partners.org (J.J. Pribaz).

Clin Plastic Surg 36 (2009) 493–505
doi:10.1016/j.cps.2009.02.010
0094-1298/09/$ – see front matter © 2009 Elsevier Inc. All rights reserved.

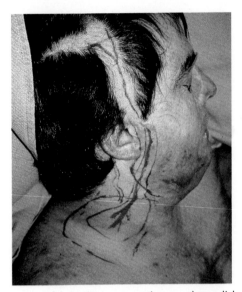

Fig. 1. In prefabrication, a nonnative vascular pedicle is used to axialize desirable tissue so that it can be transferred on that pedicle. The photo shows the planned implantation of superficial temporal vessels into an island of supraclavicular skin in preparation for future replacement of mandibular scar with optimal skin. See case example 1 for further details. (*From* Pribaz JJ, Fine N, Orgill DP. Flap prefabrication in the head and neck: a 10-year experience. Plast Reconstr Surg 1999;103:808–20; with permission.)

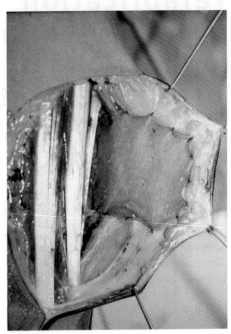

Fig. 2. A radial forearm flap is undergoing prelamination with split-thickness skin. Once the layers have healed, the composite tissue can be transferred as a preassembled unit. (*From* Taghinia AH, Pribaz JJ. Complex nasal reconstruction. Plast Reconstr Surg 2008;121:15e–27e; with permission.)

community. For example, Khouri and colleagues[3] expanded their usage of the word to describe all modes of pretransfer flap modification. Recognizing this variability may save the reader some confusion as they review the literature. This article keeps to the original description of prefabrication, as coined by Shen,[4] to facilitate clear communication among surgeons wishing to build on the technique. A more detailed historical perspective is provided later.

HISTORICAL PERSPECTIVE

The concept of vascular prefabrication traces some of its heritage to Beck and Tichy in 1930.[5] They transferred pectoral muscle to epicardium to supplement myocardial tissue perfusion in heart failure. Later groups transferred omentum to the heart with the same intention.[6] The concept was streamlined in 1946 when Vinberg[7] placed the internal mammary pedicle adjacent to coronary arteries and reported evidence of spontaneous collateralization between the two. The 1970s experienced further evolution along this trend with a series of studies demonstrating axialization of skin using demucosalized intestine and omentum in animal models.[8,9]

The first series of cases putting this concept to work in humans for reconstructive purposes was

published by Shen in 1981.[4] In this report, he coined the term "prefabrication" when describing his procedure for the precise transfer of specific tissues following implantation of facial vessels in head and neck reconstruction. Numerous reports describing incremental modifications of vascular prefabrication emerged thereafter, with a peak occurring in the late 1980s and early 1990s.[10–14]

Flap prelamination has undergone a slightly less discrete introduction and evolution. For purposes of nasal reconstruction, the technique has been implemented since at least the early 1900s;[1] reports citing Nelaton's implantation of structural cartilage grafts before staged forehead flap transfer date to that time.[16] Similar usage was repeatedly advocated by Sir Harold Gillies around the inception of modern plastic surgery.[17,18]

Contemporary groups have demonstrated impressive nasal reconstructions using radial forearm free flaps prelaminated with skin and cartilage.[15,16,19–22] Success has also been reported using mucosal grafts for prelaminating intraoral flaps, and sural nerve grafts to foster rapid sensory innervations.[23] Furnas[24] has described temporoparietal osseofascial flaps that he prelaminates with skin before transfer for palatal defects.

Overall, the reconstructive community has gravitated toward simpler, single-staged "work-horse reconstructions over the last decade.[25,26] Without demeaning the unique value of prefabrication and prelamination in certain circumstances, this trend is nevertheless probably responsible for the decreasing prevalence of such reconstructions in recent times. As is discussed at the end of this article, however, escalating interest in CTA for facial disfigurement may bring about new stimulus for prefabrication and prelamination techniques. For patients who are not candidates for facial transplantation, prefabrication and prelamination are among the most effective mechanisms available for approximating aesthetic reconstructive outcomes with autologous tissue. In the event of facial transplant failure, prefabrication and prelamination techniques are among the most effective at achieving aesthetic facial salvage.

Some clinical examples demonstrating how prefabrication and prelamination can be used to address different aesthetic goals in facial reconstruction are provided in the following section.

CLINICAL EXAMPLES
Case 1: Prefabrication Can Be Used to Import Thin, Color- and Texture- Matched Tissue into Highly Visible Facial Defects

Fig. 3A presents a 25-year-old man with a hypertrophic burn scar involving his right cheek and mandibular skin. In addition to aesthetic concerns, the patient complained of recurrent folliculitis within the scar that frequently required medical intervention.

A prefabricated flap of thin, color- and texture-matched skin was designed for eventual resurfacing of the affected area (**Fig. 3**B). Supraclavicular skin is axialized by pretransfer implantation of the superficial temporal vessels and its vascularized temporoparietal fascia.

Fig. 3C shows the vascular pedicle and fascia turned 180 degrees and fed under a preauricular skin bridge into the supraclavicular area. The arrow in **Fig. 3**C points to a thin Gore-Tex sleeve that was placed around the proximal segment of his vascular bundle to facilitate its dissection at the subsequent stage of flap transfer. The distal end of the pedicle and its fascia was implanted directly underneath skin and over a minimally pre-inflated tissue expander. Expansion was initiated on postoperative week 1 and continued weekly for 8 weeks.

At postoperative week 8, the hypertrophic skin was excised and the prefabricated supraclavicular skin was elevated (**Fig. 3**D, E). The donor area was closed primarily with minimal cervical advancement, and the prefabricated skin was transposed into the facial defect (**Fig. 3**F). Note that flap perfusion is based almost entirely on the implanted

superficial temporal system at this point, which could be demonstrated as a persistently strong pulse by Doppler examination. Trace venous congestion that was present immediately post-transfer resolved spontaneously within 72 hours.

The three-month postoperative result demonstrates a satisfactory aesthetic facial reconstruction (**Fig. 3**G).

Case 2: Prelamination Can Be Used to Import Thin, Multilaminate Tissue for Aesthetic Reconstruction of Full-Thickness Labial Defects

This 18-year-old Vietnamese man obtained charity-sponsored transportation to the United States for treatment of a prominent facial disfigurement arising from noma infection. His central face had wasted away, leaving an absent upper lip and lower nose, with atrophic extension to the cheeks bilaterally (**Fig. 4**A).

Reconstruction of the upper lip was planned using prelaminated, hair-bearing, functional submental flaps according to the markings shown. Native vascularity by the submental branches of the facial arteries would be maintained, as would innervation to the platysma by the cervical branches of the facial nerve (**Fig. 4**B).

In the first operation, the submental flaps were raised deep to the platysma and anterior belly of the digastrics, and then reclosed over a full-thickness skin graft that was apposed to the muscle. The skin graft was internally bolstered with a tissue expander. Moderate postoperative expansion was continued to thin further the submental flaps and to facilitate future primary closure of the donor site. A forehead expander was also implanted in preparation for a staged nasal reconstruction (**Fig. 4**C).

One month postoperatively, flap elevation demonstrated successful internal prelamination (**Fig. 4**D). The atrophic upper lip remnants were excised and replaced with the prelaminated submental flaps bilaterally. An Abbé flap as marked was then used to complete the reconstruction of the central part of the upper lip (**Fig. 4**E).

At the same time as the lip reconstruction, the patient's nose was reconstructed using conventional techniques. This consisted of local turn-in flaps for lining, costal cartilage grafts for support, and his pre-expanded forehead flap for coverage (also shown in **Fig. 4**E). The Abbé and forehead flaps were divided and inset 3 weeks later. All tissue survived.

Six weeks following his staged reconstruction, the patient demonstrated an acceptable aesthetic result (**Fig. 4**F). The patient returned to Vietnam without further follow-up.

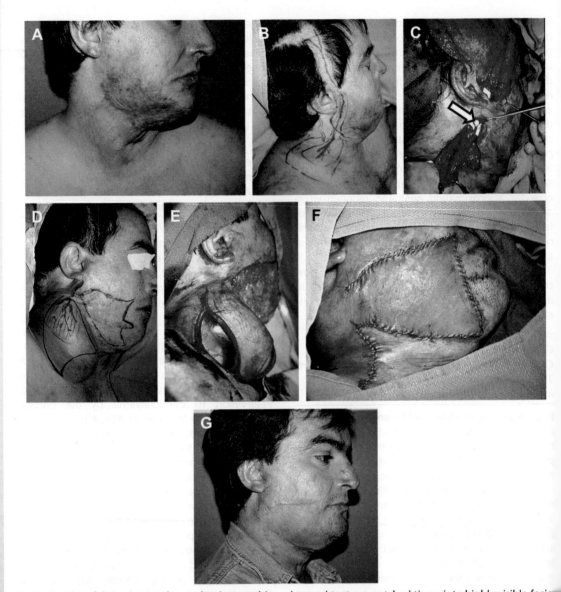

Fig. 3. (*A–G*) Prefabrication can be used to import thin, color- and texture-matched tissue into highly visible facia defects. (*From* Pribaz JJ, Fine N, Orgill DP. Flap prefabrication in the head and neck: a 10-year experience. Plas Reconstr Surg 1999;103:808–20; with permission.)

Case 3: Prelamination Can Facilitate Assembly of Composite, Three-Dimensional Flaps For Aesthetic Central Facial Reconstruction

This 62-year-old man suffered thermal injury to his face in an occupational accident (**Fig. 5**A). The disfigurement was most notable for disintegration of his lower nose, along with full-thickness cutaneous loss of his nasal dorsum, right upper lip, and his right cheek and lower eyelid.

A template was used to plan a compound reconstruction of the patient's central face within the vascular territory of his nondominant forearm's radial artery (**Fig. 5**B, C). This flap was prelaminated

with both skin and cartilage for neonasal vestibula lining and tip structure. Tie-over bolsters an internal splints were used to reinforce tip shap during initial healing.

Three weeks postoperatively, the composite fla was harvested on its native radial pedicle (**Fig. 5**D The flap assembly could then be revascularize and inset as a single unit (**Fig. 5**E). Tip lining wa supplied by local turn-in flaps of his residual dorsa nose skin. The right nasolabial fold was deepene in a minor revision performed 1 month later.

Follow-up at 6 months shows that an acceptabl aesthetic reconstruction of the patient's nose, rigi cheek, and upper lip was achieved (**Fig. 5**F).

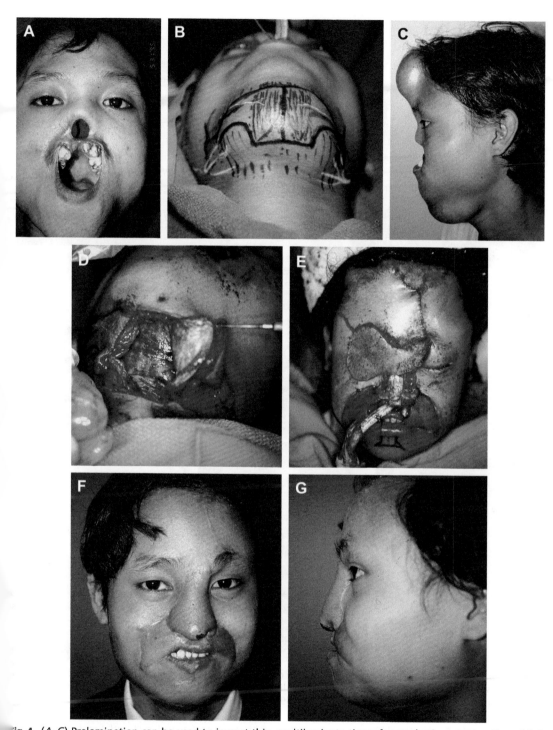

Fig. 4. (*A–G*) Prelamination can be used to import thin, multilaminate tissue for aesthetic reconstruction of full-thickness labial defects. (*From* Pribaz JJ, Fine NA. Prefabricated and prelaminated flaps for head and neck reconstruction. Clin Plast Surg 2001;28:261–72; with permission.)

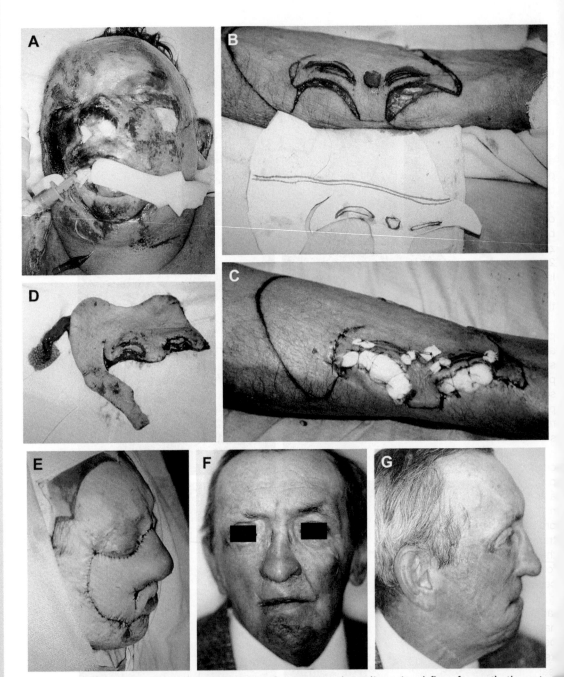

Fig. 5. (*A–G*) Prelamination can facilitate assembly of composite, three-dimensional flaps for aesthetic central facial reconstruction. (*From* Pribaz JJ, Weiss DD, Mulliken JB, et al. Prelaminated free flap reconstruction of complex central facial defects. Plast Reconstr Surg 1999;104:357–65; with permission.)

Case 4: Multiple Aesthetic Units Can Be Sequentially Reconstructed Using Prefabricated Tissue on a Single "Vascular Crane"

This 23-year-old man presented for aesthetic facial reconstruction following acute medical and psychologic stabilization for a 95% TBSA self-inflicted flame burn (**Fig. 6**A, B). Predictably, his initial closure with split grafts and cultured keratinocytes was complicated by tight skin with contractures affecting his entire body. His facial disfigurement was particularly notable for a deficiency of the upper lip, oral incompetence arising from cervical contracture, bilateral lower lid ectropion, and absent ears bilaterally. His nose remained flat and ill-defined despite prior reconstruction with forehead tissue.

Plans were made to release his neck with a free abdominal skin flap. Because of his injuries, however, all other conventional flaps including those arising from the back, forearms, and thighs were believed to be unsuitable for aesthetic facial reconstruction.

In anticipation of repetitive prefabricated tissue transfer to his upper lip and nose, the patient's descending branch of his lateral femoral circumflex artery with its venae comitantes were dissected out and transferred as a free pedicle flap to the unburned stumps of his left superficial temporal vessels (**Figs. 6**C & **6**D). The descending branch of the lateral femoral circumflex was chosen because of its long length and position deep to the zone of his thermal injury. The pedicle measured 20 cm in length and included a narrow cuff of vastus lateralis muscle around its intramuscular segment. A local triangular scalp flap was raised to cover the microanastomoses.

The distally ligated segment of the transferred pedicle was simply implanted (without any additional microanastomoses) into a small subcutaneous pocket within a relatively supple patch of supraclavicular skin. The intervening segment of exposed pedicle was partially wrapped with a postauricular skin flap, and all residual defects were covered with meshed skin grafts.

Six weeks after implantation, the prefabricated cervical skin flap was elevated on its newly implanted vascular pedicle and transferred over a revised nasal construct including costochondral rib grafts for support (**Fig. 6**E). The periphery of the prefabricated flap was congested immediately after transfer; this congestion resolved spontaneously in the ensuing 36 hours everywhere except for the folded segment at his neocolumella, which proceeded to necrose.

Three and one half weeks after transfer, the prefabricated flap was divided at the nose and revisionally inset. The bleeding end of the of the vascular pedicle was ligated, de-epithelialized for 1.5 cm at its distal end, and then reimplanted at the subgaleal level into a hair-bearing area of his left temporal region (**Fig. 6**F).

The pedicle was left implanted in the scalp for approximately 3 months while the patient underwent serial contracture releases of all four extremities. The scalp flap was delayed with two parallel incisions during one of these procedures.

The patient's second prefabricated flap was then transferred to his surgically prepared upper lip (**Fig. 6**G). Mild postoperative venous congestion again resolved within 36 hours postoperatively. The flap survived completely.

One month later the pedicle was again divided, but this time at its proximal end, to allow for a third tissue transfer by retrograde perfusion to the nasal tip (**Fig. 6**H). This tissue represented a third prefabricated flap, consisting of the temporal skin that had been rotated over the pedicle's anastomoses in the patient's first operation. The tissue was purposed to augment the previously lost columellar tissue in daisy-chain fashion. The nose was revised with pedicle excision over the subsequent 2 months.

The patient is shown 10 weeks after the final step of his aesthetic reconstruction with serially prefabricated flaps on a single pedicle (**Fig. 6**I). He is wearing a hairpiece and auricular prostheses fixated to osseointegrated temporal implants.

ADVANTAGES AND LIMITATIONS OF PREFABRICATION AND PRELAMINATION

The case examples shown provide some insight into a few of the notable advantages and limitations of prefabrication and prelamination techniques for aesthetic facial reconstruction. These are summarized in **Table 1**.

For example, evident among each case is one of the principle disadvantages of both methods of pretransfer flap modification: they necessitate at least one additional operation before that of flap transfer and inset. The minimal period between operations generally ranges from about 2 weeks with prelamination, to 8 weeks or longer with prefabrication.

The relatively protracted and staged nature of these techniques diminishes their attractiveness for patients with frailty in the face of repetitive general anesthetic or poor prognosis. These patients are obviously better served by single-staged reconstructive techniques requiring minimal convalescent time. The overarching reconstructive goal in such cases is also more heavily weighted toward achieving reliable wound closure over an ideal aesthetic result.

The temporally staged nature of pretransfer modification techniques also limits their use to cases where facial defects can tolerate a delay in reconstruction. Facial defects related to malignancy, for example, are less suited to prelaminated and prefabricated reconstructions because it is typically undesirable to postpone extirpation while flap tissue undergoing staged preparation. Although it is true that tumor excision could be performed contemporaneous with the first stage of flap prefabrication, and the defect stabilized with dressings or temporary closure until the flap becomes suitable for transfer, patients in that scenario would lose the psychologic advantage

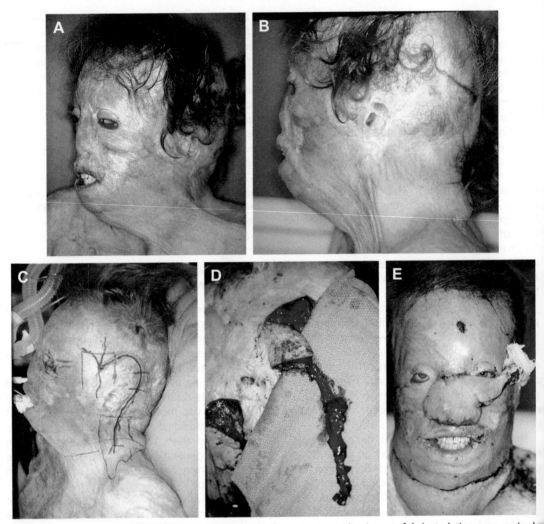

Fig. 6. (*A–I*) Multiple aesthetic units can be sequentially reconstructed using prefabricated tissue on a single vascular crane. (*From* Pribaz JJ, Maitz PK, Fine NA. Flap prefabrication using the "vascular crane" principle: an experimental study and clinical application. Br J Plast Surg 1994;47:250–6; with permission.)

of awakening from their extirpation procedure without an unreconstructed facial disfigurement.

Given the issues raised, prefabrication and prelamination techniques are probably most advantageous for addressing facial defects that are either already present, or that can be accurately predicted to be present at the time of tissue transfer. As in case examples 3 and 4, substantial burn injuries represent good beneficiaries for reconstruction using the techniques described.[1,27]

Relatively benign facial lesions that are too extensive for reconstruction using local techniques may also benefit from prefabricated or prelaminated reconstruction. Vascular malformations, congenital hairy nevi, and giant neurofibromas all fit into this category, examples of which are also available in the literature.[15,16] Excision of such lesions can be reasonably postponed until after

prefabricated and prelaminated flaps have matured. Residual facial defects following prior failed or suboptimal reconstructions also qualify.

Despite their limitations, prefabrication and prelamination techniques provide unique advantages for autologous reconstruction by significantly extending the scope of flap customizability for purposes of best approximating aesthetic goals. With vascular prefabrication, optimal tissue in terms of color and tissue can be recruited for reconstructive transfer, on a single vascular pedicle, irrespective of that tissue's native vascular supply (as in case examples 1 and 4). With prelamination, composite flaps with specialized features can be preassembled for later single-unit transfer in reconstructing intricate or multilaminate surfaces (as in case examples 2 and 3).

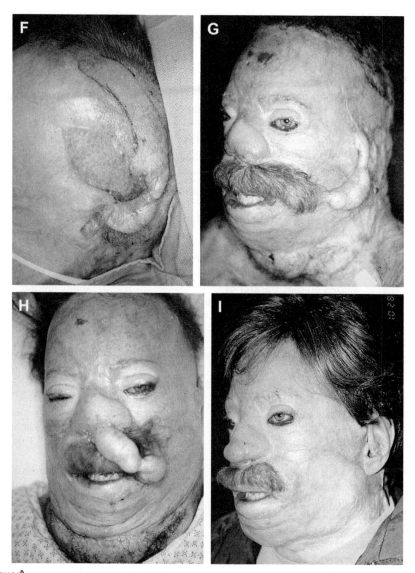

Fig. 6. (continued)

Overall, it has been shown experimentally that prefabricated flaps are more robust than random pattern flaps, but less hardy than axial pattern flaps.[28] One particular susceptibility of prefabricated flaps is their tendency toward posttransfer venous congestion. A typical appearance is shown in case example 1. This congestion presumably reflects the fact that arterial neovascularization outpaces (or outperforms) venous neovascularization. Either way, experimental and clinical investigations reveal that the tendency toward early venous congestion renders prefabricated flaps particularly vulnerable to loss if the congestion is exacerbated by a tight or folded inset.[29] Such maneuvers as delay procedures, additional native venous anastomoses, and longer periods of pretransfer incubation, however, can diminish or eliminate posttransfer venous congestion (see later).

When it comes to prelamination, an off-site preassembly can grant additional reconstructive advantage by allowing for primary flap maturation before flap transfer. Minor deformation resulting from unpredictable scar forces may then be compensated at the time of inset. It has been recognized, however, that further deformation can ensue following transfer, presumably from abrupt lymphatic interruption that causes transient edematous changes within the transferred tissue.[16] Aesthetic revisions may therefore still be required following en bloc transfer of apparently stable prelaminated tissue constructs.

Finally, prefabrication offers unique use in situations where it is practical to use a single vascular

Table 1
Advantages and limitations of prefabrication and prelamination techniques

	Advantages	Limitations
(Both)	Extended flap customizability Good for fixed and stable defects (burns, benign lesions, traumatic or congenital disfigurement)	Two or more operations required Less suitable for surgically frail, poor prognosis, malignancy
Prefabrication	Can axialize optimal tissues (color thickness, texture, composition, special features) for transfer, irrespective of native vascularity	Prone to venous congestion
	More robust than random-pattern flaps	Less robust than natively axialized flaps
	Can transfer islands of tissue without microsurgery	Decreased perfusion predictability compared with natively axialized flaps
	Can mobilize multiple tissue units on a vascular crane	Volume of recruitable tissue decreases with successive transfers
Prelamination	Allows en-bloc transfer of preassembled composite flaps Primary flap maturation precedes flap transfer	Transferability limited to native vascular territories Additional scar contracture posttransfer may still necessitate flap revisions

pedicle for importation of multiple volumes of tissue into a centripetal space. The process takes advantage of the finding that implantational neo-vascularization is repeatable, and permits pedicle recycling as a so-called "vascular crane."[30] Notably, experimental models have shown some degradation of tissue recruitability with successive transfers. As illustrated in case example 4, the process can nevertheless facilitate aesthetic reconstruction of compound facial disfigurements with multiple specialized tissues, and without multiple microvascular procedures.

TECHNICAL POINTERS

Some technical details are worth pointing out to enhance success with the previously described techniques. This is particularly true in the case of flap prefabrication.

Vascular pedicles harvested for prefabrication should include at least the artery and its venae comitantes surrounded by adventitia, but can also include fascia or muscle.[16] For thin cutaneous flaps, the pedicle is implanted directly under the skin to be recruited. Locations where optimal skin for facial reconstruction can be harvested include the cervical and supraclavicular regions.[16] Along these lines, Khouri and coworkers[31] have elaborated on the use of temporoparietal fascia with its superficial temporal vascular pedicle for the prefabrication of cervical skin flaps.

When transferring prefabricated flaps, pedicle elevation can be significantly simplified if it is wrapped in Gore-Tex or thin silicone sheeting at the time of its first exposure.[16] This is exemplified in case example 1.

As mentioned in the previous section and demonstrated in case examples 1 and 4, prefabricated flaps are prone to venous congestion immediately following transfer. Fortunately, tissue that survives congestion over the first 36 hours following transfer typically normalizes its capillary refill and proceeds to full survival.[16] Some supportive methods for minimizing posttransfer congestion include the establishment of supplemental venous drainage by including native veins with the transferred flap, or by using early postoperative chemical or biologic leeching.[16] Decreased congestion has also been observed with longer intervals between pedicle implantation and flap elevation.[16]

Tissue expansion has proved to be a useful adjunct to the process of flap prefabrication. As demonstrated in case example 1, benefits include its ability further to attenuate flap tissue for thinner reconstruction, and its facilitation of primary donor site closure following flap transfer.[32] More significantly, tissue expansion has been shown experimentally to increase the area of tissue that can be transferred successfully.[32] This last benefit has been hypothesized to result from either (1) the expander's passive role in concentrating neovascularization into the flap tissue positioned superficial to it, (2) augmented neovascularization arising secondary to the dynamic forces of expansion, (3) the vascular delay that the expander imparts along the deep surface of the flap, or (4) some combination thereof.[1]

When an expander is used, the vascular pedicle is laid directly on top of the expander, in between it and the deep surface of the tissue to be recruited. It is safe to start expansion 1 week after implantation and to continue weekly at the fastest rate tolerated, so long as the pedicle remains pulsatile by Doppler ultrasonography.[16] Should the signal become reduced during a fill, the expander is simply deflated until signal returns. Expansion can usually be continued as necessary thereafter.

Tissue expansion also can facilitate prelamination. In addition to attenuating its overlying tissue for thinner flaps and facilitating eventual donor site closure, expanders are useful for internally bolstering deep skin grafts. An example of this is demonstrated in case example 2.

RELEVANCE OF PREFABRICATION AND PRELAMINATION IN THE ERA OF COMPOSITE TISSUE ALLOTRANSPLANTATION

What is the relevance of prefabrication and prelamination for aesthetic facial reconstruction in the burgeoning era of CTA? This discussion is increasingly pertinent as acceptance of facial transplantation for the treatment of facial disfigurement gains significant momentum within today's clinical arena. Mounting experimental and clinical evidence supports the notion that CTA permits superior realization of aesthetic facial reconstructive goals than arguably any other technique available. For example, consider the achievement of Devauchelle and colleagues[33] with their first successful facial transplant recipient, Isabelle Dinoire. At 3-year follow-up,[34] it is not difficult to imagine this patient enjoying easier social reintegration than patients with similar disfigurements that may have been reconstructed according to any other technique, including those presented in this issue.

Similarly compelling aesthetic achievement with facial transplantation has been published on at least two other patients within the contemporary medical literature.[35,36] Multidisciplinary teams aimed at evaluating further application of facial transplantation are emerging at academic centers worldwide. As of this writing, a fourth facial transplantation, and the first in America, has been announced by Siemionow and colleagues to the popular press.[37] Vastly more experience with CTA for facial reconstruction is bound to follow.

One reason that CTA is so disruptive for aesthetic facial reconstruction emanates from the fact that although it is built on surgical principles intrinsic to reconstructive surgery, CTA is fundamentally different. At its best, "reconstruction" only *approximates* aesthetic ideals using similar tissues, whereas CTA can actually *mirror* aesthetic ideals using replicate tissue. If a term could be coined to encapsulate the fundamentally different nature of CTA in the process of aesthetic restoration, it might be termed "replicative surgery" rather than "reconstructive surgery."

Semantics aside, it is important to recognize that CTA is not likely to overtake traditional methods of facial reconstruction anytime soon. It is true that significant CTA hurdles are falling on many fronts; for example, growing experimental and clinical experience with facial harvest and revascularization are diminishing its technical formidability,[38,39] ethical opposition is simmering down as perceived problems with identity transfer become less acute,[40] public exposure is becoming more prominent, and organ banks are becoming increasingly collaborative in their consideration of composite tissue needs.[41] The issues surrounding immunomodulation, however, continue to loom large. For instance, it is the patient's perceived ability to tolerate lifelong immunosuppression that represents one of the most important features influencing their candidacy for facial transplantation at this time.[42,43] Furthermore, it is immunologic rejection, rather than technical failure, which represents one of the most feared potential complications of CTA. If the issue of immunotolerance could be neatly and reliably surmounted, then the general applicability of CTA for facial defects might gain significantly greater predominance. The solution to immunotolerance, however, does not appear imminent.

In the meantime, although far from perfect, conventional reconstructive techniques are likely to remain the central method of aesthetic reconstruction for substantial facial disfigurements. Among the most useful techniques are those of prefabrication and prelamination. As described and illustrated in this article, these techniques are useful because of their ability to broaden the recruitability of optimal donor tissues and to facilitate the assembly of composite tissue units. Surgically fit patients with significant facial disfigurement who are not candidates for CTA may nevertheless gain significant aesthetic improvement from prefabricated or prelaminated reconstructions. When patients are good candidates for CTA, the allotransplantation should probably proceed before exhausting other forms of conventional reconstruction, so that they can serve as

---

Box 1
Key points regarding the relationship between flap prefabrication and prelamination and CTA

For surgically fit patients who are not candidates for CTA

Flap prefabrication and prelamination are among the most powerful surgical techniques for reconstructing significant facial defects.

For surgically fit patients who are candidates for CTA

CTA should be attempted first

If CTA fails, or if rejection requires its debridement, then flap prefabrication and prelamination represent two of the most important surgical bailouts for reconstructing the resulting defect.

CTA should preferably only be done at centers that can also perform flap prefabrication and prelamination.

---

reconstructive lifeboats should the transplantation fail. If a facial CTA does fail, or if host-versus-graft complications necessitate a transplant debridement, these patients will likely be left with more problematic facial defects than that of their initial disfigurement. In such a case, prefabrication and prelamination techniques would likely rank among the most important bailout techniques available for restoring some element of facial aesthetics. For all of these reasons, units that offer CTA should ideally also offer some expertise with prefabricated and prelaminated reconstructive techniques, or at least work in collaboration with one that does. These points are summarized in **Box 1**.

SUMMARY

Prefabrication and prelamination techniques can offer significant advantage in aesthetic facial reconstruction. Specifically, they can be applied to expand the recruitment and assembly of optimal tissues for better approximation of aesthetic ideals. Some of their unique abilities are presented in this article. Advantages, limitations, and technical pointers are also provided.

Although not detracting from their unique advantages in aesthetic facial reconstruction, innovation and exposure with these techniques has slowed over the last decade. This probably relates to an increasing gravitation toward single-staged "work-horse" reconstructions, and a shifting attention toward CTA.

Facial allotransplantation may herald superior aesthetic results for facial disfigurement because of its replicative (as opposed to reconstructive)

nature. Although immunotolerance remains an elusive security, prefabrication and prelamination remain among the most effective options for severely disfigured patients seeking aesthetic improvement.

REFERENCES

1. Pribaz JJ, Fine N, Orgill DP. Flap prefabrication in the head and neck: a 10-year experience. Plast Reconstr Surg 1999;103:808–20.
2. Pribaz JJ, Fine NA. Prelamination: defining the prefabricated flap–a case report and review. Microsurgery 1994;15:618–23.
3. Khouri RK, Upton J, Shaw WW. Principles of flap prefabrication. Clin Plast Surg 1992;19:763–71.
4. Yao ST. Microvascular transplantation of prefabricated free thigh flap. Plast Reconstr Surg 1982;69: 568.
5. Beck CS, Tichy VL. Production of collateral circulation to the heart: experimental study. Am Heart J 1935;10:849.
6. O'Shaughnessy L. An experimental method of providing a collateral circulation to the heart. Br J Surg 1936;23:665.
7. Vinberg AM. Development of an anastomosis between the coronary vessels and a transplanted internal mammary artery. Can Med Assoc J 1946; 55:117.
8. Erol OO, Spira M. Development and utilization of a composite island flap employing omentum: experimental investigation. Plast Reconstr Surg 1980;65: 405–18.
9. Washio H. An intestinal conduit for free flap transplantation of other tissues. Plast Reconstr Surg 1971;48:48.
10. Hirase Y, Valauri FA, Buncke HJ. Neovascularized bone, muscle, and myo-osseous free flaps: an experimental model. J Reconstr Microsurg 1988;4:209–15.
11. Hirase Y, Valauri FA, Buncke HJ. Prefabricated sensate myocutaneous and osteomyocutaneous free flaps: an experimental model. Preliminary report. Plast Reconstr Surg 1988;82:440–6.
12. Hirase Y, Valauri FA, Buncke HJ, et al. Customized prefabricated neovascularized free flaps. Microsurgery 1987;8:218–24.
13. Hyakusoku H, Okubo M, Umeda T, et al. A prefabricated hair-bearing island flap for lip reconstruction. Br J Plast Surg 1987;40:37–9.
14. Khouri RK, Upton J, Shaw WW. Prefabrication of composite free flaps through staged microvascular transfer: an experimental and clinical study. Plast Reconstr Surg 1991;87:108–15.
15. Pribaz JJ, Weiss DD, Mulliken JB, et al. Prelaminated free flap reconstruction of complex central facial defects. Plast Reconstr Surg 1999;104: 357–66.

16. Pribaz JJ, Fine NA. Prefabricated and prelaminated flaps for head and neck reconstruction. Clin Plast Surg 2001;28:261–72.

17. Gillies H. A new free graft applied to the reconstruction of nostril. Br J Surg 1942;30:305.

18. Gillies HD, Millard DR. The principles and art of plastic surgery. 1st edition. Boston: Little; 1957.

19. Baudet J, Rivet D, Martin D, et al. Prefabricated free flap transfers. In 3rd Annual Meeting of the American Society for Reconstructive Microsurgery, San Antonio (TX), 1987.

20. Burget GC, Menick FJ. Aesthetic reconstruction of the nose. St. Louis (MO): Mosby; 1994.

21. Costa H, Cunha C, Guimaraes I, et al. Prefabricated flaps for the head and neck: a preliminary report. Br J Plast Surg 1993;46:223–7.

22. Taghinia AH, Pribaz JJ. Complex nasal reconstruction. Plast Reconstr Surg 2008;121:15e–27e.

23. Rath T, Millesi W, Millesi-Schobel G, et al. Mucosal prelamination of a radial forearm flap for intraoral reconstruction. J Reconstr Microsurg 1997;13:507–13.

24. Furnas DW. Temporal osteocutaneous island flaps for complete reconstruction of cleft palate defects. Scand J Plast Reconstr Surg Hand Surg 1987;21:119–28.

25. Disa JJ, Pusic AL, Hidalgo DH, et al. Simplifying microvascular head and neck reconstruction: a rational approach to donor site selection. Ann Plast Surg 2001;47:385–9.

26. Lutz BS, Wei FC. Microsurgical workhorse flaps in head and neck reconstruction. Clin Plast Surg 2005;32:421–30.

27. Parrett BM, Pomahac B, Orgill DP, et al. The role of free-tissue transfer for head and neck burn reconstruction. Plast Reconstr Surg 2007;120:1871–8.

28. Ono H, Tamai S, Yajima H, et al. Blood flow through prefabricated flaps: an experimental study in rabbits. Br J Plast Surg 1993;46:449–55.

29. Maitz PK, Pribaz JJ, Hergrueter CA. Manipulating prefabricated flaps: an experimental study examining flap viability. Microsurgery 1994;15:624–9.

30. Pribaz JJ, Maitz PK, Fine NA. Flap prefabrication using the vascular crane principle: an experimental study and clinical application. Br J Plast Surg 1994;47:250–6.

31. Khouri RK, Ozbek MR, Hruza GJ, et al. Facial reconstruction with prefabricated induced expanded (PIE) supraclavicular skin flaps. Plast Reconstr Surg 1995;95:1007–16.

32. Maitz PK, Pribaz JJ, Hergrueter CA. Impact of tissue expansion on flap prefabrication: an experimental study in rabbits. Microsurgery 1996;17:35–40.

33. Devauchelle B, Badet L, Lengelé B, et al. First human face allograft: early report. Lancet 2006;368:203–9.

34. Dubernard J-M, Lengele B, Morelon E, et al. Outcomes 18 months after the first human partial face transplantation. N Engl J Med 2007;357:2451–60.

35. Guo S, Han Y, Zhang X, et al. Human facial allotransplantation: a 2-year follow-up study. Lancet 2008;372:631–8.

36. Lantieri L, Meningaud J-P, Grimbert P, et al. Repair of the lower and middle parts of the face by composite tissue allotransplantation in a patient with massive plexiform neurofibroma: a 1-year follow-up study. Lancet 2008;372:639–45.

37. Altman LK. First U.S. face transplant described. In: The New York times; New York: 2008. p. A18.

38. Meningaud JP, Paraskevas A, Ingallina F, et al. Face transplant graft procurement: a preclinical and clinical study. Plast Reconstr Surg 2008;122:1383–9.

39. Wilhelmi BJ, Kang RH, Movassaghi K, et al. First successful replantation of face and scalp with single-artery repair: model for face and scalp transplantation. Ann Plast Surg 2003;50:535–40.

40. Morris PJ, Bradley JA, Doyal L, et al. Facial transplantation: a working party report from the Royal College of Surgeons of England. Transplantation 2004;77:330–8.

41. Pomahac B, Aflaki P, Chandraker A, et al. Facial transplantation and immunosuppressed patients: a new frontier in reconstructive surgery. Transplantation 2008;85:1693–7.

42. Peled ZM, Pribaz JJ. Face transplantation: the view from Harvard Medical School. South Med J 2006;99:414–6.

43. Siemionow M, Agaoglu G. Allotransplantation of the face: how close are we? Clin Plast Surg 2005;32:401–9.

Current Concepts and Future Challenges in Facial Transplantation

Benoît G. Lengelé, MD, PhD[a,b]

KEYWORDS

- Face transplantation • Functional results • Immunotherapy
- Neuropsychology • Indications • Ethics

"The face is always of an Other…" Emmanuel Levinas, philosopher (Ethique et Infini. Paris: Fayard; 1982)

In the writings of ancient Greek philosophy and, more recently, in the texts of leading contemporary thinkers, the face has always embodied the essential expression of humanity. Individual by nature and expressing each single emotion of its owner at any given moment in a unique relationship with the exterior world, the face enjoys an unequalled symbolic value in the midst of a company of animated organs as bearer of the soul. Envisaging transposing the face of one person to another, albeit in order to restore the appearance of a human being, becomes an enterprise that is audacious, provocative, and transgressive. Constrained to the esoteric world of myth and legend until the dawn of the second millenium, such an intervention nevertheless has progressively entered the spheres of mere probability rather than possibility with the advance of science.

When the first facial graft was performed in Amiens, France, on November 27, 2005,[1] this surgical event, which largely surpassed medical boundaries, raised many questions. It did not fail, and rightly so, to launch a society-wide ethical and philosophic debate.[2] Since then three facial allotransplantations (FATs) have been performed, first in Xian, China,[3] then in Paris,[4] and, more recently, in Cleveland, Ohio, in the United States.[5] Today, as emotions subside, a retrospective analysis of the results obtained from those successive clinical experiences enables an initial account of the techniques, results, and cost-benefit balance of FATs.

This article addresses four fundamental issues raised in the medical world by the principle of facial transplantation, even though this procedure has long since passed from the stage of the conceptual virtual world of yesteryear to the surgical reality of today:

- The first issue is technical and concerns the microsurgical feasibility of composite tissue transfers to the face. This opportunity is analyzed from a perspective of interest not only in the static restoration of surfaces and volumes but also in restoring the vectors of facial expression.
- The second issue is biologic and concerns the possibility of medically limiting the rejection of a composite tissue allograft (CTAG), reputedly extremely immunogenic due to its skin cover.
- The third issue is functional and neurophysiologic and raises the question of a possible integration of a facial allograft (FAG) not only in the body scheme of the recipient but also in the day-today life of facing the reality in the mirror and in the gaze of fellow human

[a] Department of Plastic and Reconstructive Surgery, Faculty of Medicine, Cliniques Universitaires Saint-Luc, Avenue Hippocrate, 10, B-1200, Brussels, Belgium
[b] Department of Experimental Morphology, Université catholique de Louvain, Tour Vésale 52.51, Avenue Emmanuel Mounier, 52, B-1200 Brussels, Belgium.
E-mail address: benoit.lengele@uclouvain.be

Clin Plastic Surg 36 (2009) 507–521
doi:10.1016/j.cps.2009.02.006
0094-1298/09/$ – see front matter © 2009 Elsevier Inc. All rights reserved.

beings. This is precisely the point where essential fears of seeing a massive transfer of the identity of the donor to the recipient, along with the organic transfer of visible nonautologous tissues, come to light. The dread of a major psychologic conflict of personality, therefore, is expected.

- The last issue is ethical and questions the legitimacy of high-risk surgery that mutilates the image of one patient who is about to die in order to pass it to one who, deprived of a face, is about to receive it at the price of the uncertainty of a future existence resulting from the risks engendered by the immunosuppressive treatment and the unknown longevity of the allograft.

Addressing these four cardinal issues and looking beyond current achievements, the author outlines the needs for further research, potential new indications, and future technical challenges concerning new FAGs.

TECHNICAL FEASIBILITY AND JUSTIFICATION OF INDICATIONS FOR FACIAL ALLOGRAFTS

Under the apparent continuity of its form and contours, the face is surgically divided into distinct anatomic units, each of which must, in principle, be the object of a separate reconstruction to be cosmetically perfectly individualized in the rebuilt face. Following this rule, each loss of facial substance limited to a single anatomic unit easily can be repaired with one or several reliable alternative restoration techniques, whose indications, advantages, and disadvantages have been described abundantly. Usually, when only one unit is missing, for example, the nose, lips, eyelids, cheeks, or forehead, it can have its contours, surface, and multitissular architecture elegantly restored with the help of autologous surrounding tissues, with steadfast morphologic results and a satisfactory cosmetic appearance. This is not always the case when a tissue defect is more substantial and concerns several adjacent anatomic units. In spite of the considerable contribution offered, in such circumstances, by microsurgical transfers, several operative procedures are then necessary to restore the bony support of the missing units and to reposition superficially, side by side, the corresponding soft tissues. Despite multiple reinterventions, the results of these daring undertakings are poor, more than often cosmetically imperfect, and nearly always incapable of reviving the dynamics of the lost facial harmony.[6] A face reconstructed in this manner invariably takes on the appearance of a mosaic of juxtaposed cutaneous units, often different in color and texture, separated by multiple scars at wound edges and robbed of the subtle movements required for the oral function and facial expressivity. Precisely because the 3-D multitissular architecture of the face is of unrivalled complexity compared with the rest of the human body, it is justifiable to turn to composite tissue allotransplantation (CTA) when loss of substance extends over several anatomic units and deprives a patient of several cardinal orofacial functions, such as competent feeding, intelligible speech, and spontaneous nonverbal expression. Experts in complex facial reconstruction have recognized the limits of the microsurgical possibilities in the domain of severe disfigurement.[6,7] In the light of these limits, FAT seems more an act of surgical humility than a pretentious action destined to spectacularly demonstrate extreme microsurgical talent. When, despite all its creativity and know-how inherited from peers, the hand of a surgeon considers itself incapable of restoring the genius of nature, is it not better, perhaps, to accept in all humility that only a loan of the genius of nature itself might enable it to further its science and art?

Anatomically, the face rests on rigid skeletal bases and assembles, narrowly schemed under the skin, the orbicular muscular rings that circle the lips and the eyelids, the multidirectional slings of the elevator and depressor muscles organized around the oral cleft, and the gravitational and antigravitational muscles of the eyebrows. Connected by the fibrous sheath of the superficial musculoaponeurotic system that coordinates their movements, each of those muscles acts on distinct adipose cushions that are distributed in cellular subcutaneous tissue, and the dynamic mask thus constituted is supported in various places by retaining ligaments that are responsible for the expressive mimic of the face. The principle of each FAT technique is first to harvest, then to transfer onto the remaining facial structures of the recipient, all those tissue elements, cut to size, without severing them from the skin surface or from the deep mucosal and periosteal planes. The surgical transposition of these structures is technically possible because of the rich vascularization of the face, which consists of several anastomotic arterial and venous networks, distributed in multiple longitudinal or transverse arcades around the oral, nasal, and palpebral clefts running between the facial, transverse facial, and superficial temporal vessels. Around the orbital region, the main arterial axes branch on terminal segmental branches of the ophthalmic arteries arising from the internal carotids. The efficiency of functional complement of that vascular network has been demonstrated clinically by the complete survival of all the soft tissues of the face after traumatic avulsion and microsurgical reimplantation on the segmental branches of the external carotid artery and their neighboring veins.[8]

In the deeper planes, this same network supplies the periosteal plate of the maxillary and mandibular arches, which therefore can be included, by careful dissection, in custom-made allografts. The latter also include, emerging from the mental, infraorbital, and supraorbital foramina (V_3, V_2, and V_1, respectively), the sensitive segmental branches of the trigeminal nerves (V) necessary to restore proprioceptive and epicritical sensitivity to the transplant. Laterally, in the parotid area, the common trunk or the segmental branches of the facial nerves (VII) are harvested depending on the muscle groups required and in the hope of restoring voluntary motricity to the face transplant.

According to these anatomic principles, there are three main segmental FAGs that can be harvested from one or more branches of the external carotid arterial network:

- The lower central FAG (type I) includes harvesting the donor's nose, lips, and chin from the cutaneous surface to the deep mucosa.[1] It is vascularized by the two facial pedicles dissected down to their emergence from the large vessels of the neck and contains all the oral cleft muscles harvested by subperiosteal elevation, from the zygomatic and maxillary bones to the mandibular rim (**Fig. 1**). These muscles are reinnervated by zygomatic, buccal, and mandibular branches of the facial nerves (VII) dissected as separate segmental rami or traced more proximally up to their common origin on the trunk of the facial nerve. The sensitive nerves of the allograft are the mental (V_3) and infraorbital (V_2) nerves exposed at the corresponding bone foramina and lengthened on their proximal course by intraosseous dissection.[1,9] This standard allograft concerns only the soft tissues of the face[1] (type IA). It may be extended laterally to the cheeks and up to the preauricular areas.[4] In the latter case it also contains the parotids and is raised on the external carotid and jugular axes and on the proximal trunk of the two facial nerves.[4] If necessary, it can extend deeper to include the middle part of the mandibular arch to restore the bone support to the chin (type IB; B = bone). In the latter transplant, the mandibular bone

segment then is vascularized by the periosteal network of the two submental arteries, which are connected in the area of the mental foramina with the inferior alveolar arteries. The submental vessels, therefore, must be included and left undamaged when the type IB graft is harvested. Consequently, the latter contains an additional skin surface corresponding to the submandibular region next to the hyoid bone.

- The mid-FAG (type II) contains the nose, upper lip, cheeks, and muscles elevating the oral cleft, equally elevated on right and left[3] facial pedicles. Although it can consist of soft tissues only (type IIA), it usually includes the anterior part of the maxillae and zygomatic arches and a variable segment of the anterior palate (type IIB). Its sensitivity is restored by the infraorbital nerves (V_2), and its motor reinnervation relies on the restored continuity of the zygomatic and buccal rami of the facial nerves (VII), if possible along with that of the buccal nerves (V_3) if tonicity to the buccinator muscles is to be restored (see **Fig. 1**). Depending on the extent of the defect to be reconstructed, the allograft may be very wide and on both sides of the midline or, alternatively, unilateral.[3] In some cases, it can be more or less extended downwards, toward the lower portion of the cheek.

- The upper FAG (type III) includes the superficial planes of the forehead, eyelids, and root of the nose and the deeper planes of the frontalis, glabellar, and orbicularis oculi muscles (see **Fig. 1**). It is raised on the two superficial temporal pedicles and on the supraorbital sensitive nerves (V_1). Deep dissection of the allograft around the palpebral sulci must include the preseptal and periosteal anastomotic vascular circle around the orbital rim to include the shunts connecting the intra- and extracranial vascular networks (see **Fig. 1**). Restoration of palpebral blink motricity is delicate but may be mediated by restoring the continuity of the frontal and zygomatic branches of the facial nerves (VII). To date, this segmental transplantation model remains theoretic, because it never has been implemented clinically.

Unlike the three composite transplants (described previously), which are segmental and linked to large functional, neurovascular territories of the face, the total facial skin allograft (type IV) is a purely tegumental transplant designed to

Type I : Lower central face

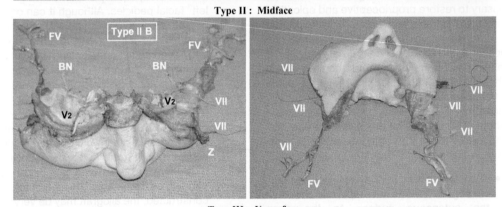

Type II : Midface

Type III : Upperface

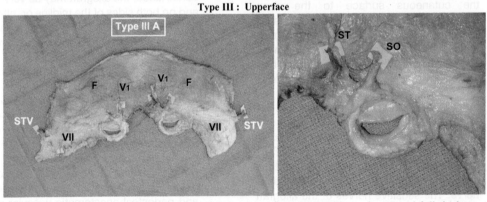

Fig. 1. Surgical classification of segmental facial CTAG. Partial face allografts are functional full-thickness transplants, which include all tissues of the lower (type I), middle (type II), or upper (type III) parts of the facial architecture. They may include soft tissues only (type n-A) or hard and soft tissue together (type n-B; B, bone). All of them are designed to match exactly the facial defect and to include all muscles, motor and sensitive nerves, and lining and to support to restore any missing functions. BN, buccal nerve (V_3); D, depressor muscles of the lower lip; F, frontalis muscles; FV, facial vessels; L, levator muscles of the upper lip; ST, SO, supratrochlear and supraorbital neurovascular pedicles; STV, superficial temporal vessels; V_1, V_2, and V_3, terminal cutaneous branches of ophthalmic, maxillary, and mandibular nerves; VII, facial nerve branches; Z, zygomatic muscles.

restore, in a single segment, the cutaneous cover of the whole facial mask and a variable portion of scalp, according to its laboratory description.[10] It is vascularized by the two facial and superficial temporal pedicles that are harvested separately or in a continuous fashion along the external carotid and jugular axes. It is pierced by three artificial orifices for the nostrils, lips, and eyelids and

can be likened to a carnival mask placed over a face, with all its deeper functional structures supposed to be intact and able to adhere to the deep surface of the FAG.[11] It does not, therefore, have any intrinsic motricity, and was not initially described as sensitive.[10,11] It seems, however technically possible to reinnervate its cutaneous surface by using a deeper dissection plane to include the three segmental terminal branches of the left and right trigeminal nerves.[12] The name, full face allograft, often suggested to describe this transplant, therefore is somewhat abusive and inexact. Although it covers a wider area than segmental allograft types I, II, or III, this theoretic transplant was devised to resurface extensive burns to the face. Devoid of any functional purpose, it does, however, constitute a partial FAG and, therefore, could be applicable to a hemiface or the whole facial cutaneous cover. In an attempt to avoid any ambiguities with regard to nomenclature, this allograft should be termed partial (type IVp) or a full (type IVf) CTAG of the facial mask.

Strictly speaking, a true full FAG (type V) ought to be performed as a multisegment or composite transplant combining the partial allograft types I, II, and III in a single block of uniform thickness. This would have to be harvested on the entire external carotid axis and the confluent jugular veins on both sides of a donor's head.[13] It would contain all the expression muscles, the common trunks of both facial nerves, and the three segmental branches (V_1, V_2, and V_3) of the two trigeminal nerves. In the deeper planes, it could involve soft tissues only, including superficial musculoaponeurotic system, with or without the periosteal plane[13] (full soft tissue FAG, type VA) or it also could include the maxillary or mandibular arches if necessary (full hard and soft tissue FAG, type VB). Although theoretically conceivable, such allografts correspond to such extensive tissular defects that they hardly ever are encountered clinically. They belong, therefore, more to the realm of virtual or conceptual surgery than practical reality.

To date, clinical experience has focused on allograft types I and II, and in the four documented cases, the composite allografts survived successfully after microsurgical transplantation.[1-5] Three were harvested from a heart-beating donor with a facial morphology comparable to the recipient's,[1,4,5] whereas one was obtained from a cadaveric donor.[3] In none of these cases was partial necrosis of any tissular transplant component reported, and peroperative hemodynamic observation of the allografts showed at all times that the transplant was fully vascularized on unilateral arterial and venous anastomoses (**Fig. 2**). Moreover, wound healing along the lines of cutaneous and mucosal sutures always was fully satisfactory. These results can be explained by the intense anastomotic collateralization of the facial architectural blood vessels (described previously). These results, achieved by four different teams, provide the first evidence of the vascular reliability of face transplants when the fundamental rules of microsurgery are observed.[1-5] Vascular anastomoses always must be performed on large-caliber vessels and should be bilateral, even when the entire transplant can survive on a single vascular axis. Attention to this rule anticipates and prevents the harmful consequences of thrombosis of one of the two arterial or venous axes supplying the transplant. When an allograft predominantly concerns a single hemiface, however, this precaution is not compulsory.[3] Only by extension of these observations to a larger group of patients can these preliminary conclusions be confirmed with regard to the reliability and primary survival of composite FAGs.

BIOLOGIC REJECTION CONTROL AND MEDIUM-TERM VIABILITY OF FACIAL ALLOGRAFTS

Having successfully passed the critical phase of immediate revascularization, the composite FAG must face the challenge of sustainable survival within the recipient's organism. This survival is immediately conditioned by the possibility of controlling biologically the rejection of all its tissular components. Initially, this immunologic challenge was considered the main stumbling block to successful FAT because of the extremely high antigenicity of its main component, skin.[14] The biologic function of skin is a barrier, with many dendritic cells in the dermis and epidermis. Early experiments in primates suggested that a higher level of immunosuppression would be necessary to prevent rejection of CTAGs lined by skin compared with solid monotissular organs in the same animals.[15] Clinical experience gathered from first-hand allografts dispelled these initial fears and showed that once the high-risk period of the first year is over, CTAG rejection could be controlled using similar or lower doses than those commonly used in renal transplantation.[16] Antigenic competition between the various tissues of composite allografts, the induction of blocking antibodies, and activation of regulatory T lymphocytes[17] were the mechanisms evoked to explain these most positive and encouraging observations, which were confirmed by the study of the first three face transplantations.

Hence, classic immunosuppression therapy advocated for the prevention of FAG rejection is no different from successfully tried and tested therapy used in visceral transplantation. Induction immunosuppression comprises infusions of antithymocyte globulin (thymoglobulin coenzyme, for 10 days) along with oral tacrolimus (TRL) a calcineurin inhibitor (target through levels, 10 to 15 ng per mL

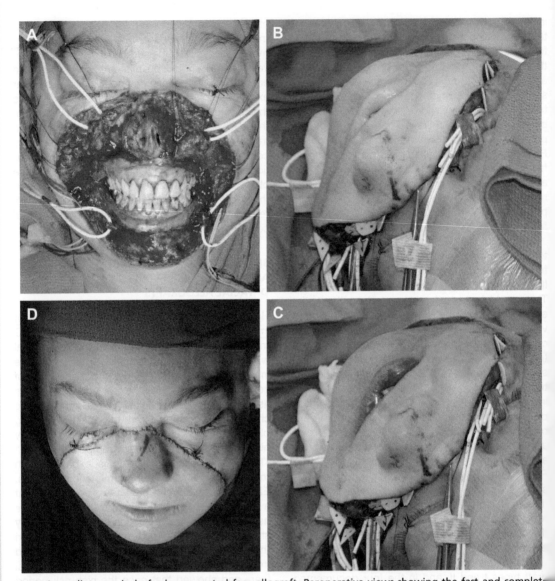

Fig. 2. Immediate survival of a lower central face allograft. Peroperative views showing the fast and complete revascularization of the allograft on a single vascular pedicle. (*A*) Recipient's face anatomic exposure; (*B*) FAG before clamps release; (*C*) FAG 1 minute after clamps release on right facial vessels; and (*D*) 6 hours later, after repair and completion of security bilateral anastomoses. Recipient sensitive nerves are tagged on white laces, recipient blood vessels are exposed on red and blue laces in both submandibular areas. Recipient muscles stump and facial nerves rami are tagged on stitches. Donor muscles are secured on small silicon rubbers to allow their identification and to prevent their retraction inside the FAG.

throughout the first month), and mycophenolate mofetil (MMF), an antiproliferative agent (2 g per day). These drugs are supplemented with prednisone, administered in rapidly decreasing doses (250 mg on day 1, 100 mg on day 2, then 60 mg/day through day 12, followed by a gradual taper). Additional medication is prescribed for cytomegalovirus and *Pneumocystis jiroveci* prophylaxis.[1,9] Maintenance therapy includes smaller doses of a combination of prednisone, TRL, and MMF (**Fig. 3**).

With the help of these therapeutic regimens, the first three FAGs reported in the medical literature were well tolerated, although all three experienced several rejection episodes with follow-up period now at 3, 2, and 1.5 years, respectively.[1–5] In the case of the first patient to have benefited from a type I transplant, two rejection episodes were reported,[1,9] at 3 weeks and 8 months postoperatively (see **Fig. 3**). During each of these rejection episodes, cytotoxic activity specifically directed against the donor's antigens could be observed

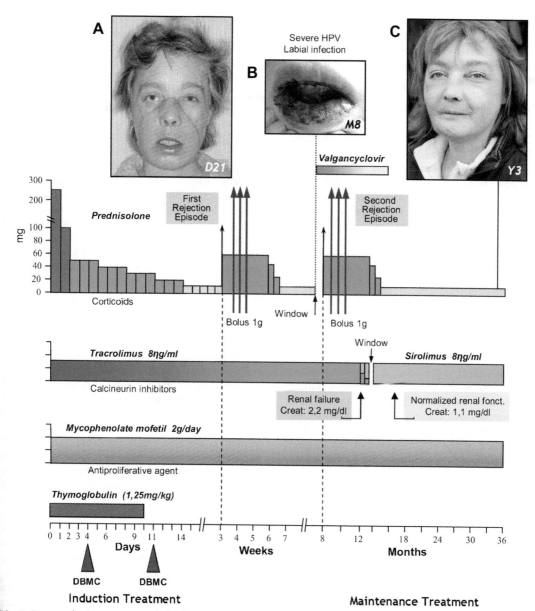

Fig. 3. Immunologic outcomes of the first partial face transplant. Color rectangles indicate the relative doses of immunosupressants used to prevent graft rejection and arrowheads show the two infusions of donor bone marrow cells (DBMC) given during induction treatment. Vertical dotted lines show the two rejection episodes. (*A*) Erythematous aspect of the graft during first rejection. (*B*) Severe human papillomavirus labial infection, just before the second rejection episode. Arrows indicate steroid boluses given to control both episodes. At M 12, a transient renal failure complicated the immunosuppressive treatment but disappeared when TRL was stopped and replaced by sirolimus. Maintenance treatment is characterized by low-doses of immunosuppressant drugs. (*C*) Appearance at 3 years.

T lymphocytes isolated in the allograft skin.[9] This activity was not observed between the rejection episodes and was found less severe and easier to reverse during the second episode. This first patient's allograft has remained immunologically silent for 33 months. Similarly, the second allograft patient (type IIB) presented with acute

signs of allograft rejection at 3, 5, and 17 months post transplantation,[3] and the third patient experienced two episodes, at 1 and 2 months postoperatively.[4]

All rejection episodes without exception were clinically diagnosed as allograft edema and erythema (see **Fig. 3**) and were then objectively confirmed by biopsies of the transplant mucosa and skin. All the biopsies were grade I or II according to the CTA rejection classification.[18] It also was invariably observed that inflammatory reactions were more intense under the grafted mucosa than under the transplant skin.[9,18] Furthermore, immunohistochemical studies showed that these specific reactions were caused predominantly by CD3+ and CD4+ lymphocytes (T-helper lymphocytes) with few CD8+ cells (cytotoxic lymphocytes).[3,9] In all cases, clinical and histologic rejection signs disappeared completely after a slight increase in TRL and MMF doses, with one or several 1g boluses of prednisone.[3,4,9] Local application of TRL ointment[19] and corticosteroid mouthwashes also were effective.[1,9]

In an unprecedented move, immunologic and therapeutic monitoring of the first FAG was performed using a radial forearm flap harvested from the donor and transplanted to a concealed area of the recipient, namely her left submammary fold.[1,9] This sentinel composite graft, which was revascularized at the same time as the main FAG, has continuously evolved biologically in strict parallelism to the latter. It constitutes, therefore, a valuable and durable skin reserve, particularly useful when iterative biopsies are required for the diagnosis and grading of rejection episodes.[9] Moreover, this sentinel graft allows the objective assessment of the effectiveness of the installed immunosuppression regimen. One further advantage of this indirect monitoring process is that it spares the surface of the main FAG, thereby preventing multiple additional wounds and scarring to the cosmetic appearance of the reconstructed face. It may be argued in opposition to this ancillary procedure, which was in addition to the main graft albeit with no increase in operating time, that it is superfluous because histopathologic monitoring of CTAG could be performed using biopsies of the oral mucosa. Bearing in mind, however, that the monitoring of most FAGs should be fanned out over dozens of years, it is likely that repeated mucosal biopsies would create thick scar tissue under this lining, rendering subsequent biopsies more difficult to interpret and possibly creating invalidating jugal adhesions through contraction.

The favorable results (discussed previously) in relation to medium-term survival of the first few FATs are encouraging and particularly remarkable when compared retrospectively to the initial survival rate of every first visceral allograft.[14] Contrary to the fears initially voiced, they show that rejection of any composite FAG may be routinely controlled with moderate doses of immunosuppressors, thereby proportionally reducing the systemic medical risks associated with them.[17] These observations, however, do not allow in the long term reliably predicting the average lifespan of the allografts, even if this likely survival rate could be extrapolated by analogy with that of other composite grafts from the study of the immunologic behavior of hand allografts over their 10-year history.[17] The risk for chronic rejection, identical to that encountered in visceral transplants, and documented infraclinically in the oral mucosa of one of the face transplant patients, remains real.[3,4] The hope to control these phenomena in the long-term relies on the use of new molecules supposedly more effective and less toxic than those currently used. Some of these promising new drugs are sirolimus, everolimus, active metabolites of FK778 and FK779, and Campath.[14] Some of these drugs have shown, during their phase III studies, that even when administered alone, they are able to reduce the use of immunosuppressors to the sole treatment of rejection episodes and even occasionally to eliminate the need for corticotherapy.[14] Definitive and sustainable biologic control of CTAG rejection will depend on the possibility of manipulating the immune system by inducing a specific state of tolerance against the donor's antigens.[20] Such a state already has been induced at an experimental level in several animal models of CTA.[21–24] In most cases, this entails the creation of a mixed hematopoietic microchimerism or simultaneous allotransplantation of allogenic stem cells, which migrate into the recipient's bloodstream and educate regulatory T cells to specifically recognize the donor's antigens, thereby increasing long-term survival rate of the composite allograft.[25–28] The absence of chronic rejection in most hand transplant patients stems from this phenomenon, as stem cells are supplied by the simultaneous transplantation of allogenic bone marrow within the bones of the distal forearm. The demonstration of CD4+ D25+ FOXp3+ regulatory T cells in the transplanted skin suggests that the donor's hematopoietic stem cells, originating from the vascularized bone graft, migrated there to exert their beneficial effector influence.[29] This observation formed the basis for the addition, at treatment induction on days 4 and 11, of two infusions of hematopoietic stem cells harvested from the donor's bone marrow to the immunosuppression therapy of the first face transplant patient.[1,9]

At follow-up, however, only one of the many analyses of medullary chimerism suggested at month 2 that 0.1% of the bone marrow cells were donor derived.[9] Yet the presence of a microchimerism susceptible of being correlated with the induction of allograft immune tolerance is classically defined by the threshold value of 1%.[20,25] Although the current results of this clinical trial are not convincing, further research in this area is advocated to develop, on sound objective scientific grounds, tolerance induction protocols that will provide similar results to those observed in several experimental animal models[21–28] or even in certain clinical series reported in solid organ transplantation.[14] There can be no doubt that the future of face transplantation will be conditioned considerably more by progress in the realm of induction of specific sustainable biologic immunotolerance than by surgical factors alone.

FUNCTIONAL RECOVERY OF FACIAL ALLOGRAFTS AND NEUROPHYSIOLOGIC REINTEGRATION WITHIN THE BODY SCHEME

In the author's opinion, a CTA cover to the facial frame is justifiable only if it is a genuine face allograft (ie, a full transfer of all the dynamic players in orofacial function).[1,2] Beyond the undoubted cosmetic benefits of surface and volume restoration in reconstructing extensive defects, it is the possibility of bringing back to life several autonomous functions in the anatomic units transferred that firmly grounds the definitive legitimacy of face transplantation. In addition to its cosmetic aspect, the FAG attains the full status of a genuine organ transplant.[30] It is for this reason that a distinction is made between segmental functional transplants types I, II, or III and the facial mask allograft type IV. In terms of anatomy and neurology, full-thickness allografts are all conceived to enable restoration of all essential sensitive and motor pathways for a balanced relational life characteristic of full facial function.

The observations collated during postoperative follow-up of the first three FAGs reported in the literature[1,3,4] have demonstrated that this ambitious goal could be attained. In all probability, assisted by the neurotrophic effect of TRL, regeneration of sensitive nerves enabled the allografts to recover first their thermalgesic sensitivity, and subsequently their discriminative sensitivity, between the fourth and sixth postoperative months.[9] In relation to motricity, the restoration of facial muscular function is a slower process that can be attained only through intensive physiotherapy initiated as early as the first week after transplantation.[1] When the neuromuscular repairs concern healthy stumps, the restoration of labial contact in a type I allograft may be secured at first partially, then completely between the sixth and eighth postoperative months.[9] From then on, patients recover a normal orbicular function that enables them to feed competently and to emit occlusive phonemes perfectly when speaking. The smile, incomplete at 4 months post transplantation, becomes progressively symmetric between months 10 and 14 and acquires its normal and spontaneous characteristics at approximately 1.5 years (Fig. 4). One even more remarkable feature is that the prolongation of dissociated physiotherapy on each of the grafted muscles also enables patients to progressively recruit, for the dissociative mimicry of expressions, the lip elevator muscles to express joy and happiness or those muscles lowering the lips and chin to convey hesitation, sadness, pain, or bitterness.[9] Concomitantly, after the appearance of a wide range of multidirectional expressive movements, the skin of the FAG, initially smooth and motionless, recovers its natural folds that spontaneously generate cutaneous creases and dynamic adipose cushions, particularly in the philtral, mental, and nasogenian areas (see Fig. 4). Such motor functional results have never been observed or reported in secondary surgical repair of facial paralysis, not even when resorting to reinnervated autologous muscle transfers.

In correlation with these spectacular sensitive and motor modifications, iterative functional MRI showed, after stagnation of atrophied cortical images of the face for the first 3 postoperative months of the first FAG patient, unquestionable signs of a reorganization of the body image at 4 months (ie, at the exact time of full restoration of the allograft's objective epicritical sensitivity).[9] In parallel with re-expansion of the cortical area corresponding to the face, momentarily invaded by the hand territory during the disfigurement process, reconstruction of the cerebral homunculus is accompanied, in neuropsychologic terms, by an unconscious reappropriation of the allograft in spoken language. At first the patient uses the definite article, "the nose, the lips" to describe the allograft's anatomic components, but then spontaneously starts to use the possessive form "my nose, my lips." This phenomenon unquestionably demonstrates that FAG genuinely reintegrates the body scheme at approximately 8 months postoperatively, as it becomes again a dynamic, sensitive, and reactive interface with the outside world. In this fashion, face transplantation perfectly demonstrates, despite its many constraints, its undeniable superiority over conventional autologous reconstruction techniques in disfigurement, the cosmetic results of which are much poorer and the functional consequences always unsatisfactory. Furthermore, it may be added that this type of surgery, although major, produces its multiple results and benefits within a single operation time, with no donor site prejudice.[1]

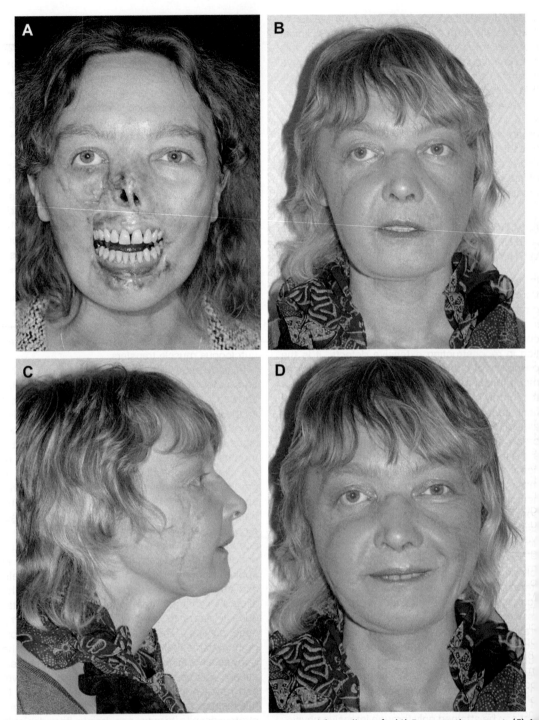

Fig. 4. Cosmetic and functional outcomes of the first lower central face allograft. (*A*) Preoperative aspect; (*B*) 1 months' postoperative frontal view at rest, showing nearly complete passive lip occlusion; (*C*) profile view emphasizing the quality of contour restoration; and (*D*) smiling appearance, with restoration of multidirectional motions and natural skin plicature.

ETHICAL ISSUES REGARDING THE COST-BENEFIT BALANCE AND RESTORED IDENTITY

Although they seem to justify enthusiasm, the results of the first FATs should not play down that at this stage they are beneficial to only a few patients, follow-up is not yet very long, and many uncertainties remain as to the future of FAT. Face transplantation still is seen as a clinical trial and raises many questions, which not only are medical but also of an extremely profound ethical nature.[30,31] In deontologic practice, every medical gesture, ordinary or innovative, cannot be justified unless the real benefits it offers to patients are considerably more substantial than the potential damaging effects.[32] Yet in the ethical debate that preceded and followed the announcement of the first FATs, many experts estimated their cost-benefit balance as dangerously negative.[2,30–33] The first argument in favor of this negative evaluation is grounded on the potential life-threatening risks to the grafted patients inherent in lifelong immunosuppression imposed to treat a nonvital problem. The second argument addresses the problematics of restored chimeric identity linked to FAG and the potential major psychologic conflict for the recipient.

Concerns about the risks for systemic complications as a result of immunosuppression[32,33] have to be understood in the light of those risks being extrapolated from literature data concerning solid organ transplantation. Many clinicians assumed that the dose of drugs required to control CTAG rejection would probably, because of the high antigenicity of the skin, be significantly higher than that usually prescribed to guarantee the survival of visceral transplants.[34] Now, 80% of renal allografts develop infections and 40% of the postgraft mortality is the result, in this group of patients, to bacterial, viral, or fungal opportunistic infections.[14] Moreover, TRL is nephrotoxic and diabetogenic.[34] The steroids induce other well-known general complications, such as hypertension (15%), osteoporosis (10%), avascular necrosis of the hip (8%), and cataracts (22%).[35] Taken together, immunosuppressants significantly increase the occurrence of skin cancer (14%–20%) and lymphoproliferative disorders (2%–10%) with global incidences varying from 12% to 68% according to the series and immunosuppressant regimen.[14] It seems, however, that these risks extrapolated from retrospective studies of renal transplant patients may not apply to the population of CTA recipients. In a retrospective study, Baumeister and colleagues[36] showed that the number of infectious and organotoxic complications of immunosuppressants was lower in patients who had

CTAG in comparison with patients who had renal transplant, as was the incidence of skin cancer (3% at 5 years) and lymphoma (1%). This observation, which can be explained by the fact that the majority of CTA recipients are young and have no associated comorbidity factors, puts these initial fears into perspective.[14,36] It also suggests that face transplant patients may, contrary to the initial assumption, have less general and systemic morbidity linked to immunosuppression than renal transplant patients.

Caution, however, is required in these deductive conclusions. In two of the first face transplant patients, one of two reported rejection episodes was induced after the decrease in immunosuppression because of a local human papillomavirus viral infection in one case and cytomegalovirus sepsis in another.[4] Furthermore, the first face transplant patient is reported to have suffered from transient renal failure as a result of the nephrotoxicity of TRL[9] (see **Fig. 3**). These clinical facts indicate that it remains crucial in the future to be able to dispose of new substitution immunosuppressants, less toxic than the previous generation, to guarantee the continued existence and the further development of face transplantation.[14,32] Finally, in the long term (discussed previously) all hopes of evening out the CTA cost-benefit balance lie in the expected success of experiments aimed at attaining long-lasting immunologic tolerance of the allografts, the survival of which would no longer require any corticosteroid support.[36]

In a correct evaluation of the cost-benefit balance of facial transplantation, the benefits should not be underestimated. The cosmetic and functional grounds have been discussed previously (see **Fig. 4**). They show that, in restoring the essential functions of relational life, such as eating, speaking, and nonverbal expression, FAG essentially is an organ graft.[37] Even if all visceral functions linked to the face are not indispensable to physical survival, all its symbolic functions, profoundly human, are essential for the psychic and social survival of each individual. Reducing the face to a simple image, as some experts do, merely shows a fundamental ignorance of the psychologic problems of dealing with disfiguration and of the profound inner suffering endured by these patients and those around them. By restoring the symbolic and eminently social functions of the face, facial transplantation is an incommensurable life-giving gesture. Thus, it is no different in any other aspect from a kidney transplantation that removes the daily constraints of hemodialysis or from a pancreas transplantation that temporarily curtails the practical constraints of insulin therapy. The only difference between those three transplantations, which all aim to improve quality of life, lies in that, like a hand transplant, a FAG is immediately visible, whereas the kidney and the pancreas are deeply buried and hidden beneath an abdominal scar.

The immediate and permanent visibility of an FAG is the source of the last ethical issue. This is in relation to the potential ambiguity of the image of self that is restored to a patient thanks to the allograft.[30,31] At the psychologic level, weakened by the disfigurement, that image ambiguity, where, in the mind of the recipient, the allograft remains linked to death, can engender a severe conflict of personality, the harmful consequences of which have been highlighted by the dramatic outcome of the first single hand allograft.[38] Morphologically, however, several virtual imaging[39] and anatomic cadaver[40] studies have shown that the face, when reconstructed by an allograft, although it acquires a mixed image of donor and recipient, retains the main characteristics of the recipient's previous appearance, which is essential for recognition by others. These data have been confirmed clinically by the first receivers of FAGs, who proved capable of recognizing themselves in their new image when looking in a mirror.[1,3,9] At a functional level, the authors have shown, in the prospective neurocognitive assessment of the patient, that her face graft, connected by motor and sensitive nerves to her own brain, had fully recovered, up to the scale of its cortical reorganization at MRI, the role of an autonomous and individual interface with the outside world. Even though the aspect of a recipient's face can never be identically restored by an FAG, a patient recovers not only an anatomic singularity through the operation but also a functional individualization that animates the new face depending on the patient's own feelings. Compared with hand grafts,[16,17,38] the phenomenon of neuropsychologic capture of FAG occurs more rapidly as a transplanted face is not constantly under the eyes of the recipient, so that the "dead," insensitive period, where the allograft does not exist in the relational life, is reduced to the 2 to 3 months necessary for the start of the restoration of sensitivity.[9] With a smile restored, the allograft then definitely belongs to the new individual human history that keeps it alive. In a technical sense, this neurologic fact underlines the cardinal importance of the sensitive and motor nerve anastomoses in ensuring the full success of FAT.[1] The psychologic background of the recipient and close psychiatric support required before and after the transplantation, therefore, are no less important.[31,32] Strict selection of potential recipients, informing them thoroughly, preparing their families, and ensuring their compliance with the rules of follow-up and therapeutic constraints are the last essential conditions to make this undertaking a success.[41] Consequently, every new facial transplantation becomes a unique multidisciplinary challenge that solicits as much intuitive intelligence of the medical team as the different technical skills they embody. All the failures reported in CTA registries have been found attributable to errors of judgment or to the lack of precautions taken regarding the four control parameters (described previously).[17,41]

FUTURE PERSPECTIVES AND CONCLUSIONS

The first facial transplantations, performed only recently, have projected the dreams of science fiction into the real world of science, turning an ancestral myth of humanity related to the image of facial chimera into surgical reality. Spurred by the considerable progress in the field of experimental immunology, these first experiences have shown that, from now on, grafting a face becomes an accessible surgical challenge and that, contrary to previously voiced fears, it is possible to prevent rejection of the composite FAG with the assistance of conventional immunosuppression therapy using small doses of steroids. The functional and neurocognitive results achieved demonstrate the indisputable integration of reinnervated transplants within the body scheme of the recipient patients and the restoration in each of them of a psychologically and socially well-established individual identity.

With these encouraging preliminary data that have partially extinguished the ethical controversy surrounding the principle of FATs, the medical world must move forward, albeit with care. The new field of progress opening engenders many research perspectives that are not only surgical in nature:

- First, in the technical domain, although many anatomic problems already have been solved, the reliability of total facial transplantation remains to be verified by clinical human evidence. Extending the surface of segmental transplants, grouping them in a single multisegmental graft (eg types I and II), and attaching vascularized bone supports to their deep layer do not present any major obstacles. The main barrier to the application of such extensive grafts in resurfacing severe facial burns stems from the irreversibility of the damage created during preparation of the face for the graft should revascularization or immediate tolerance of the transplant fail

Traumatic full-thickness facial defects involving several anatomic units of the face, particularly in young and healthy patients, remain, until further investigations, the best indications for the procedure. For reasons of risk-benefit balance, disfigured and already immunosuppressed patients constitute another target population.[42] Some benign tumors and possibly extensive vascular malformations are alternative indications.[4] Less pure than those related to heavy trauma cases, these indications pose the crucial question of whether or not, strategically, their surgical resection should be performed in a dissociated manner from the reconstructive gesture or, alternatively, at the same time as transplantation.

- Subsequently, in the realm of immunology, all future efforts must focus on the development of new combinations of immunosuppressant drugs with fewer, less harmful side effects and on the efficient clinical induction of lasting immune tolerance.[20–23] It is on this last and absolute condition that indications for FAT one day may be extended to the treatment of major substance loss after cancer exeresis.[7] Although these conditions etiologically are unfortunately the most frequently encountered in daily practice, they remain formally excluded from every CTA protocol because of the major risk for tumor recurrence induced by immunosuppression.[14,34]
- Finally, in the field of neuropsychology, the many questions that fed the controversy and the extensive public debate surrounding the legitimacy of FAT have caused the scientific community to ponder the symbolic value of the face and the considerable importance it has in the life of each one of us. Going back to the founding myths of the history of humanity, this reflection brings reconstructive surgeons back to the true dimension of their real mission at the bedside of the sick. Plastic and creative, their noble task consists, first and foremost, of listening, empathy, and compassion. Faced with the intolerable physical and moral suffering of disfigurement, the transgression sometimes represents, at the price of a controlled risk, a duty of humanity (**Fig. 5**).

Half a century ago, while painting his famous *Minotaur and Dead Mare*, in which oddly, the

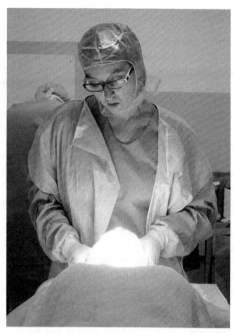

Fig. 5. *Pietà anatomica;* photo by Cédric d'Hauthuille, MD, harvesting team member of the world's first FAT. Ethics and compassion are inherent to any gesture in face transplantation. The restitution of the donor's face image after graft harvesting is a major duty of respect to the donor and the family.

Minotaur, half man, half bull, has a chimeric face, the artist Pablo Picasso evoked the resolutely transgressing character of his art when he wrote, *"I paint against those that have come before me. Not to contradict or betray the works of my great masters, but to raise them up to a new life. You don't have to incessantly repeat what was. You have to create, in the light, what will be tomorrow."* Similarly, CTAs have opened up a new universe of creativity for plastic surgeons in which patients themselves no longer are the only potential donors of tissue transfers necessary for reconstruction. Today's fellow human beings are able to offer a new source of functional made-to-measure transplants that one day may be either more or less extensive than those of today. This creative power that aspires using the achievements of autotransplantation microsurgery to roll back the boundaries of repair surgery with allotransplants is colossal. Consequently, it invests surgeons with new responsibilities of conscience.[43] On that road where progress sometimes oversteps the boundaries of reason and quantification, permanent questioning while acting is a privilege. Similarly, humility remains in the thought that directs the gesture, a duty of elegance[2] that possibly can add to its result a supplement of soul and, thus, humanity.

SUMMARY

Once confined to the universe of ancient myth and legend and subsequently the phantasmagoric world of cinema, facial allotransplantation has become a surgical reality. Rendered possible thanks to significant progress of fundamental science, the first successful segmental human face transplants have demonstrated that FAGs are reliable, that their rejection can be prevented by low-dose immunosuppression, and that their neurologic recovery enables all oral and expressive functions of the face to be restored. Moreover, in response to ethical initial objections, the clinical facts have shown that the risk-benefit balance is acceptable in the medium term, that at the neurocognitive level the allograft is reintegrated in the body scheme of the recipient, and that it does not engender a donor identity transfer. In light of these recent advances, this article presents a carefully reasoned classification of FAGs and discusses the resulting different technical, immunologic, and ethical challenges that may lie ahead.

ACKNOWLEDGMENTS

The personal reflections recorded in this article are the result of the synthesis of a multidisciplinary and multicentric project performed by the Department of Experimental Morphology at Université catholique de Louvain; the Department of Maxillofacial Surgery, CHU-Amiens (B. Devauchelle, S. Testelin, and S. Dakpe); the Department of Transplantation, University of Lyon (J.M. Dubernard, L. Badet, E. Morellon, and A. Sirigu); and the Department of Plastic Surgery, Harvard Medical School (J. Pribaz and B. Pomahac). The author thanks the staff of the Experimental Morphology Department for their invaluable technical and practical assistance and Dr. Claire de Burbure and Richard Craddock for revising the manuscript.

REFERENCES

1. Devauchelle N, Badet L, Lengelé B, et al. First human face allograft: early report. Lancet 2006; 368:203–9.
2. Lengelé B, Testelin S, Cremades S, et al. Facing up is an act of dignity: lessons in elegance addressed to the polemicists of the first human face transplant. Plast Reconstr Surg 2007;120(3):803–6.
3. Guo S, Han Y, Zhang X, et al. Human facial allotransplantation: a-2 year follow-up study. Lancet 2008; 372:631–8.
4. Lantieri L, Meningaud JP, Grimbert P, et al. Repair of the lower and middle parts of the face by composite tissue allotransplantation in a patient with massive plexiform neurofibroma: a 1-year follow-up study. Lancet 2008;372:639–45.
5. Doctors detail first U.S. face transplant. Available at: http://www.usatoday.com/news/health/2008-12-17-face-transplant_N.htm. Today-Accessed December 21, 2008.
6. Pribaz JJ, Finc N, Orgill DP. Flap prefabrication in the head and neck: a 10-year experience. Plast Reconstr Surg 1999;103:808–20.
7. Cordeiro PG. Frontiers in free flap reconstruction in the head and neck. J Surg Oncol 2008;97(8):669–73.
8. Wihelmi BL, Kang RH, Movassaghi K, et al. First successful replantation of face and scalp with single-artery repair: model for face and scalp transplantation. Ann Plast Surg 2003;50:535–40.
9. Dubernard JM, Lengelé B, Morelon E, et al. Outcomes 18 months after the first human partial face transplantation. N Engl J Med 2007;357: 2451–60.
10. Siemionow M, Agaoglu G, Unal S. A cadaver study in preparation for facial allograft transplantation in humans: part II. Mock facial transplantation. Plast Reconstr Surg 2006;117(3):876–85.
11. Butler PE, Clarke A, Hettiaratchy S. Facial transplantation. A new gold option in reconstruction of severe facial injury. BMJ 2005;331:1349–50.
12. Siemionow M, Papay F, Kulahci Y, et al. Coronal-posterior approach for face/scalp flap harvesting in preparation for face transplantation. J Reconstr Microsurg 2006;22(6):399–405.
13. Baccarani A, Fallmar KE, Baumeister SP, et al. Technical and anatomical considerations of face harvest in face transplantation. Ann Plast Surg 2006;57(5) 483–8.
14. Madani H, Hettiaratchy S, Clarcke A, et al. Immunosuppression in an emerging field of plastic reconstructive surgery: composite tissue allotransplantation. J Plast Reconstr Aesthet Surg 2008 61(3):245–9.
15. Lee WPA, Yaremchuk MJ, Pan YC, et al. Relative antigenicity of components of a vascularised limb allograft. Plast Reconstr Surg 1991;87:401–11.
16. Dubernard JM, Owen E, Herberg G, et al. Human hand allograft: report on first 6 months. Lancet 1999;353:1315–20.
17. Lanzetta M, Petruzzo P, Vitale G, et al. Human hand transplantation: what have we learned? Transplant Proc 2004;36:664–8.
18. Kanitakis J, Badet L, Petruzzo P, et al. Clinicopathologic monitoring of the skin and oral mucosa of the first human face allograft: report on the first eight months. Transplantation 2006;82:1610–5.
19. Gruber SA, Shirbacheh WV, Jones JW, et al. Local drug delivery to composite tissue allografts. Microsurgery 2000;20:407–11.
20. Fehr T, Sykes M. Tolerance induction in clinical transplantation. Transpl Immunol 2004;13:117–30.

21. Siemionow M, Agaoglu G. Allotransplantation of the face: how close are we? Clin Plast Surg 2005;32(3):401–9.

22. Siemionow M, Demir Y, Mukherjee A, et al. Development and maintenance of donor-specific chimerism in semi-allogenic and fully major histocompatibility complex mismatched facial allograft transplants. Transplantation 2005;79(5):558–67.

23. Siemionow M, Agaoglu G. Tissue transplantation in plastic surgery. Clin Plast Surg 2007;34(2):251–69.

24. Lee WP, Rubin JP, Bourget JL, et al. Tolerance to limb tissue allografts between swine matched for major histocompatibility complex antigens. Plast Reconstr Surg 2001;107:1482–90.

25. Mathew JM, Miller J. Immunoregulatory role of chimerism in clinical organ transplantation. Transplantation 2001;28:115–9.

26. Bartholomew A, Sturgeon C, Siatskas M, et al. Mesenchymal stem cells suppress lymphocyte proliferation in vitro and prolong skin graft survival in vivo. Exp Hematol 2002;30:42–8.

27. Siemionow M, Zieliniski M, Ozmen S, et al. Intraosseus transplantation of donor-derived hematopoietic stem and progenitor cells induces donor-specific chimerism and extends composite tissue allograft survival. Transplant Proc 2005;37:2303–8.

28. Siemionow M. Impact of donor bone marrow on survival of composite tissue allografts. Ann Plast Surg 2008;60(4):455–62.

29. Eljaafari A, Badet L, Kanitakis J, et al. Isolation of regulatory T cells in the skin of a human hand-allograft, up to 6 years posttransplantation. Transplantation 2006;82:1764–8.

30. Wiggins OP, Barker JH, Martinez S, et al. On the ethics of facial transplantation research. Am J Bioeth 2004;4:1–12.

31. Agich GJ, Siemionow M. Until they have faces: the ethics of facial allograft transplantation. J Med Ethics 2005;31(12):707–9.

32. Morris P, Bradley A, Doyal L, et al. Face transplantation: a review of the technical, immunological, psychological and clinical issues with recommendations for good practice. Transplantation 2007;83:109–28.

33. Rohrich RJ, Longaker MT, Cuningham B. On the ethics of composite tissue allotransplantation (facial transplantation). Plast Reconstr Surg 2006;117:2071–3.

34. Vasilic D, Alloway RR, Barker JH, et al. Risk assessment of immunosuppressive therapy in facial transplantation. Plast Reconstr Surg 2007;120:657–68.

35. Veenstra DL, Best JH, Hornberger J. Incidence and long-term cost of steroid-related side effects after renal transplantation. Am J Kidney Dis 1999;33:829–39.

36. Baumeister S, Kleist C, Dohler B, et al. Risks of allogeneic hand transplantation. Microsurgery 2004;24:98–103.

37. Siemionow M, Sonmez E. Face as an organ. Ann Plast Surg 2008;61(3):345–52.

38. Dubernard JM, Burloux G, Giraux P, et al. Three lessons learned from the first double hand transplantation. Bull Acad Natl Med 2002;186:1051–62.

39. Pomahac B, Aflaki P, Nelson C, et al. Evaluation of appearance transfer and persistence in central face tranplantation: a computer simulation analysis. J Plast Reconst Aesth Surg; in press.

40. Siemionow M, Agaoglu G. The issue of "facial appearance and identity transfer" after mock transplantation: a cadaver study in preparation for facial allograft transplantation in humans. J Reconstr Microsurg 2006;22(5):329–34.

41. Tobin GR, Breidenbach WC 3rd, Pidwell DJ, et al. Transplantation of the hand, face, and composite structure: evolution and current status. Clin Plast Surg 2007;34(2):271–8.

42. Pomahac B, Aflaki P, Chandraker A, et al. Facial transplantation and immunosuppressed patients: a new frontier in reconstructive surgery. Transplantation 2008;85(12):1693–7.

43. Sacks JM, Keith JD, Fisher C, et al. The surgeon's role and responsibility in facial tissue allograft transplantation. Ann Plast Surg 2007;58(6):595–601.

Index

Note: Page numbers of article titles are in **boldface** type.

A

ABCD rule, 329–330
Acral lentiginous melanoma, 331
Actinic cheilitis, 325
Actinic keratosis, 325
    hypertrophic, 325
    spreading pigmented, 325
Allografts, facial. See *Facial allograft(s).*
Allotransplantation, complete tissue, relationship of
    prefabrication and prelamination in, 503–504
Anel test, 401
Aplasia cutis congenital, 364, 368

B

Basal cell carcinoma, 335
    background of, 319–320
    classification of, 320
    clinical presentation of, 320–321, 322
    differential diagnosis of, 321
    excision of, and reconstruction of alar area using
        forehead flap, 444–449
    histology of, 321–322
    Mohs' micrographic surgery for, 322, 323–324
    morpheaform, 321
    of scalp, resection and resurfacing in, 360
    therapeutic algorithm for, 323
    treatment of, 322–323
Blue nevus, 328
Bowen's disease/intraepithelial carcinoma, 326
Burn injury, of forehead, scarring from, resurfacing
    in, 361

C

Calvarial defect, complex full-thickness, wound
    closure in, 373–375
Canthus, lateral, functional anatomy of, 380, 381
    reconstruction of, 391–393
    medial, functional anatomy of, 380–381
    reconstruction of, 393–394
Cervicofacial flaps, anterior-based, for reconstruction
    of defects of cheek, 463–466
    posterior-based, for reconstruction of defects of
        cheek, 466–467, 468, 469
Cervicopectoral flaps, anterior-based, for
    reconstruction of defects of cheek, 467–468, 469
    posterior-based, for reconstruction of defects of
        cheek, 468–470

Cheek, contour and outline of, 461, 462
    defects of, analysis of, 462–463, 464
        reconstruction of, 350–352
            angle rotation cheek flap for, 465–466, 467,
                468
            anterior-based cervicofacial flaps for,
                463–466, 467–468, 469
            deltopectoral flap for, 472
            free flaps for, 472–474
            maximizing results of, **461–476**
            platysma musculocutaneous flap for,
                470–471
            posterior-based cervicofacial flaps for,
                466–467, 468, 469
            posterior-based cervicopectoral flaps for,
                468–470
            prefabricated flaps for, 474–475
            supraclavicular flap for, 471–472
        reconstruction of, aesthetic facial unit principles
            in, 462, 463
Cheek flap, angle rotation, for reconstruction of
    defects of cheek, 465–466, 467, 468
Columellar lining, restoration of, options for, 436, 437,
    438–441
Cutaneous horn, of hand, 325, 326

D

Dacryocystography, 401
Dacryocystorhinostomy, in blocked lacrimal duct,
    399, 401
Deltopectoral flap, for reconstruction of defects of
    cheek, 472
Dye disappearance test, 401

E

Ear, cancer of, radiation therapy in, 340
Endoscopy, nasal, 401
Eyelid(s), aesthetic reconstruction of, **379–397**
    anthropometric norms of, 379, 380
    cancer of, radiation therapy in, 339–340
    defects of, etiology of, 382
        reconstruction of, 347–349
    functional anatomy of, 380–382
    lower, full-thickness defects of, 385–389, 390
    lymphatic drainage of, 381
    reconstruction of, 382–391
    support of, and dynamics of, 382

Clin Plastic Surg 36 (2009) 523–526
doi:10.1016/S0094-1298(09)00053-4

Moving?

Make sure your subscription moves with you!

To notify us of your new address, find your **Clinics Account Number** (located on your mailing label above your name), and contact customer service at:

E-mail: elspcs@elsevier.com

800-654-2452 (subscribers in the U.S. & Canada)
314-453-7041 (subscribers outside of the U.S. & Canada)

Fax number: 314-523-5170

Elsevier Periodicals Customer Service
11830 Westline Industrial Drive
St. Louis, MO 63146

*To ensure uninterrupted delivery of your subscription, please notify us at least 4 weeks in advance of move.

Moving?

Make sure your subscription moves with you!

To notify us of your new address, find your Clinics Account Number (located on your mailing label above your name), and contact customer service at:

E-mail: elspcs@elsevier.com

800-654-2452 (subscribers in the U.S. & Canada)
314-453-7041 (subscribers outside of the U.S. & Canada)

Fax number: 314-523-5170

Elsevier Periodicals Customer Service
11830 Westline Industrial Drive
St. Louis, MO 63146

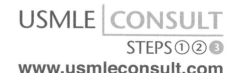

Printed and bound by CPI Group (UK) Ltd, Croydon, CR0 4YY

03/10/2024

01040353-0002